Moss Medicine

"This richly informed and deeply researched book opened my eyes to clinical possibilities from a source I wasn't previously aware of. Reading it inspired recognition of the huge number of moss species, which offer hope for novel medical treatments. This book discusses the research supporting new solutions for medical conditions, with particularly strong support for potential in dealing with both cancer and infectious diseases. I really enjoyed the fascinating chemical, medical, historical, and cultural insights that underlie the different uses of moss. I cannot recommend this book highly enough for those interested in nature-based therapeutics or traditional medicines and looking for inspiration."

Peter Silverstone, MD, FRCPC,
professor of psychiatry, University of Alberta

"I am both inspired by and grateful for Robert's focus on medicinal mosses. As a practicing herbalist, I am deeply intrigued by their history, medicinal potential, and the immense role they play in the sacred web of life on our planet."

Chad Cornell, integrative herbalist and founder of
The Hollow Reed School of Healing Arts & Herbals

"As a medical doctor and ecology enthusiast, I loved this book, especially the wonderful introductory chapter that offers a wise perspective. I appreciate a book written by a holistic systems thinker that compiles an exhaustive reference that appeals to those concerned with a planetary, or one-health, approach to living."

Raquel Feroe, MD,
Alberta Medical Association

Moss Medicine

Indigenous Wisdom & Modern Pharmacology

A Sacred Planet Book

Robert Dale Rogers, RH(AHG)

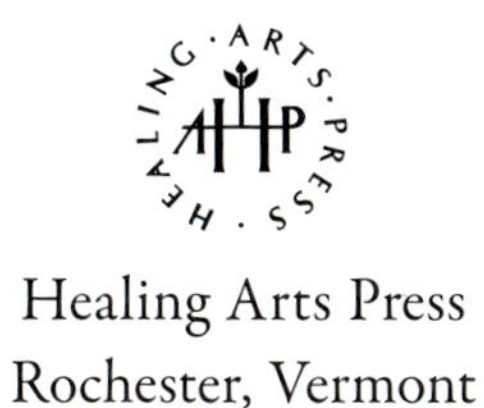

Healing Arts Press
Rochester, Vermont

Healing Arts Press
One Park Street
Rochester, Vermont 05767
www.HealingArtsPress.com

Healing Arts Press is a division of Inner Traditions International

Sacred Planet Books are curated by Richard Grossinger, Inner Traditions editorial board member and cofounder and former publisher of North Atlantic Books. The Sacred Planet collection, published under the umbrella of the Inner Traditions family of imprints, includes works on the themes of consciousness, cosmology, alternative medicine, dreams, climate, permaculture, alchemy, shamanic studies, oracles, astrology, crystals, hyperobjects, locutions, and subtle bodies.

Note to the reader: *This book is intended to be an informational guide. The remedies, approaches, and techniques described herein are meant to supplement, and not to be a substitute for, professional medical care or treatment. They should not be used to treat a serious ailment without prior consultation with a qualified health care professional.*

Cataloging-in-Publication Data for this title is available from the Library of Congress

ISBN 979-8-88850-099-6 (print)
ISBN 979-8-88850-100-9 (ebook)

Printed and bound in China by Reliance Printing Co., Ltd.

10 9 8 7 6 5 4 3 2 1

Text design by Virginia Scott Bowman and layout by Kenleigh Manseau
This book was typeset in Garamond Premier Pro with Acumin Pro Wide, Frutiger Lt Std, and Minion Pro used as display typefaces.

To send correspondence to the author of this book, mail a first-class letter to the author c/o Inner Traditions, One Park Street, Rochester, VT 05767, and we will forward the communication, or contact the author directly at **SelfHealDistributing.com**.

This book is dedicated to Laurie Szott-Rogers, my loving companion. Her beauty, wisdom, patience, and support have encouraged this Green Man to enjoy all the colors of the universe.

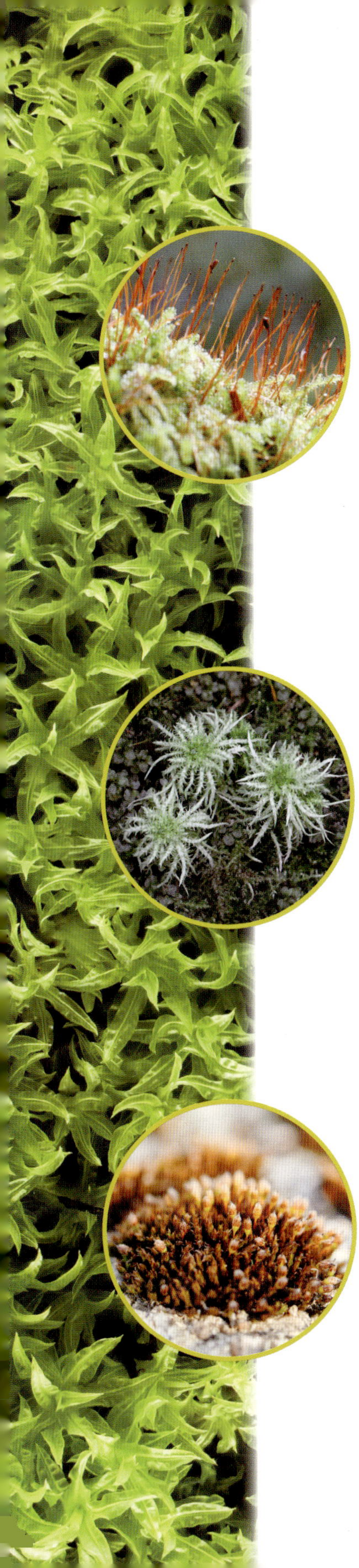

Contents

Liverwort, hornwort and moss:
Hearty land plants you may come across.
Found on logs, stones and trees,
They won't dry out or freeze,
And bryologists study this dross!

JAY BAILEY

Foreword

by Seán Pádraig O'Donoghue

Most people who have even dabbled in herbalism are familiar with the phenomenon of "the green curtain." To the untrained eye, a forest or field looks like a single green curtain onto which all of our assumptions about the plant world and wildness are projected. Once you come to know even a few individual plants, that green curtain dissolves and is replaced by a complex interdependent community of living beings, each with its own nature, its own virtues, its own ecological niche.

The green curtain slowly drops—first you learn to recognize the great trees, then the understory, and soon the green curtain has fallen to the ground. There it remains.

Once the green curtain has fallen entirely to the ground, the newly trained eye can see the fungi and the soil and the saprophytic plants. But oddly, for many of us, the soft-bodied green beings that grow on stones and roots remain a somewhat uniform green carpet that we simply call "moss." We are certainly at some level intellectually aware that the green carpet consists of a number of different species, but even to most herbalists they tend to blend into uniformity—not because they are all the same in any way, but because we have not come to know them individually. This book helps to shift that thought process.

Reading this book I learned that bryophytes—mosses, liverworts, and hornworts—are some of the oldest plants in the world. Widely varied and widely distributed, they are vital parts of the ecosystems that most of us inhabit.

I cannot think of a better guide to the strange and wonderful world of the bryophytes than Robert Rogers. Like many herbalists of my generation, I first discovered Robert's brilliant and eclectic mind through his work on medicinal fungi. Before I encountered Robert's writing, the only fungi in my personal materia medica were reishi and psilocybe. Along with mycologist Paul Stamets and a handful of others, Robert introduced many herbalists to the magnificent diversity of medicines that the fungal world provides to people (and to ecosystems).

In this book, Robert opens the world of bryophytes for the curious reader in much the same way. In the trademark fashion that will be familiar to readers of some of his sixty or so other books, Robert examines each species from the lens of many fields of knowledge, sharing information from the realms of medical research, folklore, ethnobotany, bioremediation, homeopathy, and essences. Together, these perspectives create a comprehensive picture of unique beings and their role in relation to humans as well as to the rest of life.

For herbalists, homeopaths, naturopaths, and flower essence practitioners (and perhaps some open-minded medical doctors), this book will provide a host of new medicines to consider bringing into the work of helping people in their quest for physical, emotional, and spiritual health. For naturalists it will provide new ways of looking at some fascinating plants in their ecosystems. For readers from every walk of life it will bring a deep appreciation of some of our most ancient wild kin, along with the inspiration to protect and nourish the places where they grow.

Seán Pádraig O'Donoghue

Seán Pádraig O'Donoghue is an herbalist, poet, and teacher living in western Maine. He is the author of three books: *The Forest Reminds Us Who We Are: Connecting with the Living Medicine of Wild Plants*; *Courting the Wild Queen*; and *The Silver Branch and the Otherworld: Forest Magic and Plant Allies.*

Acknowledgments

I especially wish to thank Janice Glime (2007, 2017, 2022), P. Cianciullo et al. (2022) and Christian Bailly (2023) for their stellar academic scholarship and contributions. I am also deeply indebted to Yoshinori Asakawa and colleagues and their 842 research publications. What an amazing academic career!

And thank you to Richard Grossinger, Ashley Kolesnik, Courtney B. Jenkins Mesquita, Lisa P. Allen, Margaret Jones, and Kayla Toher for helping bring this book into full form at Inner Traditions.

A special thank you to Alan Rockefeller, Graham Steinruck, and Drew T. Henderson for their generous contribution of outstanding bryophyte photographs.

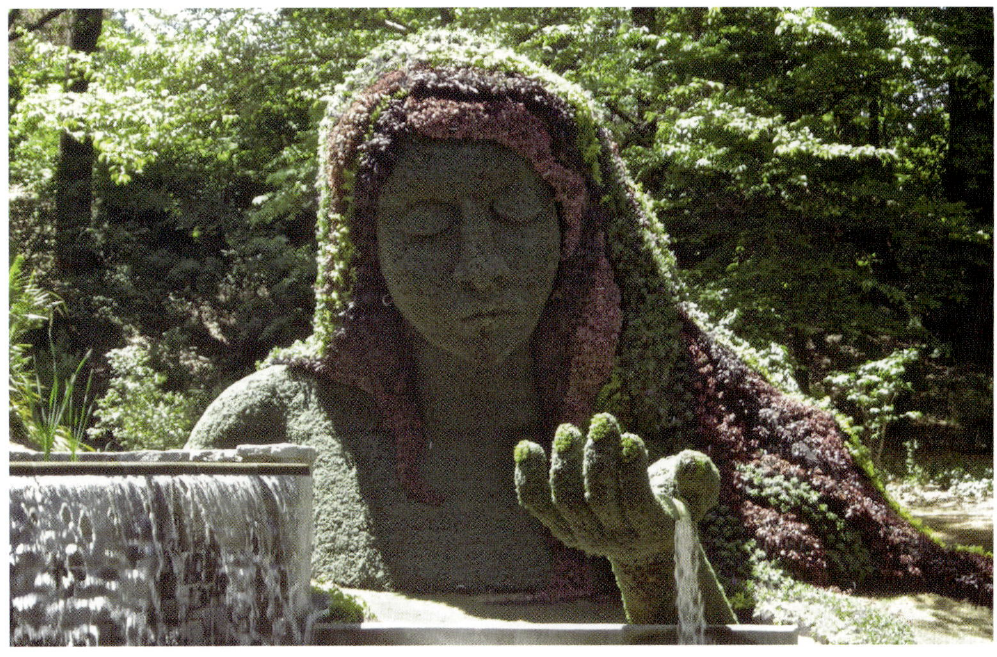

Moss Woman at the Atlanta Botanical Garden
Photo by Robert Dale Rogers

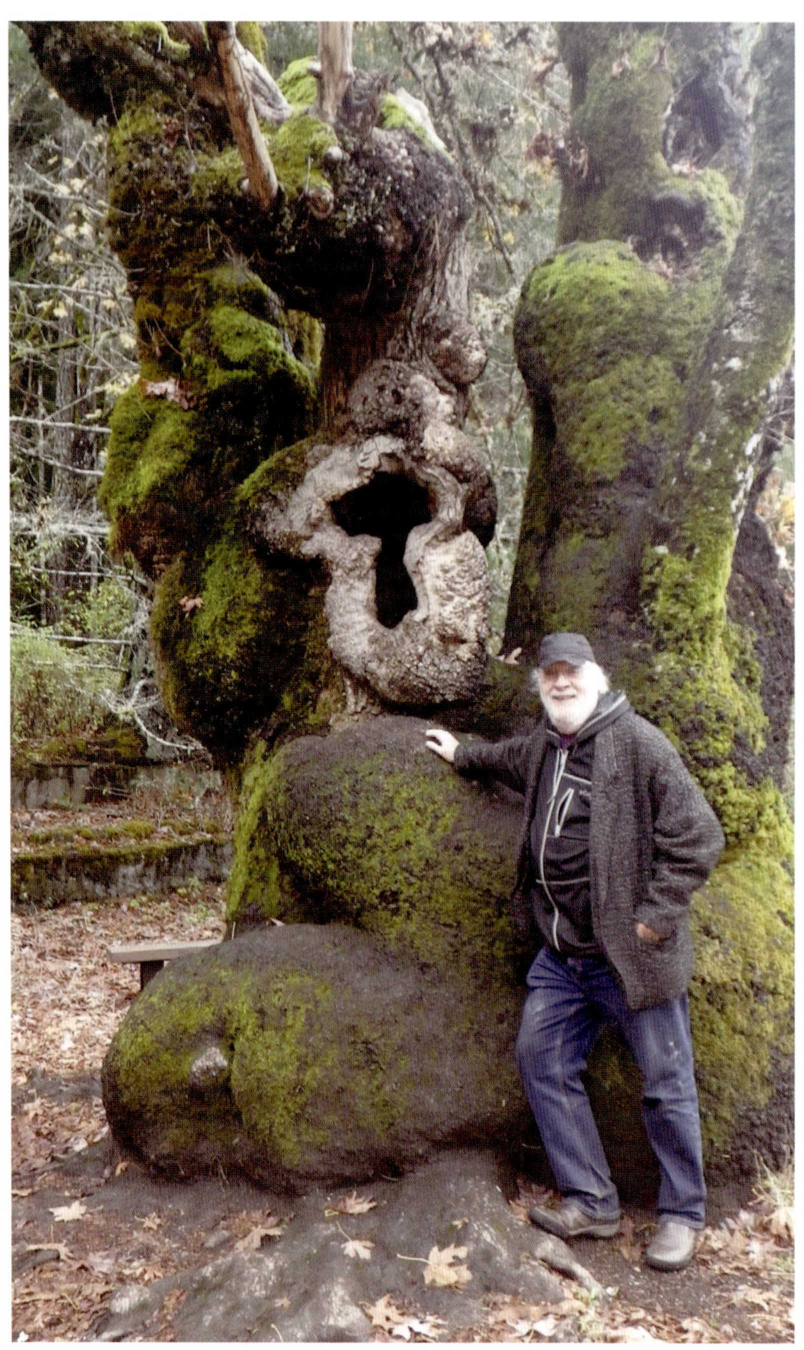

Robert Dale Rogers with moss-covered tree

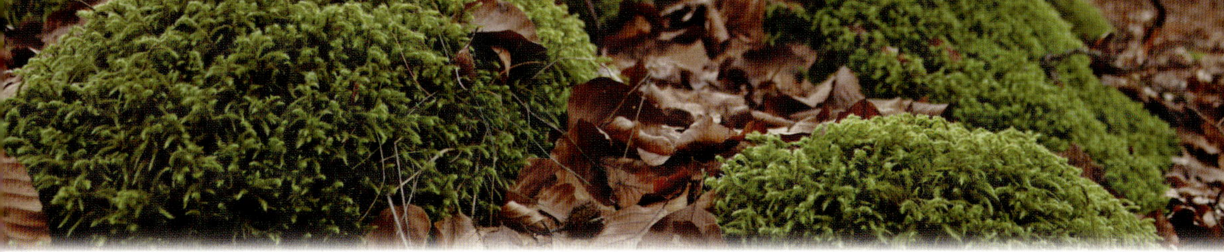

INTRODUCTION
Evolving from the Ancients

This is the forest primeval.
The murmuring pines and the hemlocks,
Bearded with moss, and in garments green.

Henry Wadsworth Longfellow

Bryophytes, which include mosses, liverworts, and hornworts, are the second-largest group of land plants after angiosperms, and among the oldest. Worldwide, there are some 14,000 species of leaf mosses (Bryophyta), more than 6,000 species of liverworts or liver mosses (Marchantiophyta), and 300 species of hornworts or foliage mosses (Anthocerotophyta) (Chandra et al. 2017). Note that *wort* is from the Middle English *wyrt*, for "root," "herb," "plant." A checklist by Söderström et al. (2016) suggests the total of both liverworts (Marchantiophyta) and hornworts (Anthocerotophyta) includes 7,486 species in 398 genera and 92 families. This number is decidedly low, as other authors suggest closer to 24,000 species worldwide.

The word *bryophyte* is derived from the Greek *brúon*, meaning "tree moss," and *phutón*, meaning "plant." The common name *moss* can be misleading. Spanish moss (*Tillandsia usneoides*), for example, belongs to the Bromeliaceae family, while reindeer moss is a lichen, spike moss a *Selaginella* spp., clubmoss a lycophyte, and Irish moss a seaweed.

There is controversy on the use of the plural *moss* versus *mosses*. The former is widely used by myself and the general population, but the scientific community deems only *mosses* as acceptable. The use of moss as a mass noun is to indicate a singular instance of its uniform nature (e.g. the *moss* blankets the rock) whereas *mosses* as a plural count noun is used to indicate various species/types of mosses. Both usages are grammatically correct, but it would make sense that

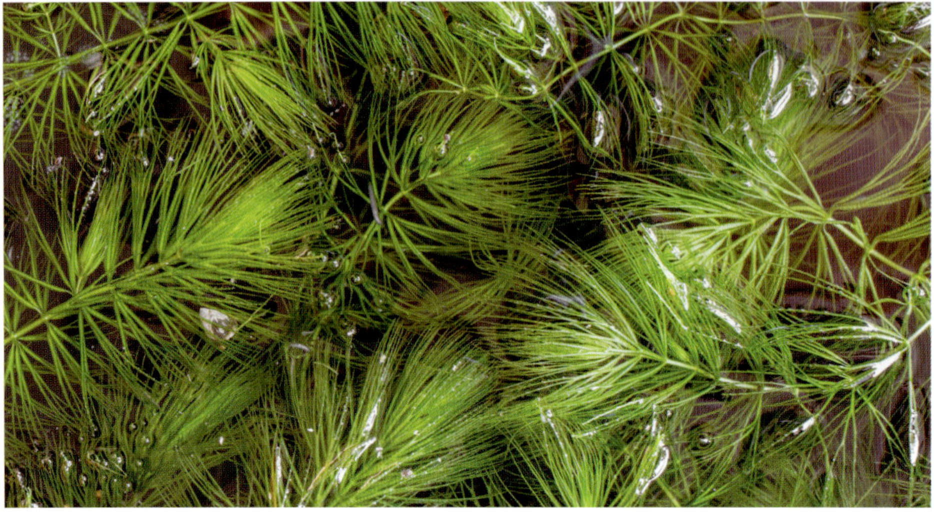

Ceratophyllum demersum (Rigid Hornwort)
Photo by Alan Rockefeller

mosses is used more often by the scientific community because they would be more inclined to identify and classify the little beings. Consider *moose*, which is used in both singular and plural senses. But the plural of *mouse* is *mice*. Oh well, such is the English language. . .

Bryophytes are distinguished by having no vascular tissue and no roots. They derive moisture from the air like a paper towel, absorbed from a leaf surface the thickness of which is only one cell, and they also extract nutrients from the air.

Hornwort is derived from the hornlike shape of the hornwort sporophyte, which is the multicellular diploid phase (Frangedakis et al. 2022).

They are found on all continents in a wide range of climates, ranging from deserts to polar regions. Access to moisture is a limiting factor to growth.

Most bryophytes remain hidden from humans simply because of their less noticeable domains. That may be a good thing, as where they grow does influence their flavonoid content. In one 2017 study (Wang, Cao et al.), it was shown that the flavonoid concentration in ninety samples of bryophytes varied from 1.8 mg/g to 22.3 mg/g. The study also showed that the flavonoid content in liverworts was generally higher than in mosses, with acrocarpous mosses (mosses with an upright growth pattern) higher in flavonoids than pleurocarpous species (mosses with a prostrate growth pattern). Bryophytes growing at low light levels exhibit the highest levels of flavonoids, and those of aquatic species the lowest. Also, the flavonoid content of low-latitude species was higher than those growing at higher latitudes.

The term *ethnobryology* was first coined by botanist Seville Flowers (1957) in a paper on their use by the Gosiute of Utah. Bryophytes, which have strong antimicrobial activity, have been widely used in traditional medicine for thousands of years for a variety of health conditions, including treatment of the liver, skin, and cardiovascular system. A study by Harris (2008) suggests the medicinal use of bryophytes has been explored mostly by Indigenous peoples of North America (28% of all species) as well as by Traditional Chinese Medicine (27% of all species). In China, for example, 40 species of bryophytes are used for medicine, while in India 22 species (but only those growing in Himalayan regions) are used. Oddly, there is no record of bryophyte use in Ayurvedic medicine.

Celtic traditional medicine, as recorded in the antique 1861 Welsh (Cymry) book *The Physicians of Myddfai: Meddygon Myddfai*, mentions using the river startip liverwort, *Scapania undulata* (Wagner et al. 2020). In a promising study by the National Cancer Institute, the antitumor properties of 123 mosses, 13 liverworts, and 1 hornwort was assessed (Spjut 1986). The research continues.

And yet, by and large, byrophytes are largely ignored by the medical community despite growing evidence of their ability to alleviate a number of chronic conditions. Perhaps this is partly because bryophytes do not produce flowers or seeds, drawing little attention from most botanists.

As a retired clinical herbalist, my interests lie in their medicinal potential for restoring human and animal health, as well as their potential to assist in the survival and well-being of our planet. The study of bryophytes is over a century old, but it's only been in the last 40 years that we have seen a tremendous accumulation of information on their chemistry and potential medicinal uses.

As with lichens, there has been a decline in bryophyte cover and richness, which is an indicator of our changing environment, in particular the heavy metal content in air pollution. Many people have heard of Oetzi, the Neolithic Tyrolean Iceman. His frozen body was uncovered in 1991 when retreating glaciers exposed him to hikers in the Austrian-Italian Alps. Along with his body was the discovery of 75 or more subfrozen bryophyte fossil species, including ten liverworts. Today, only 21 of these bryophytes grow in the same area (Dickson et al. 2019). At present, bryophytes are mainly used more prosaically as material for seed beds, fuel, food, pesticides, nitrogen fixation, gardening, construction, clothing, furnishing, packing, and soil conditioning.

THE PEATLAND PURIFIER

Mosses sequester carbon, one of their many gifts. *Sphagnum* spp. mosses, for example, soak up massive amounts of carbon dioxide, far exceeding the rate of sequestration by all the rainforests in the world combined according to bryophyte expert Annie Martin (2015). Peatlands contain as much carbon as is present in Earth's entire atmosphere, sequestering between 198 and 502 billion tons of carbon. Peat moss, especially sphagnum mosses, covers 85% of the province of Quebec, some 11.6 million hectares. One half square meter of moss sequesters one kilogram of carbon dioxide. Put another way: mosses sequester 6.43 billion tons of carbon annually from the atmosphere, or six times the carbon from altered lands (cultivated, agricultural lands) (Eldridge et al. 2023). And consider that mosses cover 9.4 million square kilometers of Earth's surface!

As one example of the great potential of bryophytes, Green City Solutions, a German company, utilizes the dust-cleansing properties of mosses to purify urban air. They have developed several products, including something called City Tree, which cleanses air for 100,000 people every hour, removing 82% of fine dust and cooling the returned air by up to 4.5° F / 2.5° C. Their larger units, City Breeze and Wall Breeze, are currently in development.

Sphagnum moss communities host numerous microorganisms, including microbial polyesterases. Work by Müller et al. (2017) identified six novel esterases, which were isolated, cloned, and heterologously expressed in *Escherichia coli*. The enzymes hydrolyzed not only common esterase substrates, but also polybutylene adipate terephthalate, or PBAT, a common material used in biodegradable plastics. The widespread use of synthetic polyesters requires the development of new sustainable technology solutions to enable recycling.

There is currently a fear that peat bogs are contributing to the rise in methane, but this has been debunked by recent findings (Wilson et al. 2016). Peat moss regenerates quickly, is easily harvested, has a low sulphur content, and its heating value is superior to wood. Moreover, peatlands, when drained and neutralized of acidity, are prolific producers of leaf and root vegetables. Over 100,000 acres throughout Canada are currently under agricultural use, supplying a large amount of produce for Toronto and Montreal. In Germany, sphagnum farming is replacing drainage-based peatland agriculture to help tackle downstream pollution and climate change (Vroom et al. 2020).

On the other hand, the destruction of peatlands, bogs, and fens by the petroleum industry has created a unique ecological and environmental

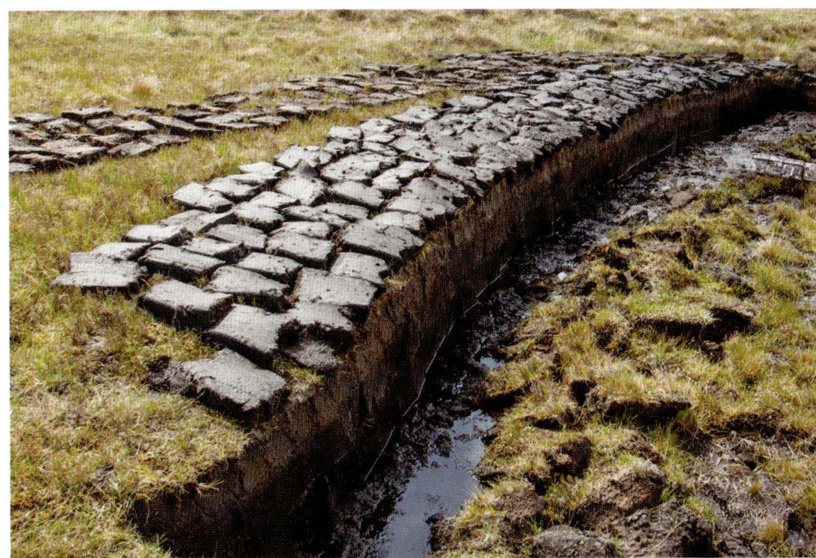

Peat moss harvest in Scotland

challenge. The re-creation of wetlands after their destruction by Athabasca oil sands companies in northeastern Alberta, Canada, will require the rapid cultivation of mosses, including fast-growing *Sphagnum* species. Fortunately, clonal in vitro cultivation of various species, including blunt-leaved bogmoss, *Sphagnum palustre*, is greatly increased some ten- to thirtyfold with the additions of sucrose and ammonium nitrate (Beike et al. 2015). These kinds of advances in biotechnology can help prevent the exploitation of wilderness mosses while also advancing the production of unique compounds for natural health and pharmaceutical benefit.

Peat moss is a valuable commodity that is used primarily in dry form as a soil conditioner. In nineteenth and early twentieth century Europe, peat was heavily pressed into round button shapes and a design was stamped into it. Peat moss is a very good medium for germinating jack pine and stimulates the growth of tamarack (larch) seedlings. It is used by florists and horticulturists to start cuttings and propagate orchids.

Alberta, my home province, has 103,000 square miles of peatland, or over 16% of its land base. The provincial peat moss industry produces over $33.5 million in sales annually, with three quarters shipped to the United States. On the Observatory of Economic Complexity website, Canada-wide, the annual figure in 2023 was about $490 million. In Canada, it seems that there is more energy in native peat than in the forest and natural gas reserves. The United States imports about 98% of Canadian peatmoss production.

A University of Exeter investigation shows that "global warming will cause peatlands to absorb more carbon—but the effect will weaken as warming increases, new research suggests" (University of Exeter 2018). The destruction of peatlands is an ecological disaster. The world's largest peat bog in Siberia, equal to the size of Germany and France combined, is thawing for the first time in 11,000 years (Martin 2015). As a result, untold levels of carbon dioxide are being released into the atmosphere. When peatlands are destroyed, they release up to two billion tons of carbon dioxide annually.

There is some good news to offset these revelations in the discovery that bryophyte spores are triggered into germination by smoke. A 2023 study (Yusup et al.) found that smoke enhanced the germinability of one-year old spores and considerably increased germination of spores naturally buried in peat for more than two hundred years. The study suggests that an increase in wildfires may lead to shifts in species dominance, which in turn may affect long-term carbon sequestration in peatlands. And in yet another bit of good news, some hornworts have been found to halt the growth of toxic blue-green algae by sucking up the nitrates, nitrites, and ammonia-based fertilizers.

THE EVOLUTION OF BRYOPHYTES

Let's now take a look at the three categories of bryophytes, their similarities and their differences.

Mosses emerged at the end of the Mesozoic era and existed on Earth approximately 264 million years before flowering plants (Altuner 2008). About five hundred million years ago, what are now today's land plants diverged from a common ancestry—the bryophytes and tracheophytes (the latter being vascular plants, including lycophytes, ferns, gymnosperms, and angiosperms). A fossil identified as *Hepaticites devonicus* is the thallus of a small leafy liverwort that lived approximately 400 million years ago (Hueber 1961). According to Britannica, an even older liverwort fossil dating from 473 to 471 million years ago was unearthed in northern Argentina.

Three different hypotheses are presently being considered for how bryophytes evolved some 450 million years ago. The first one suggests that they descended from the green alga Chlorophycean line. This is based on the protonemata of bryophytes being structurally similar to algae (Turmel 2020). The second hypothesis suggests that a green, unicellular algae may have evolved into a plant adapted to moist soil environments, and these plants, which possess the female reproductive organ archegonium found in mosses and ferns, may also be ancestors of the Chorophyceae algae line (Altuner 2008). A third theory suggests that bryophytes evolved from primitive vascular plants (Schofield 2001). Vermeulen (2011) speculates, "[It] is interesting in consideration of mosses own ancient heritage from algae, bypassing the more common developmental route that gave plants vascular structure and a root system, both of which mosses lack."

Some liverworts have been found preserved in amber, a fossilized tree resin. Work by Heinrichs et al. (2015) identified 23 fossil species of liverworts preserved in Baltic amber and dating from the Eocene epoch 35–50 million years ago. To put this in perspective, the dinosaurs had been extinct for about ten million years before their appearance. Notably, the term *Eocene* derives from the ancient Greek term for "dawn," referring to the early development of modern fauna. However, this pales in comparison to liverwort like fossils found in rocks in Oman that date back 460 million years (Wellman 2003), a discovery that predates fossils of mosses and hornworts by hundreds of millions of years. Adding to this body of prehistoric evidence, mats of fossilized liverworts were uncovered in a quarry in New York State that date back 380 million years (Hernick 2008), while in China, a rare liverwort fossil has been found to date back 411 to 407 million years (Guo et al. 2012).

CHARACTERISTICS OF MOSSES, LIVERWORTS, AND HORNWORTS

Mosses, liverworts, and hornworts differ in several ways:

	Mosses	Liverworts	Hornworts
complex oil bodies in leaf cells		x	
fused leaves		x	
thalloid		x	x
leafy	x	x	
ventral rank of leaves	x	reduced/absent	
lateral leaves with lobes		x	forked
pointed leaves	x		
smooth edged leaves	x		
spiral leaves	x		
seta*	x	soft, hyaline and short-lived	
peristome	x		

*Bristle or hairlike structures

CHARACTERISTICS CONTD.

	Moss	Liverwort	Hornworts
elaters**		x	
complex chemistry		x	
rhizoids	multicellular	unicellular	unicellular

**Spirally twisted, hygroscopic threads among the spores

Most liverworts have opposite round leaves that do not spiral. An exception are the *Homalia* species, which has round leaves and no sharp point on the tip. Note that a magnifying glass or 10x jeweler's loupe is essential for exact identification.

Hornworts have unique traits not found in other plants. These include their zygote development, which is longitudinal. The sporophyte stage in hornworts differs from mosses and liverworts in terms of lacking a seta (a bristle or hairlike structure), and it continually produces spores upward from a basal

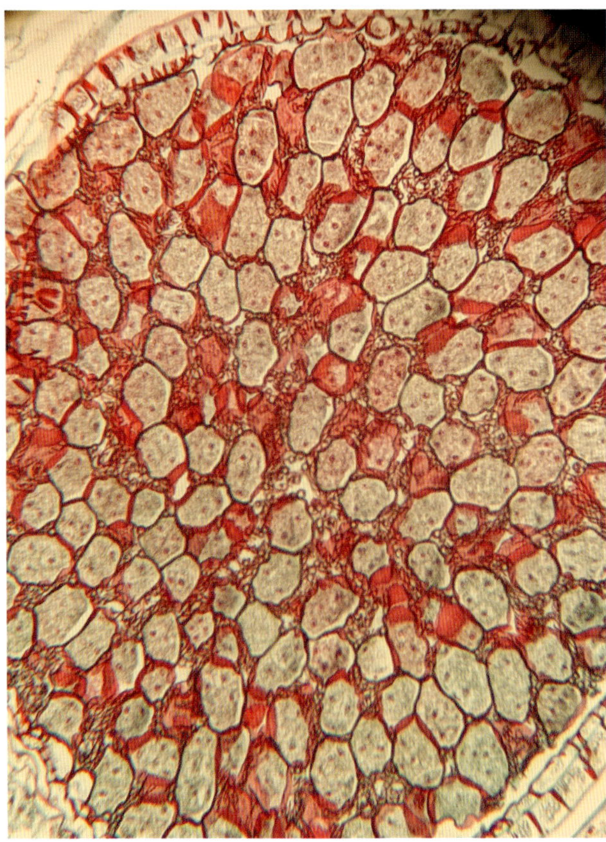

Pellia sporophyte under magnification

meristem.* Hornworts have only a single or few chloroplasts per cell. Some species contain a pyrenoid in chloroplast, also found in algae, but not in other land plants. They form symbiotic relationships with endophytic cyanobacteria (a type of gram-negative bacteria) and various fungal partners and possess one of the highest RNA editing rates of land plants (Frangedakis et al. 2022).

Numerous studies show that bryophytes have antibacterial, antiviral, antifungal, and anticancer activities. In so doing they have the potential to address the skyrocketing rates of cancer and the numerous strains of drug-resistant microbials prevalent today. Liverworts, hornworts, and mosses harbor fungal endophytes that are gaining increased interest from researchers for their ability to address these health concerns. The term *bryendophytes*, a portmanteau of *bryophyte* and *endophyte*, now refers to this important and productive source of biota possessing unique medical compounds (Stelmasiewicz et al. 2023, "Bioactive Compounds").

Bryophytes are a rich source of volatile terpenoids, with activities that are phytotoxic, antimicrobial, anticancer, antifungal, anti-inflammatory, antiparasitic, insecticidal, and piscicidal, to mention just a few benefits. The essential oils of bryophytes are antiviral and neurotrophic; they inhibit nitric oxide production and tubulin polymerization, relax the muscles, and are liver X-receptor alpha agonists and liver X receptor beta antagonists, among other activities (Asakawa and Ludwiczuk 2013). In many cases, some 10% to 15% of the compounds in bryophytes still have not been identified (Valarezo et al. 2020), suggesting unlimited potential health benefits as interest in these plants grows, and as we shall soon discover in the coming chapters.

Mosses, liverworts and hornworts contain salicin and its derivatives for protection from herbivores and microbes, as well as hormonal regulation for reproduction and growth (Whiteman 2023). It may surprise many readers that humans and other animals circulate small amounts in their bloodstream, mostly coming from diet.

In the chapters that follow we will examine the health potentials of bryophytes. We will consider traditional uses, modern medicinal applications, various water and alcohol extractions, and essential oil production.

*A type of plant tissue consisting of undifferentiated cells capable of cell division.

AUTHOR'S NOTE ON HOW THIS BOOK IS ORGANIZED

As you read ahead, you'll notice that the bryophytes (mosses, liverworts, and hornworts) are organized by genus. Each genus has a list of species by their common names found in that genus (such as "Magellanic Bogmoss") as well as groups of names in plural (such as "Feather Mosses"). For more prominent genera, a green box contains descriptions of the geographic range, habitat, practical uses, and medicinal applications of a number of species in that particular genus. Each species does not necessarily have every attribute presented in the summary, but collectively the species in that genus share these characteristics.

In each blue box is a description of a notable essence from that particular genus, including its emotional gifts and guidance bestowed. A recommendation of where to find the essence is also given where applicable.

At the end of the book you will see a comprehensive list of bryophytes by their common names. If you happen to know a particular moss, liverwort, or hornwort in your area by its common name, you can look up the common name in the list to see the bryophyte's Latin binomial. Then use the first part of the binomial, the genus, to flip to that section in this book. And if you are as passionate about mosses, liverworts, and hornworts as I am, you may review this list frequently to become familiar with the names. Enjoy!

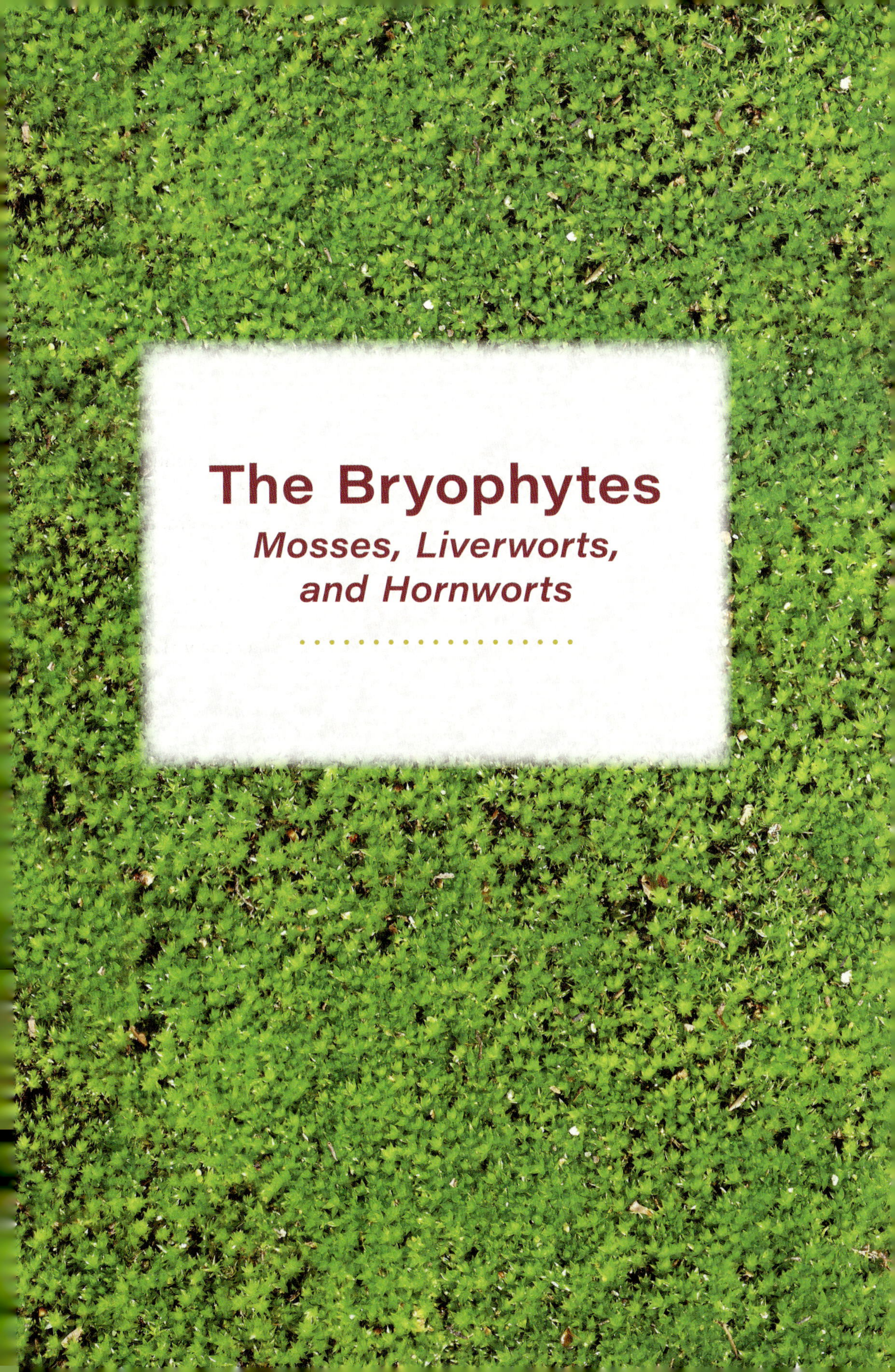

The Bryophytes

Mosses, Liverworts, and Hornworts

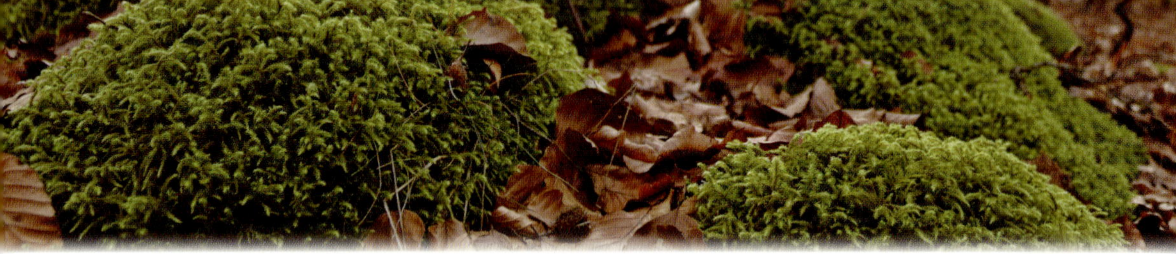

1
Mosses

Bryophyta

The sacred Virgin's well, her moss most sweet and rare against infectious damps.

Michael Drayton, *Poly-Olbion*

[Moss appears] where the cosmic forces bring to life only the uppermost layer of the Earth and where the life of Earth itself is reduced to a minimum. The mosses spread a tundra carpet all over the Earth and build a second plant world under and among the normal vegetation . . . Mosses are closely related to the mineral earth. They are a kind of transition stage between dead mineral and live plant, as can be seen by those species which continue to grow above whilst becoming peat below . . . A single moss plant would be an absurdity, for only in a mass, a carpet, are they a viable whole.

Gerbert Grohmann

The word *moss* derives from the Old English *mos*, meaning a bog or the vegetation growing in it. It stems from the Latin *muscus*, and further back, to the Indo-European *meu*, meaning "damp."

The interior of mosses is rich in algae and other life. According to Robin Wall Kimmerer, professor at the SUNY College of Environmental and Forest Biology and the founding director of the Center for Native Peoples and the Environment, "One gram of moss from the forest floor, a piece about the size of a muffin, would harbour 150,000 protozoa, 132,000 tardigardes, 3000 springtails, 800 rotifers, 500 nematodes, 400 mites and 200 fly larvae" (Kimmerer 2003).

Mosses are incredibly hardy, surviving dry conditions and then recovering

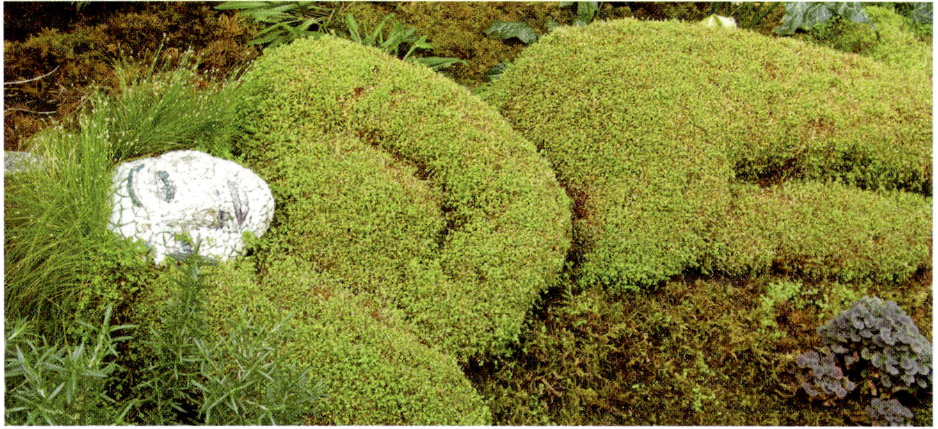

Moosfräulein, "moss woman"
Photo by Robert Dale Rogers

with moisture. *Cryptobiosis* is a term that describes the reversible state of being whereby metabolic processes cease. This allows for periods of survival under intense or adverse climate conditions. A 2017 study (Cannone et al.) found moss surviving in Antarctica after six centuries of glacial burial. After the retreat of the glacier, some of the moss survived and returned to a metabolic state. The genetic pathways involved may have implications for the fields of medicine, agriculture, biodiversity, and space exploration.

Tardigardes, or water bears, provide a fascinating comparison with mosses in this regard. These micro-animals were first discovered in 1773 by German zoologist Johann A. E. Goeze, who called them "little water bears"; a few years later, Italian biologist Lazzaro Spallanzani named them *tardigrada*, meaning "slow walkers." Like mosses, which shrink when desiccated, water bears can reduce to one-eighth their former size, known as a tun state, wherein they can survive for years and withstand extreme environmental conditions, in the state, known as anabiosis.

Water bears in this state can survive temperatures down to 0.008 degrees above absolute zero (-459.4° F / -273° C) and only revive—also like mosses—when exposed to water. Water bears can survive temperatures of -4° F/-20° C for up to thirty years and withstand ionizing radiation hundreds of times stronger than lethal to humans.

Mosses have long been used in medicine, with early citations in European literature dating back to the sixteenth century. Cultures around the world, including India and China, as well as Indigenous healers from North America, have also made use of mosses for healing.

Interest in moss medicine diminished greatly in the 1880s due to the emergence of pharmaceutical medicine but has recently revived thanks to the work of countless diligent scientists and researchers as well as practitioners of various forms of natural healing.

HISTORIAL USES OF MOSS IN EUROPE

In mosses . . . strength is mingled with humility, gentleness, and charm, with elemental essence, reflecting the gladness of wind, sun and rain.

JOHN BLAND

Like their blue-green algae ancestors, mosses have no roots and must therefore absorb water and nutrients from the air. Water moves osmotically from cell to cell, thus the diminutive size of the organisms. On the other hand, the tiniest piece of moss can regenerate into another moss. The ball mosses, for example, have modified stems that break off like tumbleweeds to start life in a new geographic location.

A fascinating use of bryophytes arose in the 1500s and involved moss growing on the skulls of the dead. This form of medicine, *Muscus ex Cranio Humano*, or skull moss, was described by the Victorian dramatist Douglas Jerrold as "Newgate Moss," or "the periwig of a dead cranium." The first mention of skull moss, however, was by the Swiss physician Paracelsus, also known as Philippus Aureolus Theophrastus Bombastus von Hohenheim (1493–1541). In his book *Die Grosse Wundartzney* (1536), he mentions "*das mies auf den toten kopfen*," "moss from the skull of the dead." Around this same time, the physician, botanist, and herbalist Jacobus Theodorus, known as Tabernaemontanus (1525–1590), considered the father of German botany, published *Nuew Kreuterbuch* (roughly "New Herb Book") in 1588, which was reprinted several times. In a 1590 edition there is an image of a human skull with moss growing on its surface. Later editions record that medics and apothecaries would place human skulls in damp places so they could be overgrown with moss, which "crawl back and forth like a long rough worm" (Duffin 2022). Tabernaemontanus's suggested use for dried and powdered skull moss was for bleeding. Flemish physician and botanist Rembert Dodoens (1517–1585) recorded that decoctions of skull mosses were useful for mitigating heavy menstrual flow in women, stopping nosebleeds, and mixing into a variety of unguents and astringent oils (Dodoens 1557). English herbalist John Gerard (1545–1612) published an English translation of Dodoen's work in 1597, resulting in Gerard's *Great Herball.* He used an image produced earlier by Tabernaemontanus with the following text:

> This kind of Mosse is found vpon the scull or bare scalpes of men and women, lying long in charnell houses, and other places where the bones of men are kept together: it growth very thicke, white, like vnto the short Mosse vpon the trunkes of olde Oakes: it is thought to be a singular remedie against the falling euill, and the Chincough in children if it be powdered, and then gluen in sweet wine, for certaine daies together (Gerard 1597).

Chincough was the term used then to refer to whooping cough or pertussis.

In those days it was believed the vital force exited the body through the skull at the time of death. Some believed that the cranium of those hanged was especially therapeutic due to the vital force being trapped there for up to seven years; this vital energy was transferred to the growing moss.

Philosopher, statesman, and all-around Renaissance man Francis Bacon (1561–1626) weighed in on the availability of skull moss, suggesting Ireland was a good source due to the heaps of unburied dead there.

A preparation called weapon salve was an ointment that contained skull moss, often combined with human fat, powdered mummy, man's blood, linseed oil, oil of roses, and bole armoniack. Oddly, the ointment was kept in a box, and a stick was used to collect blood from a wound to be stuck into the ointment. The actual wound was bound with linen and washed each morning with the patient's urine. It was believed that weapon salve could heal remotely over great distances as well (Duffin 2022). Astrologer and alchemist John Dee (1527–1609) claimed:

> [This concoction] can heal patients at a thirty-mile distance. Instead of applying the medicine directly to the wound, the medical practitioner needs to apply it to the bloodied weapon that caused it, or, in its absence, an object made from a similar material to the weapon after it has been dipped into the wound. More extraordinary still, the medicine requires various ingredients extracted from corpses: skull moss, human fat and blood, and powdered mummy (Drieshen 2024).

Skull moss was best harvested when "the Moon is in the Increase in the House of Venus, when she is in Pisces, Taurus or Libra" (Duffin 2022).

The main use of skull moss, however, was in the treatment of epilepsy and nervous afflictions. *Homalothecium sericeum*, a moss commonly found growing on walls in England and Ireland, was collected to be grown on skulls for this medical purpose. Various combinations were added, including peony, elk hoof, coral, amber, and emeralds, all ground into a powder. Other ingredients included frankincense, dragon's blood, Armenian bole, terra sigillata ("medicinal earth"), gypsum, "prepar'd frogs," and hare pelage. English physician William Salmon (1644–1733) suggested skull moss for the treatment of bleeding following amputation of a limb.

Mosses conjure up all kinds of emotions. They are associated with antiquity and aging, beauty, quiet, cemeteries, seclusion, loneliness, retrospection, and death. German and Norse "moss folk" were said to resemble the Greek dryads, the "little people" living in the forest. The Grimm Brothers described these moss people as clad in moss, hanging out in dark forests, usually hollow trees, or dwelling in a bed of moss. Female moss people were known as *moosfräulein*, "moss ladies," and their queen was called *Buschgroßmutter*, "Shrub Grandmother." They are reminiscent of Irish leprechauns in that they borrow things but are also helpful to humans. A gift of caraway bread was said to anger them. During plagues and epidemics the moss folk would show people medicinal herbal cures.

> *And the moss hung down from the branches,*
> *Without any companion it grew there uttering joyous leaves of*
> *dark green,*
> *And its look, rude, unbending, lusty, made me think of myself.*
>
> Walt Whitman

My friend and colleague Dr. Jim Butler founded the Elemental Life Form Encounters Project (ELFEN) many years ago, collecting stories on elementals, nature spirits, fauns, wood nymphs, little people, elves, and fairies from around the world. I have no personal experience of such little people, but on a recent trip to Reykjavik, Iceland, I came across many people willing to share their stories of the diminutive folk. While driving down a busy, straight highway, it suddenly took a wide turn around a pile of rocks and then resumed. When I inquired later, I was told that little people lived in the rocks, and the powers that be ordered the detour to appease the populace.

JAPANESE MOSS GARDENS

The Japanese have a deep appreciation of bryophytes and have long cultivated moss and lichen gardens. The word *shibusa* describes the venerable quality of refinement they instill in a setting. Common hairy cap moss, *Polytrichum* species, is the most widely used species in these moss gardens, alternating with *Pogonatum* species.

The most famous moss garden in the world is Kyoto's Saiho-ji, also known as Kokedara, which means "Moss Temple." A World Heritage Site to which tourists must apply in advance to gain access, the temple and garden was founded and restored by Zen priest and garden designer Musō Soseki in 1339. The main pond is shaped like the Chinese character *kokoro*, which means "heart." The garden has over 120 different types of moss spread out over 18,000 square meters. "Going through the garden is like weaving through a soft felt of different tones of green, gold and bronze" (Nordström 2019).

In Kyoto alone there are 1,700 temples where gardens reflect traditional Japanese culture in displays of trees, rocks, and especially mosses (Nordström 2019). In addition, quasi-indoor pocket moss gardens known as *tsubo-niwa* are common sights in courtyards and at the entrances of private homes. References to moss are found in a form of classical Japanese poetry known as *waka* and in Zen Buddhist writings going back a thousand years.

The Portland Japanese Garden and the Bloedel Reserve on Bainbridge Island, both in Washington State, are two great examples of North American

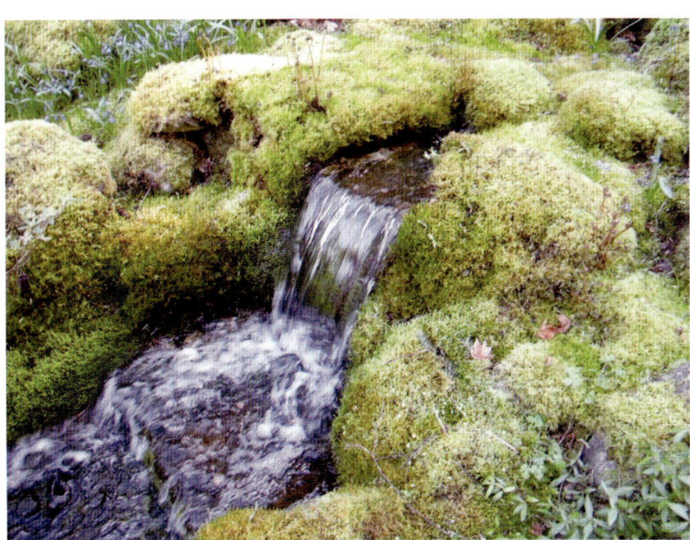

Waterfall at Japanese moss garden in Butchart Gardens
Photo by Robert Dale Rogers

moss gardens. My personal favorite is the Japanese moss garden at the Butchart Gardens on Vancouver Island. My friend and herbal colleague Tony Oakworth lives a few blocks from this amazing spot, which we've visited together. This magnificent garden was started in 1906, when Jennie Butchart, with the assistance of Japanese landscape expert Isaburo Kishida, began shaping the former rock quarry.

Moss-covered boulders are the astute landscaper's prize find, with half moss and half exposed rock considered ideal.

THE LAWN CONTROVERSY

The North American obsession with growing grass lawns is an ecological disaster. According to the U.S. Environmental Protection Agency, lawn care, including golf courses, use one-third of the public water supply. This is roughly nine billion gallons daily! It is estimated that 80% of American households have grass lawns covering some 28 million acres, with 21 million acres being private lawns. Americans spend $40 billion annually to maintain their grass lawns, with an average of 150 hours of labor. And those noisy, smelly gas lawnmowers, weed wackers, and leaf blowers use 200 million gallons of fuel, adding to air pollution, not to mention the environmental impact of fertilizers, pesticides, fungicides, and herbicides. Gas-powered lawnmowers emit ten to twelve times more hydrocarbons than cars and trucks; weed wackers twenty-one times more. One hour of lawn mowing equals 43 hours of driving a car (Martin 2015).

In contrast to the wasteful practice of growing grass lawns it is estimated that a mat of moss measuring 60 by 80 cm turns one kilogram of carbon dioxide into one killogram oxygen annually. Overall, algae, liverworts, and mosses sequester some 14 billion tons of CO_2 and fix 50 billion tons of nitrogen annually (Elbert et al. 2012). Moss gardens also invite beneficial insects, frogs, and other endangered species. Deer do not eat moss, which is an added bonus in many neighborhoods. Other uses of moss include erosion control, flood mitigation, and water filtration of oil, detergents, dyes, and remediation of heavy metals and pharmaceutical seepage. Some of the more common varieties of mosses used in moss landscaping are *Polytrichum commune* and *Bartramia pomiformis*.

Moss lawns are great for the environment and do not require mowing. They rarely require weeding, don't use fertilizers, and can grow on low-nutrient soil. A small velvet carpet moss lawn absorbs more carbon than 275 mature trees, produces oxygen, but requires periodic watering.

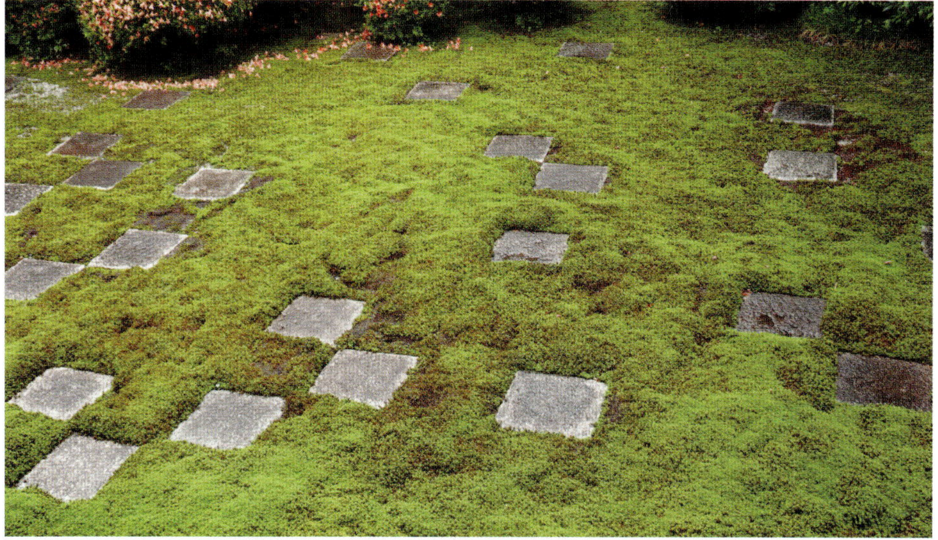

A moss lawn

Unfortunately, not all people appreciate the spread of moss into their pristine Kentucky bluegrass. Hardware stores stock chemicals like ferrous sulphate to kill mosses: Moss-Out, Moss-B-Gone, Moss-B-Ware (for roofs and walks), and MossEx. When sprayed with any of these products the moss will turn black within a few days.

GARDENING WITH MOSS

In some regions, moss roofs are a beautiful and ecological choice. Simply cover the existing roof with plastic and then mould layers of peat soil before transplanting the moss. This works best where the roof is in partial shade and protected from severe winds and direct sunlight. This will add considerable weight, and you may wish to consult an architectural engineer before any large project.

To propogate many species of moss to make a moss garden, you can make a moss milkshake.

Moss Propagation Milkshake

Take moss and place in blender with a litre of buttermilk/water and quick pulse to a green froth. You are not making a smoothie, just making the moss into a sticky paste.

Next, paint a thick coating of this mixture onto rocks in order to yield a moss garden within two years. Other recipes use yogurt (one part yogurt to seven parts water), egg whites, brewer's yeast, etc. I personally find mixing dry pieces of moss in beer works great.

Optional: Add some polymer crystals or powder, available at nurseries, which helps by absorbing water and producing a slimy gel.

You can create more moss if your garden already contains mosses, by brushing this liquid on rocks, or sprinkling moss powder. The best time is spring or fall, during cooler, humid weather. You can purchase sphagnum peatmoss blocks to which spores easily adhere. You can later cut to desired shape. And don't forget to water as growth begins.

However, Martin (2015) is not a big fan of moss milkshakes. She favors taking moss fragments and then water them for at least the first month. I especially like her living moss walls, which are grown horizontally, then placed upright when mature. Office and home moss walls add a unique green vibrancy. For rock walls, she suggests masonry glue or two parts epoxy to keep the mosses in place.

Alum will create the right soil pH for moss growth. If your soil is quite alkaline, the addition of sulfur or aluminum sulfate can adjust the pH to around pH 5, which is ideal. For example, if your soil is pH 7 (neutral) you would need less than two kilograms of sulfur per 30 square metres to obtain optimal level.

THE POPULAR, MULTI-FUNCTIONAL SPHAGNUM MOSS

The uses of sphagnum moss, commonly called peat moss, one of the most widely known forms of moss known to us today, can be traced back to *The Annals of Loch Cé* (Hennessey 1871, 2012), which notes its use for wounds suffered in the Battle of Clontarf, near Dublin, Ireland, in 1014 AD.

In Germany in 1882, a peat worker was unable to treat his open fracture skin wound on his forearm, so he stuffed it with dry sphagnum, and when a doctor examined it ten days later it had healed. The two species mainly used were *Sphagnum papillosum* and *S. palustre*.

Sphagnum has traditionally been woven with wool in northern Europe. Throughout the world, peat moss has been used for its absorbent and insulation properties, in pillows, mattresses, furniture, doormats, toilet paper, and as moisture absorbers between summer and storm windows. The Anishinabe, a group of culturally related Indigenous peoples in the Great Lakes region of Canada and the United States, used *Sphagnum dusenii* in sleeping mattresses (Smith 1932). The Saomi (Sámi) of northern Scandinavia used sphaghum moss in baby cradles and for diapers and menstrual pads, according to Linnaeus in his 1737 work *Flora Lapponica*. It was the first disposable diaper material because of its absorbency (sphagnum moss is capable of retaining twenty times its weight in water) as well as its disinfecting properties. Other Indigenous peoples mixed green sphagnum moss with animal fats to treat cuts. Sphagnum moss was possibly used by various Indigenous women as a contraceptive "sponge" to obstruct sperm.

The Cree of Saskatchewan and Alberta call the moss used for diapers *askiyah*, and they also use it for wiping, much like paper towels are used today. It was traditionally used to clean babies of mucous and blood after birth. The Chipewyan people further north call it *tth'al* and distinguish between the red and green varieties. The white variety is used for baby diapers, toilet paper, and menstrual pads.

Ground moss in general is known in Cree as *astâskamkwa*, while green peat moss in particular is called *maskwoskwa*. Russell Willier, a noted Cree healer, uses it on cuts and infected skin, as well as for baby diapers. It is traditionally combined with animal fat to treat skin problems. Red peat moss is applied directly to cuts or skin infections, while the green type is considered better for diapers, since the red type, probably *Sphagnum capillifolium*, is considered too irritating for babies.

The Dena'ina people of Alaska use red sphagnum for any injury involving swelling, broken bones, blood poisoning, or serious ear or eye problems. It is boiled, and the afflicted area is held over the steam that results, with the moss then placed on the skin. An ointment can also be made by mixing the dried moss with animal or bird fat to treat cuts. For ear troubles, hot rocks are surrounded by wet red sphagnum in a birch bark container and then placed on the patient's head so that the steam enters the ears. *Sphagnum magellanicum*, commonly called Magellan's peatmoss, is soaked in cold water and applied to treat headaches and lung problems; as well as used for sanitary napkins and diapers. Interestingly, a moss sanitary napkin introduced in 1991 by pharmaceutical giant Johnson & Johnson did not have initial consumer interest (Martin 2015).

Pink sphagnum (*Sphagnum divinum*) is preferred by Indigenous peoples around the Great Lakes area, while *S. nemoreum* syn. *S. capillifolium*, a type of red sphagnum, is avoided due to skin irritation and diaper rash.

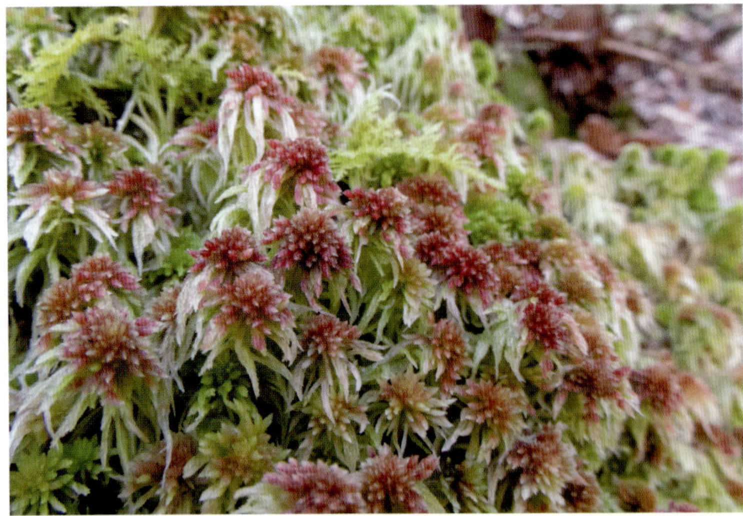

Sphagnum nemoreum (Acute-Leaved Bogmoss)

Wet sphagnum moss was sometimes put on hot coals to smoke meat or leather.

The Crow of southern Montana know sphagnum moss as *bee ma ga sut che*, while the Nlaka'pamux of British Columbia know it as swamp moss or creek moss. The Gwich'in, of the Mackenzie Delta in northwestern Canada, used *nin'*, or sphagnum moss, for some of the same purposes. The wet moss was used for washing dishes and wiping off fish tables or put in a jar of water as a houseplant. For diapers it was first hung in the lower branches of black spruce trees to dry and to let the bugs crawl away. Special houses to store the dried moss for winter diaper use were built of black spruce saplings bent to form a bent dome as for sweat lodges and tied together with split black spruce roots. The walls were filled in with spruce saplings stuck into the ground to form a dense wall. Boughs were placed on the ground, and then the dried moss was heaped on top.

An unusual traditional use in places where moss, known as *uske* or *muskak* by the Cree, is plentiful is for building moss houses. These houses were built of blocks of moss cut in the fall just after it starts to freeze. In the spring, the blocks were stored until the next fall, when the good ones would be reused. The blocks measured three feet by one foot wide and eight inches thick and were packed between peeled poles that came together at the top. For a large, three-family home, twenty poles would be required, and it would take about one week to construct.

A fireplace was built in the middle, and gravel stones were built up about one foot to serve as a footing. As the ground thawed, more stones were placed on the platform. If the moss house was built carefully, the smoke from the fireplace would linger about six feet above people's heads. Smaller moss houses were sometimes built along trap lines.

In China, sphagnum moss is traditionally used as a binder for iron and as a supplement for piglets that are often born anemic. Europeans used the powder or burnt ashes of sphagnum moss as a germicide. During World War I it was used as surgical dressing on the battlefield. Toward the end of the war, about one million pounds of dressings per month were used. These dressings were cooler, softer, retarded bacterial growth, and were more absorbent than cotton, absorbing three to four times as much liquid three times faster.

Sphagnum moss puts hydrogen ions into the water in exchange for cations of calcium, magnesium, and sodium. The addition of hydrogen makes the water more acidic, making bogs and fens more so in this direction. This natural acidity contributes to sphagnum's antimicrobial activity. The pH of water at the edge of a sphagnum bog may be 4.3, the equivalent of dilute vinegar. Work by Varley and Barnett (1987) cites evidence from controlled testing that the amount of wound area covered by new epidermis doubled using sphagnum dressing compared to none.

Laplanders use the moss in children's cradles.

The use of sphagnum moss for spinning material has been attempted in Sweden to produce cloth and clothing. It is manufactured into the inner soles of hiking boots to absorb moisture and odors. The Vikings used mosses to pack soft leather slippers.

Sphagnum is used today to clean up heavy metals, PCPs, and toxic wastes, including oil spills and dyes. It is very effective at removing nitrogen (96%) and phosphorus (97%) from rivers and wastewater. It absorbs up to twelve times its weight in petrochemical spills. Many bryophytes are hydrophobic and lipophilic, meaning they repel water and absorb oils. The hummock species, *Sphagnum. fuscum*, *S. capillifolium*, and *S. rubellum*, can remove biofilms from pools, reducing the need for chemicals by 90%.

In the past, sphagnum moss has been used to make alcohol, various chemicals, paper, paraffin, naphtha bricks, life preservers, gunpowder, fireworks, paint, insulation, and charcoal. One of the most valuable byproducts of peat moss is a wax with a relatively high melting point—peat yields 9.4% of a crude wax with a melting point of 163.4° F / 73° C. One factory near Minsk, Russia, produces a mineral wax from peat for use in leather polishes, crayons, and plastics. A cream is also made for the treatment of eczema, ulcers, and burns.

Peat mosses are burned in the distillation of Scotch whiskey, giving a distinct smoky taste to single malt varieties. In some whiskeys the grains are first steeped in water from a sphagnum peatland during the malting stage. These include the Ardbeg, Highland Park, Octomere, Laphroaig, and Talisker brands. The smoky flavor is derived by drying the malt over a peat fire.

Some thirty-five years ago, I visited Wales and took in the Eisteddfod, an annual celebration of song, poetry, and dance, as well as imbibing in alcohol. One evening I stayed at a local hotel with a small bar downstairs. Only those with a room could drink into the night, and a few locals took advantage of me by buying too many single malt scotches to sample so they also could drink. Some were very peaty, if that is the correct term.

Various mosses have been used worldwide to pack fruit and mushrooms for shipment. In Great Britain, mosses were used as temporary stuffing for taxidermy and to pack bomb sights during World War II. In other parts of Europe, moss helped protect against the sharpness of blades and daggers during shipment.

In Japan various soil-free mosses were used to hold ancient silk garments.

Indigenous peoples of Japan, Alaska, and Siberia used moss for funerals. In Siberia, mosses were used to fit together birch bark sheets to line the roof of tombs, some over 2,500 years old.

The Guanche mummies from the Canary Islands, dating back to 1380, were found with *Exsertotheca intermedia* syn. *Neckera intermedia* in their abdominal cavities.

Sphagnol, a tar-like pitch substance derived from sphagnum, was isolated in 1899 and added to ointments and medicated soaps until the 1960s. Each soap bar contained 15% pure sphagnol. It was also used in ointments, shaving soap, and even suppositories. It is very useful for external application in cases of eczema, psoriasis, skin itching, mosquito bites, hemorrhoids, chilblains, acne, and scabies. It is very similar to Cade oil, which is dry distilled from juniper wood, in its use. The soap was used during both World Wars by the British Red Cross to treat facial wounds (Glime 2017).

Sphagnan, a pectin-like polysaccharide, was isolated from sphagnum moss in 1983 and was found to inhibit bacterial growth and remove ammonia from microbial environments.

MEDICINAL USES OF MOSSES

Traditional Chinese Medicine (TCM) uses about 40 species of bryophytes to treat illness of the cardiovascular system, skin, burns, tonsillitis, bronchitis, tympanitis, and cystitis.

Mosses contain biologically active compounds that protect them from pathogenic fungi and other microorganisms as well as insects, slugs, and other predators. This biochemistry helps mosses make up for their lack of thick bark or protectant cuticles. An extract of *Rhodobryum giganteum*, giant rose moss, for example, has been shown to increase aorta blood flow by up to 30% in animal studies (Alam et al. 2015).

In general, mosses contain polyunsaturated fatty acids that have been found to prevent atherosclerosis and cardiovascular disease, reducing collagen-induced thrombocyte aggregation and lowering triacylglycerols and cholesterol in blood plasma (Radwan 1991).

Mosses show great potential, mainly in vitro, against a variety of cancer cell lines. A 2009 investigation tested 219 moss extracts against human epithelial/cervical (HeLa) cancer cells and identified 41 extracts acting on cell division in various manners (Krzaczkowski et al). Moss compounds also provide adjunctive benefit to chemotherapy drugs, reducing predictable side effects and improving survival rates. Also, they contain compounds that act synergistically with today's antibiotics, helping fight drug-resistant bacterial infections, thereby saving lives. These community and hospital-acquired infections are the third leading cause of death in North America.

Mosses do not contain the abundance of beneficial volatile oils found in their cousins, the liverworts. The most common monoterpenoid found in mosses is citrocitral, with α-and β-pinene, limonene, α-terpineol, and camphor often present.

An exploration of homeopathic remedies derived from mosses has been restricted until fairly recent times. Generally, the new and proven bryophyte remedies address issues of vulnerability, smallness, and insignificant or shy personalities, where the person may feel helpless and unable to deal with difficulties and therefore retreats. They may also display a quality of devotion and giving to others at their own expense.

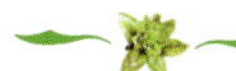

ABIETINELLA

Fir Moss   Pine Branched Moss   Spruce Tree Feather Moss

The name of the genus *Abietinella* and the species name *abietina* both derive from the Latin *abies*, meaning "fir," and *tina*, implying a likeness or resemblance.

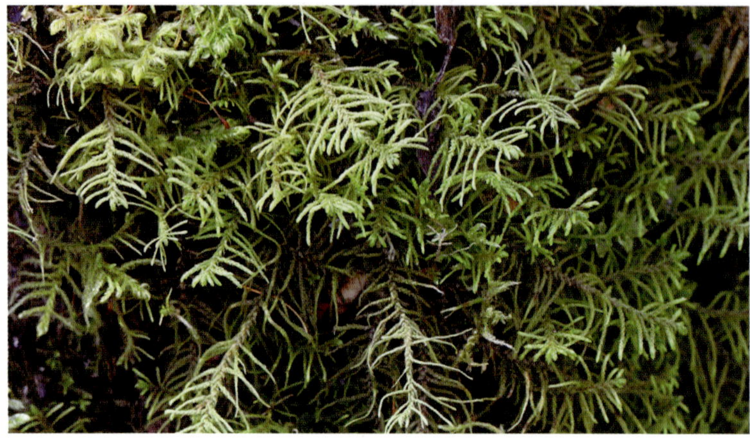

Abietinella abietina (Fir Moss)

The common names of *Abietinella abietina* derive from this plant's somewhat erect, conifer-shaped appearance.

A 2022 study evaluated ethyl acetate extracts of this and four other mosses on 5-fluorouracil–resistant (5-FU) colorectal cancer lines (HCT116 and HT29) (Özerkan et al.). All five bryophytes were found to be cytotoxic. Another recent study found methanol extracts cytotoxic to epithelial/cervical (HeLa) and ductal breast cancer (T47C), and water extracts active against just the latter (Vollár et al. 2018). This moss also shows antifungal activity against *Trichoderma viride*, *Penicillium ochrachloron*, *P. funiculosum*, and *Aspergillus flavus* (Bukvicki, Veljic et al. 2012).

AEROBRYIDIUM

Air Moss

Aero derives from the Greek *aër*, meaning "air," and *bryidium*, meaning "moss-like." *Aerobryidium filamentosum* syn. *Neckera filamentosa* mosses are used in TCM for clearing heat, relieving toxicity, and healing burns. The mosses are known as *mao niu xian* in Mandarin.

AEROBRYUM

Air Moss

The genus name derives from the Greek *aër*, meaning "air," and *bryon*, "moss."

Lanosum, in *Aerobryum lanosum*, means "woolly," referring to the texture of moss hair.

Aerobryum lanosum was traditionally decocted in goat urine and applied externally to burns (Chandra et al. 2017).

ALLENIELLA

Neckera Mosses

Alleniella genus belongs to the Neckeraceae family, and was first described in 2011 by S. Olsson, Enroth and D. Quandt.

Besser's neckera moss, *Alleniella besseri* syn. *Neckera besseri*, is found in the northeastern United States and in Tennessee, Missouri, Kentucky, and Arkansas, as well as parts of Europe. The moss is cytotoxic to one or more hormonal cancer cell lines. Vollár et al. (2018) selected 42 bryophytes, including *Neckera besseri*, and did 168 water and organic extracts. The researchers then screened for activity against cervical epithelial adenocarcinoma (HeLa), ovarian (A2780), and invasive ductal breast (T47D) cancer cell lines. Ninety-nine of the extracts derived from 41 species, including *Alleniella besseri*, exerted more than 25% inhibition of at least one of the cancer cell lines at 10 µg/mL. Both methanol and water extracts were inactive against ovarian cancer cell lines. Only 19 samples of 15 taxa showed moderate antibacterial activity, with *Staphylococcus aureus* and MRSA the most susceptible.

Flat neckera or glistering feather moss (*Alleniella complanata* syn. *Neckera complanata*) was found in the colon of Oetzi, the ice man. *Alleniella complanata*, exhibits antioxidant activity (Yayintas et al. 2019). The fresh moss can be applied to blisters (Lubaina et al. 2014).

AMBLYSTEGIUM

Crawling Feather Moss Creeping Feather Moss

The genus name is derived from the Greek *ambly*, meaning "blunt," and *stege* or *stegeon*, "roof" or "lid," which describes the conical form of the plant's lid, or operculum. Creeping feather moss, or crawling feather moss (*Amblystegium serpens*, is traditionally used to heal external injuries and staunch bleeding (Harris 2008). The moss exhibits both antimicrobial and antiproliferative activity (Motti et al. 2023).

A 2018 study (Vollár et al.) found methanol and water extracts cytotoxic to epithelial/cervical (HeLa), ovarian (A2780), and breast (T47D) cancer cell lines, while the water extract showed activity only against the breast cancer

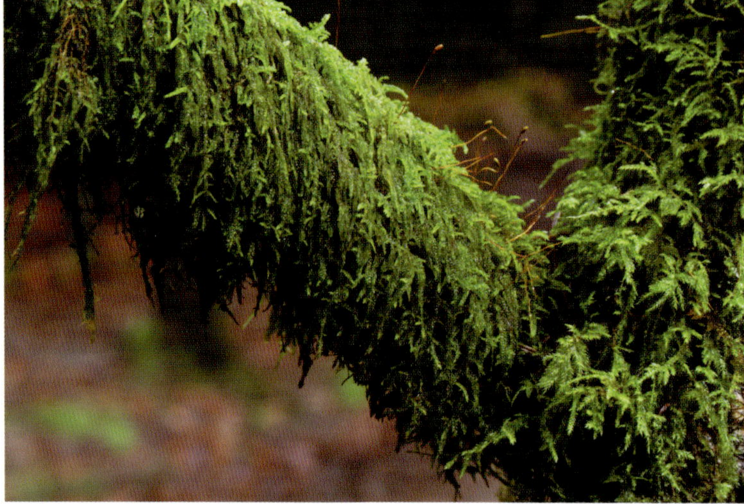

Amblystegium serpens (Creeping Feather Moss)

line. Extracts were also seen to inhibit the gram-negative bacterium *Moraxella catarrhalis*. The species name *catarrhalis* derives from the Greek *catarrh* (i.e., mucus), "to flow down." Catarrh, an inflammation of the mucous membranes, can be a serious infection in children under two years of age as well as in the elderly, particularly since the *Moraxella* bacterium has developed resistance to standard treatment via antibiotics like penicillin, ampicillin, amoxicillin, and tetracycline; as well, and further complicating matters, elderly people may suffer from preexisting respiratory issues or COPD (chronic obstructive pulmonary disease).

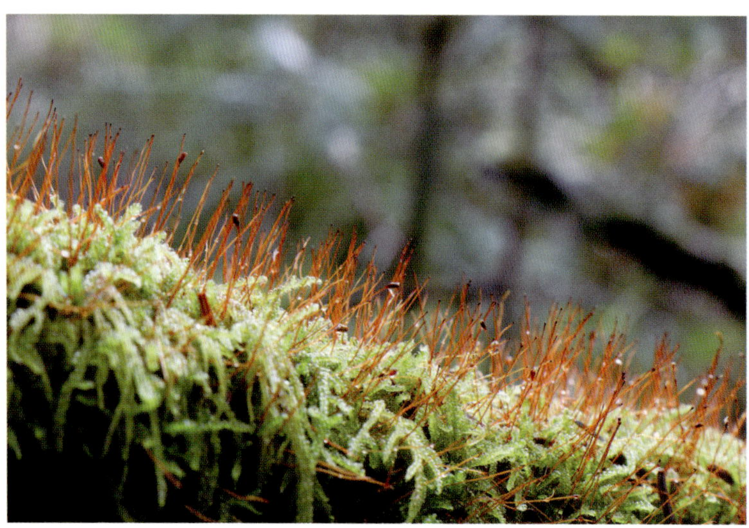

Amblystegium serpens (Creeping Feather Moss)

ANDREAEA

Black Rockmoss   Rough Rockmoss

The *Andreaea* genus is comprised of 78 accepted species. Black rockmoss, *Andreaea rupestris*, also called rough rockmoss, is a dark brown species, one of the thirty moss species found clinging to the clothing of the Neolithic Tyrolean Iceman Oetzi (see page 3), which also included two of the *Neckera* genus. These mosses were low woodland species, suggesting the Iceman traveled north from Italy, and not south from Austria (Dickson et al. 1996).

ANITRICHIA

Hanging Moss   Pendulous Wing-Moss

The genus name derives from *anti*, "opposite," and *trichia*, "filaments." This is actually a misnomer in that the processes alternate with, and are not opposite to, the outer teeth (Dixon 1954). Work by Önder (2021) found *Antitrichia californica*, found in western North America, has a high phenolic content as well as a high metal-chelating capacity.

Hanging, or pendulous wing moss (*Antitrichia curtipendula*), is sometimes mistaken for a lichen when hanging from tree branches. Its older names are scarce anchor tooth and short hanging odd tooth. The moss is found widely throughout western North America, and temperate parts of western Europe.

The essential oil of this moss was investigated by Yücel (2021). The major components are nonanal (19.96%) and tetracecanal (20.23%) which exhibit antioxidant and antimicrobial activity.

ANOECTANGIUM

Beardless Mosses

The genus name *Anoectangium* may derive from the Greek *anoikto*, meaning "open," and *angion* "a vessel."

Two-colored beardless moss (*Anoectangium thomsonii* syn. *A. bicolor*) was one of 39 species tested for activity on the neurotransmitter enzyme cholinesterase. It is well-known that the neurotransmitter acetylcholine is found in many plants, including bryophytes. Work by A. Gupta et al. (2001)

found that the *Anoectangium* moss showed the highest cholinesterase activity. Inhibition of acetylcholinesterase is a possible route of protecting and treating human neurodegenerative conditions such as Alzheimer's and Parkinson's diseases.

Ethanol extracts of clear beardless moss, *Anoectangium clarum*, demonstrated the inhibition of pathogenic bacteria *Escherichia coli*, *Salmonella typhimurium*, and *Bacillus subtilis*, in descending order of efficacy (Bishnoi et al. 2016). Earlier work by Bishnoi (2015) examined the potential antifungal activity against the pathogens *Aspergillus niger*, *Fusarium solani, and Trichoderma viride*. At a concentration of 4%, the various solvent extracts, including ethanol, exhibited better results than the antifungal medication fluconazole.

ANOMODON

Tail Mosses

The genus name derives from *a*, "not," and *nomo*, "law" or "rule"; or *anomos*, "anomalous," and *odön*, "tooth." In both cases the meaning is "an abnormal peristome." This name is erroneous, however, as it supposes the processes arose from between the outer teeth and not, as they do, from an inner membrane (Dixon 1954). Older English names include spriggy odd tooth moss and yellow-striped silk thread moss. The German name wolf's paw refers to the appearance of the dried moss.

Long tail moss, *Anomodon viticulosus*, also called rambling tail-moss is one of the six mosses found in the gastrointestinal tract of Oetzi, the Tyrolean Iceman. Why? It is inconclusive, as they are not edible, nor do they give sustenance. Perhaps small pieces adhered to ingested food or water.

Work by Colak et al. (2011) found that methanol extracts of *Anomodon. viticulosus* inhibit the bacteria *Staphylococcus aureus*, *Saccharomyces cerevisiae*, *Candida albicans*, and *Escherichia coli*. Methanol extracts show modest cytotoxicity against epithelial/cervical (HeLa) and breast (T47D) cancer cell lines and can inhibit the growth of gray mold (*Botrytis cinerea*) (Nedeljko et al. 2019). The ethanol extract was only active against *Saccharomyces cerevisiae*.

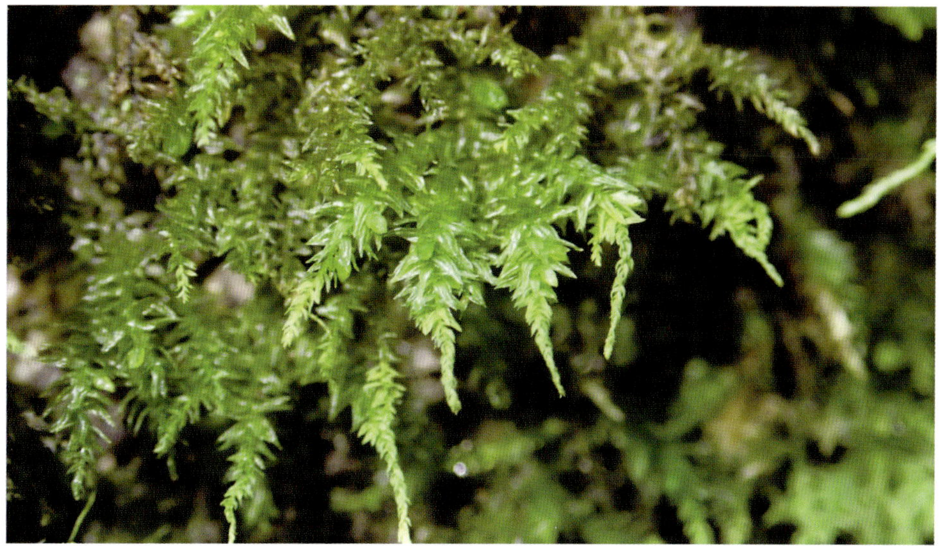

Anomodon giraldi

Homeopathy

In homeopathy, the main themes of long tail moss, from *Anomodon viticulosus*, involve attachment and distance; the former is desired, but the person is too vulnerable to seek it, thus very sensitive in relationships.

As a result they can be distant, reclusive, or fleeing; they want to be alone or else they become aggressive. The person feels not seen or appreciated. Sexual abuse or trauma may be involved. In addition, depression and PMS were found in two case histories. Physically there may be a feeling of shortened tendons in hands and feet, as if constricting to form a claw, and muscle pain.

The recommended dose is 30c to 200c.*

ARCHIDIUM

Ohio Archidium Moss

The *Archidium* genus is comprised of about 35 species. Ohio archidium moss, *Archidium ohioense*, possesses anti-inflammatory secondary metabolites (Ayinke et al. 2015).

---

*Case histories by Britta Dähnrich and Martin Jakob are found in Narayan Verlag's *Mosses and Ferns* (2021–22). A complete proving is found in *The Fairylike Mosses* by Jan Scholten (2018).

ATRICHUM

Big Star Moss
Queen Catherine's Moss
Smooth Cap Moss
Starburst Moss
Undulated Hair Moss
Undulating Catharinea

Geographic Range: North America, Central America, South America, West Indies, Europe, Asia, Africa, Australia

Habitat: fen margins; shaded areas; wet banks along streams,

Practical Uses: moss lawns

Medicinal Applications: antibacterial, anticancer, antifungal, antioxidant

The genus name is derived from *a*, "lacking," and *trichos*, "hair," in reference to the hairless appearance of the calyptra (Dixon 1954) that gives this moss one of its common names, smooth cap.

Work by McCleary and Walkington (1966) found eighteen mosses with antibiotic properties, including *Atrichum* species as well as *Dicranum*, *Funaria* (syn. *Mnium*), *Polytrichum*, and *Sphagnum* species. These five mosses were the most active against both gram-positive and gram-negative bacteria.

Long smooth cap moss (*Atrichum androgynum*) produces an oxidative burst of hydrogen peroxide during rehydration (Mayaba et al. 2002), perhaps to protect against bacteria and fungi. This reactive oxygen species production is also quite useful in breaking down the cell walls of pathogens but is also a pathway to the destruction of cancer cell walls.

Big star or starburst moss, (*Atrichum undulatum*) inhibit nine bacteria except *Klebsiella aerogenes* (previously known as *Enterobacter aerogenes*) and *Escherichia coli*. The former bacterium is drug-resistant and can create serious and even deadly infections in immune-compromised individuals. In Britain the moss is known as Queen Catherine's moss, undulating Catharinea, and more commonly undulated hair moss.

Two mosses, *Atrichum undulatum* and *Physcomitrella patens*, and one liverwort, *Marchantia polymorpha*, were cultured and collected from the wild, then extracted with DMSO to test activity against a range of fungi (Sabovljevic et al. 2011). Activity was noted against the fungal pathogens *Aspergillus versicolor*, *A. fumigatus*, *Penicillium funiculosum*, *P. ochrochloron*, and *Trichoderma viride*. The bryophytes grown in culture had greater antifungal activity than those collected from the wild, which is somewhat surprising. At the same time, however, it was found in the same study that wild-growing moss possessed more antibacterial activity.

Activity was noted for *Atrichum undulatum*, the liverwort *Marchantia polymorpha* subsp. *ruderalis*, and the moss *Physcomitrium patens* against the bacteria *Escherichia coli*, *Pseudomonas aeruginosa*, *Salmonella typhimurium*, *Listeria monocytogenes*, *Bacillus cereus*, *Micrococcus flavus*, *Staphylococcus aureus*, and *Enterobacter cloacae* Sabovlijevic et al. 2011. The latter bacterium can create infections in neonatal intensive care units, resulting in meningitis and death. Also, the use of urinary catheters in hospital settings has resulted in antibiotic-resistant strains. Recent work by Yang, Hong et al. (2022) suggests the bacterium may also play a role in calcium oxalate stone formation (such as kidney stones).

Atrichum undulatum mosses possess strong antioxidant activity (Chobot et al. 2008). Recent work by Saxena and Yadav (2018) examined the antibacterial and antifungal activity of water and alcohol extractions. No inhibition was found against *Proteus mirabilis*, a life-threatening, hospital-acquired bacteria, or the fungi *Aspergillus fumigatus*; however, both water and alcohol extracts showed significant inhibition of *Klebsiella pneumoniae*, *Salmonella typhi*, and *Escherichia coli*. Another study (Vollár et al. (2018)) found that three solvent extracts of *Atrichum undulatum* exhibit cytotoxicity against epithelial/cervical (HeLa), ovarian (T47D), and especially ductal breast (A2780) cancer cell lines.

Martin (2015) notes the moss is strongly recommended for a moss lawn with high foot traffic. In some regions with sufficient moisture, its rapid growth will achieve full coverage in less than a year.

Homeopathy

In homeopathy, starburst moss, from *Atrichum undulatum*, is indicated for those who feel dark and hopeless, as if trapped in a tunnel. There is great despair and crying out, as well as nightmares.

The recommended does is 12c to 30c.*

Emerald Dagger Moss Essence

This essence from *Atrichum androgynum* anchors cosmic light into the first layer of DNA. Emerald Dagger Moss "Re-vivifies, upgrades and aligns DNA, bringing it into energetic alignment with the higher vibrational resonance of *Homo cosmicus* and the Path of the Priestess

*Initial proving by Jan Scholten. Case study by Britta Dähnrich found in Narayana Verlag's *Mosses and Ferns* (2021–22).

and Priest." It creates a powerful magical linkage and connection with the Sacred Altars of the West and the places of true emotional well-being.

First Light Flower Essence of New Zealand produces No. 161.

AULACOMNIUM

Bog Bead-Moss
Bud-Headed Groovemoss
Ribbed Bogmoss
Thread Mosses

The genus name is derived from *aulacos*, meaning "furrow," and *mnion*, "moss," together referring to the plant's striate capsule (Dixon 1954).

Bog bead-moss or ribbed bogmoss (*Aulacomnium palustre*) is usually found on the edge of bogs, black spruce forests, fens, and near waterfalls. In Virginia, robins have been observed using this moss to build nests, suggesting this species' other common names, thread moss and swelling thread moss. It is a very spongy moss with a neon green or chartreuse color (Martin 2015). Another species, swollen moss or turgid thread moss (*Aulacomnium turgidum*), also called mountain groove moss, can regenerate after being covered with ice for over four hundred years.

Antimicrobial and anticancer activities of *Aulacomnium* spp. were screened. Ethanol extracts contain caffeic acid; 7,8-dihydroxy-5-methoxycoumarin-7-β sophoroside; ferulic acid; atraric acid; 4-hydroxybenzoic acid; and minor amounts of benzoic compounds. It is unusually rich in L-tryptophan amino

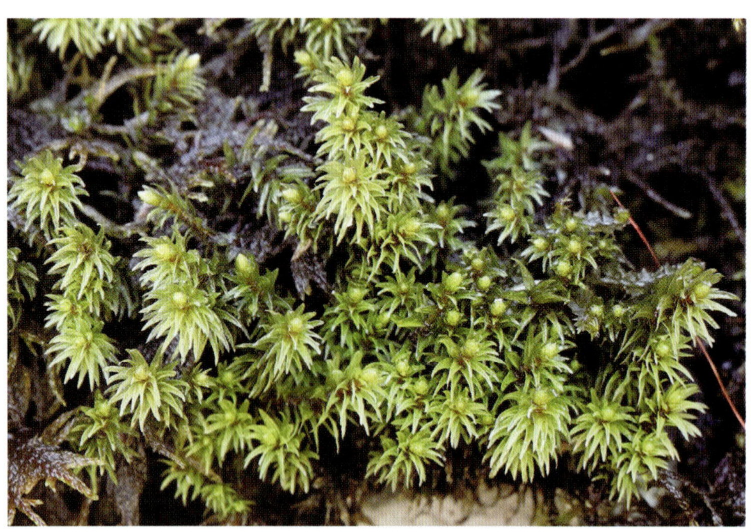

Aulacomnium palustre (Bog Bead-Moss)

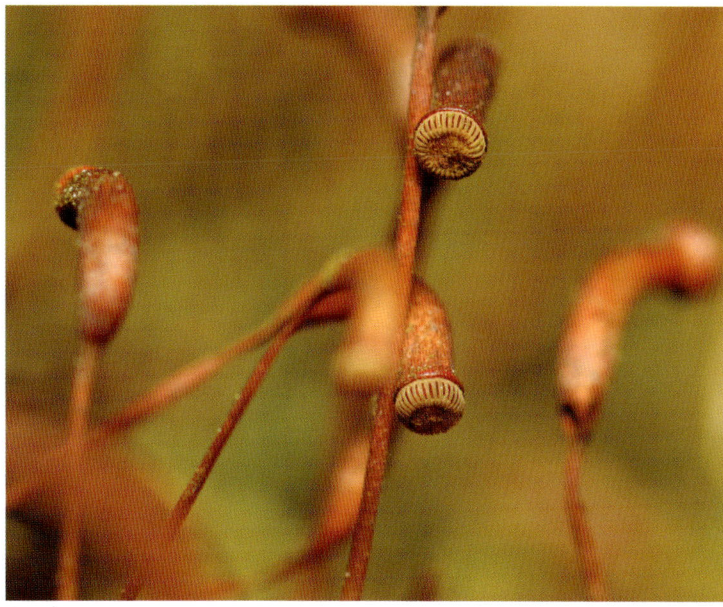

Aulacomnium androgynum (Bud-Headed Groovemoss)

acid. Antiproliferative activity against a panel of four microbes and six cancer cell lines was weak (Klavina et al. 2015).

Homeopathy

The homeopathic remedy from *Aulacomnium palustre* is indicated for people who have suffered a traumatic experience with a hopeless situation and no escape. A feeling of drowning may present.

The recommended dose is 30c to 200c.*

BARBELLA

Beard Moss Pendulous Barbella

The genus *Barbella* is a member of the Meteroiaceae family, distinguished by their axillary hairs.

Pendulous barbella or beard moss, *Barbella pendula* syn. *Neodicladiella pendula*, hangs downward from trees, appearing at first glance as a lichen. It is imperiled or vulnerable in Louisiana and Mississippi and should not be harvested commercially. The moss is also found in Mexico and Asia.

This moss contains significant amounts of vitamin B_{12}, and when fed to

*Case study by Christina Ari, in Narayana Verlag's *Mosses and Ferns* (2021–22).

puppies and chickens it caused no noticeable side effects, according to Sugawa (1960). The author notes that metformin, taken by millions of people for pre-diabetes, reduces levels of B_{12} in the blood, thereby increasing blood sugar levels. This information is not widely shared with patients, leading to many unnecessary and premature prescriptions for insulin. Many physicians and pharmacists are not aware of this predictable side effect.

BARBULA

Beard Mosses Sheaf-Leaved Screwmoss

The genus name *Barbula* derives from the diminutive form of the Latin *barba*, meaning "beard," alluding to the fuzzy-looking peristome (Dixon 1954). There are 101 accepted species.

Methanol extracts of lesser bird's claw beard moss or sheaf-leaved screwmoss, (*Barbula convulata*) inhibit the pathogens *Listeria monocytogenes*, *Escherichia coli*, *Bacillus cereus*, and *Pseudomonas aeruginosa* (Abdel-Shafi et al. 2017). The benzene and methanol extracts exhibited significant antiviral activity against zucchini yellow mosaic virus, an aphid-borne pathogen that damages commercially important food crops such as zucchinis, pumpkins, watermelons, squash, melons, and cucumbers.

Twisted teeth beard moss, *Barbula indica*, is found worldwide, including a few eastern states where it is imperilled. It is traditionally brewed in India as a tea to treat intermittent fever and is used externally as a warm pelvic compress to treat dysmenorrhea (Lubaina et al. 2014).

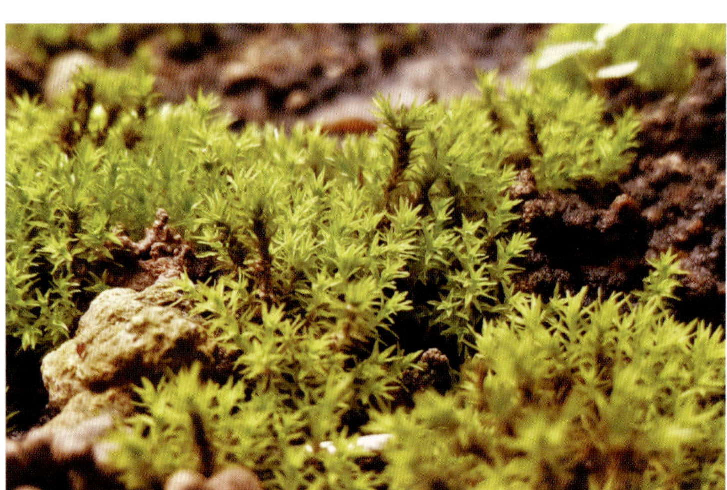

Barbula unguiculata (Common Beard Moss)

Common beard moss or bird's claw beard moss (*Barbula unguiculata*) was used externally by the Seminole of Florida for fever and body pain (Sturtevant 1954; Chandra et al. 2017; Azuelo et al. 2011). Some older British names include clawtip twisted beardlet and dwarf screwmoss.

BARTRAMIA

Apple Mosses

Geographic Range: worldwide, especially in humid climates

Habitat: acid soil, rocky ledges, and slanted hillsides with lots of shade and moisture

Practical Uses: construction, horticulture, indicators of water pollution

Medicinal Applications: antibacterial, antianxiety, cardiovascular, epilepsy, nervine

The genus *Bartramia* is named in honor of the American Quaker and botanist John Bartram (1699–1777). His contemporary, Swiss botanist Linnaeus, said Bartram was the greatest natural botanist in the world—high praise indeed from someone who truly believed himself to be the greatest. Bartram started the eight-acre Bartram's Garden in 1728, the first botanical garden in America, located about three miles from the center of Philadelphia. Along with Benjamin Franklin, Bartram was a cofounder of the American Philosophical Society in that city. Bartram claimed to have been influenced by German botanist Johann Jakob Dillenius (1684–1747). He is credited as saying, "Before Dr. Dillenius gave me a hint of it, I took no particular notice of mosses but looked upon them as a cow looks at a pair of new barn doors" (Martin 2015).

There are 57 accepted species of *Bartramia* found worldwide, with at least ten in North America. Straight-leaved apple moss, *Bartramia ithyphylla*, has been used traditionally in Traditional Chinese Medicine for calming the nerves, irregular heartbeat, epilepsy, apoplexy, and suppressing fear (Du 1997). Note that the species name *ithyphylla* derives from the Greek *ithyphallikos*, meaning "straight" or "erect phallus," icons of which were carried in ancient festivals of Bacchus. It likely also refers to the rigid position of the dry leaves, or phylla. The bioflavonoid pattern of *Bartramia ithyphylla* has been isolated and identified and were found to contain a new bioflavonoid unknown in the family (López-Sáez et al. 1995).

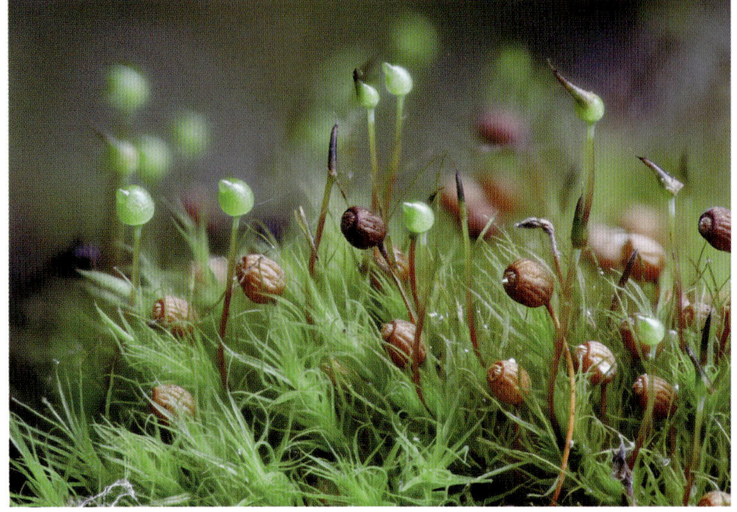

Bartramia pomiformis (Common Apple Moss)

Common apple moss, *Bartramia pomiformis*, possesses some murine leukemia (P-388) antitumor activity as well as activity using the astrocytoma assay that measures both cytotoxicity and microtubule inhibition.

The species name *pomiformis* is from the Latin, meaning "apple-shaped," alluding to the small, green, apple-shaped spore capsules that turn red when ripe. Older common names include apple-shaped Bartram, cushion apple moss, and pear-capsule bead moss.

Seven flavonoids were isolated from *Bartramia pomiformis* and four other moss species: apigenin, apigenin-7-0-triglycoside, lucenin-2, luteolin-7-0-neohesperidoside, saponarine, vitex, and the bioflavonoid bartramiaflavone. The latter compound inhibits *Pseudomonas aeruginosa*, a gram-negative bacterium that can cause disease in plants and animals (Basile et al. 1999). Some of the mosses investigated showed significant inhibition of the pathogens *Enterobacter cloacae*, *E. aerogenes*, and *Pseudomonas aeruginosa*, all gram-negative bacteria. *Enterobacter cloaceae* (formerly *Klebsiella aerogenes*) bacteria may play a role in calcium oxalate stone formation and is a multidrug-resistant organism. A recent study by Chou et al. (2023) found this species is associated with a greater risk of 30-day mortality as a result of bloodstream infections.

An ethanol extract of this moss exhibited modest activity against *Bacillus subtilis* (Russel 2010). The flavonoid luteolin 4'-Neohesperidoside (L4N) inhibits four antibiotic-resistant bacteria, including MRSA, *Klebsiella pneumoniae*, fosA-positive shiga toxin producing the *Escherichia coli* serogroup O111 (STEC 0111), and *Bacillus cereus*. Significant synergistic activity with pharmaceuticals was noted. For example, gentamicin, combined with *Bartramia* spp., was effective against gram-negative bacteria, and vancomycin was effective against *Bacillus cereus*. Moreover, in vivo evaluation showed significant decrease in *Klebsiella pneumoniae* and STEC shedding and colonizing. Renal and pulmonary lesions in lab animals were remarkably enhanced, with significant decreases in bacteria-infected tissue. A study by El-Shiekh et al. (2023) suggests L4N as a potential substitute or adjuvant for traditional antibiotics.

Kang et al. (2007) found that the activity of extracts of the moss that inhibit *Staphylococcus aureus* were enhanced by UV-A light irradiation.

BESTIA

Bestia Moss

Bestia derives from the Latin or Old Spanish *bestia* meaning "beast."

This genus, which has seven species, is named in honor of George Newton Best (1846–1926), an American bryologist, moss expert, and second president of the Sullivant Moss Society, which is now known as the American Bryological and Lichenological Society. No medicinal attributes have been found to date.

BRACHYTHECIASTRUM

Rough-Stalked Feather Moss Rough-Stalked Ragged Moss Velvet Feather Moss

Brachy means "short" or "stout," *theca* is from the Greek for "vessel," and *astrum* is Latin for "star."

Rough-stalked ragged moss, or rough-stalked feather moss, *Brachytheciastrum rutabulum*, contains phenols that exhibit antioxidant activity (Pejin and Bogdanovic-Pristov 2012).

Velvet feather moss, *Brachytheciastrum velutinum*, was investigated by Vollár et al. (2018). The researchers found various solvent and water extracts exhibited cytotoxicity against epithelial/cervical (HeLa), ovarian (T47D), and breast cancer (A2780) cell lines. Older common names are apt descriptions of the appearance of this moss: matted feather moss and fine leaf verdant moss.

This moss contains four phenolic acids (4-O-caffeoylquini, 5-O-caffeoylquinic, caffeic acid, and ellagic acid) and three flavonoids (apigenin-7-O-glucoside, luteolin, and apigenin) (Jockovic et al. 2008).

BRACHYTHECIUM

Cedar Moss
Feather Mossess
Pale-Leaved Thread Moss
Rough Foxtail Moss

Geographic Range: Britain, Ireland, North America

Habitat: lawns and hedge bases next to intensively managed arable fields; lowlands, woodlands

Practical Uses: moss lawns, wound dressing

Medicinal Applications: antibacterial, anticancer, antifungal, antimicrobial, antipyretic, antispasmodic

The genus name derives from the Greek *brakhys* and the Latin *brachy*, meaning "short," and the Greek *theca* or *thekion*, for "short," "fat," "capsule," or "vessel," suggesting a container where spores are stored.

Unspecified *Brachythecium* species have been used in China to treat fever and induce detoxification (Harris 2008).

Whitish feather moss, or pale-leaved thread moss, *Brachythecium albicans*, has been steam-distilled. The two main components are nonanal (41%) and 4,4-dimethyl-*E*-2-pentene (6.6%) (Özdemir et al. 2010).

Brachythecium buchananii methanol extracts contain gallic, hydroxyl benzoic, sinapic, vanillic, chlorogenic, ferulic, and cinnamic acids; catechol; and phloroglucinol (Greeshma et al. 2016). Phloroglucinol is an organic antispasmodic compound used to treat colic and spastic digestive and renal, urinary, and biliary tract pain. It relaxes smooth muscles by inhibiting voltage-dependent calcium channels without the anticholinergic side effects common to most antispasmodics. A recent double-blind, placebo-controlled randomized trial by Jung et al. (2021) compared the effectiveness of oral intake of phloroglucinol to a placebo taken fifteen minutes before an esophaogastroduodenoscopy (a diagnostic endoscopic procedure that visualizes the upper part of the gastrointestinal tract). Seventy-one patients were in each group, but those taking phloroglucinol showed better outcomes, with significantly suppressed gastrointestinal peristalsis. Greeshma and Murugan (2018) found that *Brachythecium buchananii* exhibits remarkable antifungal activity.

The moss *Brachythecium campestre* syn. *B. calcareum* syn. *B. leucoglaucum* possesses antimicrobial inhibition (Yayintas and Yapici 2009).

The main component of the essential oil of *Brachythecium salebrosum*, commonly called smooth stalk feather moss or yellow feather moss, is n-nonanal (66.3%) (Kahriman et al. 2009).

Work by Özdemir et al. (2009) identified n-nonanal (66.3%), as well as n-octanol (3.1%), n-heptanal (2.7%), hexa-hydro-farnesyl acetone (3.1%), and minor amounts of n-decanal and β pinene.

Rough-stalked ragged feather moss, *Brachythecium rutabulum*, was probably used in a similar manner as sphagnum moss in Europe for wound dressing, at least between 1651 and 1731 (Drobnik and Stebel 2017). In those days it was known as *muscus terrestris en hortensis*, roughly "ground moss in the garden." Older common names used in Britain include rake-shaped feather moss and oven rake moss. In North America it also goes by the names rough foxtail moss or cedar moss. It is a common lawn moss. During photosynthesis it deposits calcium carbonate.

Brachythecium rutabulum, yet another moss also called rough-stalked ragged moss, is cytotoxic to one or more hormonal cancer cells lines. Vollár et al. (2018) selected 42 bryophytes and did 168 water and organic extracts. The researchers then screened for activity against cervical epithelial (HeLa), ovarian (A2780), and invasive ductal breast (T47D) cancer cell lines. From the tested families, Brachytheciaceae and Amblystegiaceae provided the highest number of antiproliferative extracts, with the extracts derived from 41 species exerting more than 25% inhibition of at least one of the cancer cell lines at 10 μg/mL. Only 19 samples of 15 taxa showed moderate antibacterial activity, with *Staphylococcus aureus* and MRSA the most susceptible.

Ethanol extracts of *Sciuro-hypnumpopuleum* syn. *Brachythecium populeum,* called matted feather moss, along with *Brachythecium rutabulum,* were tested on

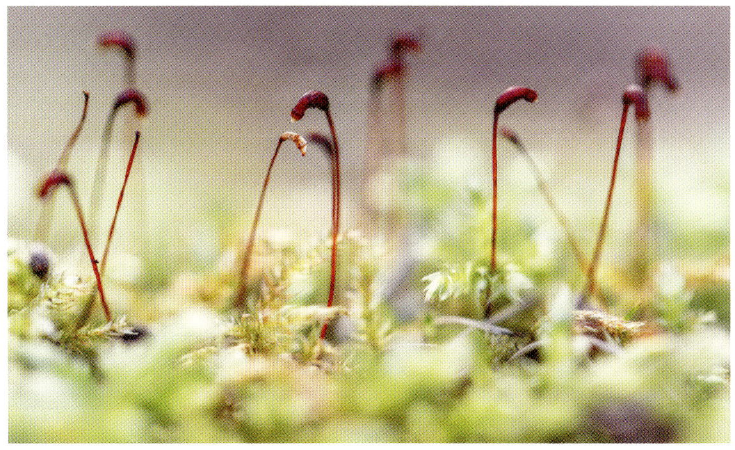

Brachythecium rutabulum (Cedar Moss)

five gram-positive and six gram-negative bacteria, and eight fungi: *Micrococcus luteus, Bacillus subtilis, Bacillus cereus, Enterobacter aerogenes, Escherichia coli, Klebsiella pneumoniae, Proteus mirabilis, Pseudomonas aeruginosa, Staphylococcus aureus* (including MRSA), *Salmonella typhimurium*, and *Streptococcus pneumonia*. Five *Aspergillus* species were also included in the investigation, as were the fungi *Candida albicans, Cryptococcus albidus*, and *Trichophyton rubrum* (Singh et al. 2007). *Cryptococcus albidus* has been found in 62.5% of homes of people suffering summer-type hypersensitivity pneumonitis. Immunoglobulin A (IgA) and immunogloblin M (IgM) antibodies are involved (Miyagawa et al. 2000).

Homeopathy

In homeopathy, rough-stalked feather moss *Brachythecium rutabulum* relates to an altered sense of time, childishness, and insecurity. There is a tenseness about doing things properly for others and not for oneself; resistance and stubbornness; feeling blocked and alone in a group; wanting to save the Earth; deep knowledge; exhaustion; and unstructured chaos with a sense of falling into a dark hole.

The recommended dose is 200c.*

BRAUNIA

Red Branch Moss

In Mexico, red branch moss, *Braunia secunda*, is decocted and used as a wash on the head to relieve headaches (Hernandez-Rodríguez et al. 2020). The moss grows at elevated locations in Mexico as well as in Arizona, New Mexico, and Texas.

BREUTELIA

Bottlebrush Moss

The genus is named in honor of the German bryologist Johann Christian Breutel (1788–1875), who was a member of the religious society of the Moravian Brethren, one of the oldest Protestant denominations of Christianity, and was anointed a bishop in that church in 1853. He collected mosses, algae, lichens, and ferns from 1814 until his passing. He traveled abroad, collecting specimens with his wife in the West Indies and South Africa.

*Case study by Britta Dähnrich and Martin Jacob in Narayana Verlag's *Mosses and Ferns* (2021–22), based on previous work by Jan Scholten in *The Fairylike Mosses* (2018).

Breutelia subdisticha syn. *B. rivalis* exhibits antioxidant activity (Téllez-Rocha et al. 2021).

Valarezo et al. (2018) gathered, steam-distilled, and identified 94 constituents in six mosses found in Ecuador. Breutelia tomentosa contains as its major constituents epi-zonarene (8.7%) and α-selinene (6.7%).

BRYOANDERSONIA

Spoon Moss Worm Moss

Spoon moss or worm moss, *Bryoandersonia illecebra*, is found on rock substrates and hardwood tree bases, on either acid or alkaline soils. The genus was named in honor of Lewis Anderson (1912–2007), a botany professor at Duke University and co-author of *Mosses of Eastern North America*. This makes sense, as this moss is endemic to the region.

The species name is from the Latin, meaning "alluring" or "attractive."

BRYOERYTHROPHYLLUM

Red Beard Moss

The genus name is derived from *bryon*, "moss," *erythros*, "red" (in reference to the brick-red color of most species), and *phyllos*, "leaf." Red beard moss, *Bryoerythrophyllum rubrum*, for example, has bright red stems.

Work by Özerkan et al. (2022) evaluated ethyl extracts of this and four other mosses (*Abietinella abietina, Homolothecium sericeum, Tortella tortuosa, Syntrichia ruralis*) on 5-fluorouracil-resistant colorectal cancer lines (HCT116 and HT29). All five bryophytes were found to be cytotoxic.

BRYUM

Bryum Mosses Sidewalk Moss Thread Mosses

Geographic Range: Antarctica, Asia, Great Britain, North America

Habitats: urban settings, around small animal burrows, living hardwoods and rotting logs, streamsides, wet rock crevices, fens, wet heaths, marshes

Practical Uses: landscaping, bryoremediation

Medicinal Applications: antibacterial, anticancer, antifungal, antipyretic, anti-rhinitic, bone-setting, vulnerary

Bryum derives from the Greek *bryon*, "moss." The name may also derive from *bruein*, meaning "to swell, sprout, or burgeon." It is a large genus, at one time containing over 1000 species, but today reduced to 265 accepted species.

Bryum species have been long used traditionally in North America for healing wounds, burns, and bruises, or placed under splints when setting fractures (Harris 2008).

Silver bryum, *Bryum argenteum*, is probably the most common urban moss, found on rooftops and growing through cracks in sidewalks. It is a compact silver moss that lacks chlorophyll in the upper leaves. Older English names include catkin-stemmed silver bryum, silvery thread moss, and silver web tooth moss. Its hardiness makes it a suitable candidate to place around outdoor stepping-stones.

It enjoys urban settings where nitrogen sources are plentiful. Fire hydrants frequented by dogs provide a source of nitrogen, as do pigeon droppings on apartment balconies. In the wild, this moss will be found outside the burrows of prairie dogs and lemmings. It is being studied in Antarctica to measure the effect of ozone radiation. This moss is a major bonsai ground cover.

In India, *Bryum argenteum* is used for its antipyretic, anti-rhinitic (sinus), and antibacterial activity (Alam et al. 2015). Traditional American medicine and Traditional Chinese Medicine use this moss for its antipyretic and antifungal activities. The plant is also useful as an antidote for rhinitis or nose inflammation with bacterial involvement. It contains the interesting compound, scutellarein-7-glucoside, which decreases IL-6 production, suggestive of anti-inflammatory activity.

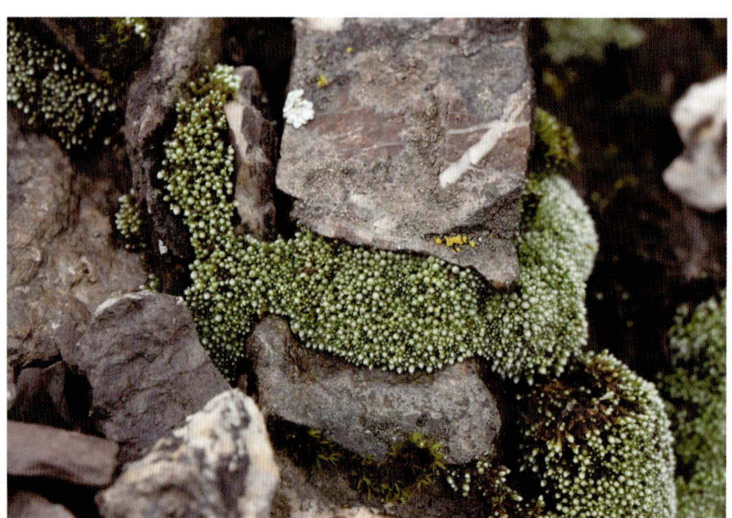

Bryum argenteum (Silver Bryum)
Photo by Graham Steinruck

Work by Sabovljevic et al. (2006) found ethanol extracts of *Bryum argenteum* inhibit a variety of bacteria and fungi, including *Escherichia coli*, *Bacillus subtilis*, *Micrococcus luteus*, *Staphylococcus aureus*, *Aspergillus niger*, *Penicillium ochrochloron*, *Candida albicans*, and *Trichophyton mentagrophytes*. Solvents of various mosses, including *Bryum argenteum*, were found to exhibit antifungal activity against *A. niger*, *Fusarium moniliforme*, and *Rhizoctonia bataticola* (Bodade et al. 2008). The latter fungus contains a lectin that induces apoptosis and inhibits metastasis in ovarian cancer cell lines SKOV3 and OVCAR3 (Hegde et al. 2021). It also causes mung bean root rot, a devastating disease that can cause crop yield loss up to 60%.

Fusarium moniliforme is a widespread fungal pathogen that damages rice, oats, wheat, corn, barley, and soybean crops. The mycotoxic fumonisins in this pathogen are a common contaminant that induces equine leukoencephalomalacia and porcine pulmonary edema. In parts of the world the contamination of corn via this pathogen is associated with higher-than-average incidences of esophageal cancer (Norred 1993).

On the other hand, this fungus is best known for its ability in the lab to produce large amounts of gibberellins, which are plant hormones that regulate various developmental processes, with significant beneficial applications in agriculture and horticulture. The fungus also produces bikaverins, a reddish pigment produced by various fungal species, that inhibits *Leishmania brasiliensis*, a protozoa parasite. Ethanol extracts of *Bryum argenteum* exhibit activity against *Escherichia coli*, *Klebsiella pneumoniae*, *Proteus vulgaris*,

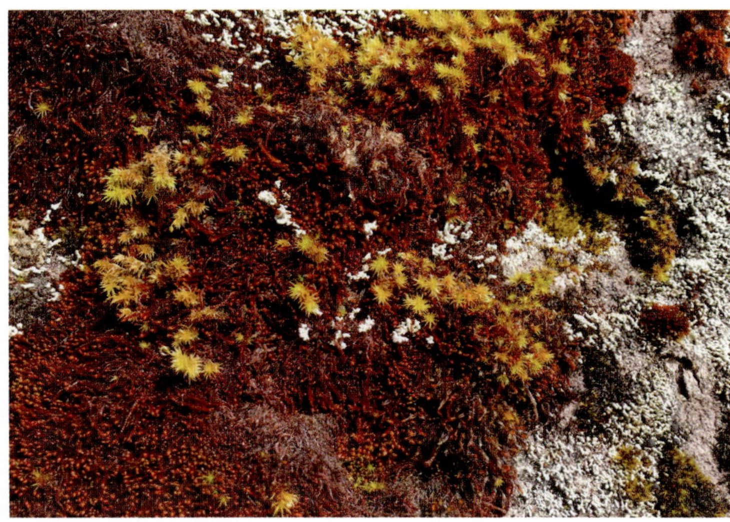

Bryum rubens (Red Bryum)

Pseudomonas aeruginosa, and *Staphylococcus aureus*; distilled water extracts also inhibited *Escherichia coli* at about one-half the rate of ampicillin (Karpinski and Adamczak 2017).

This 2017 study of *Bryum argenteum* by Karpinski and Adamczak found significant inhibition of *Streptococcus pyogenes*, *Staphylococcus aureus*, *Escherichia coli*, *Enterococcus faecalis*, and *Klebsiella pneumoniae*.

Work by Vollár et al. (2018) found solvent extracts of 42 moss species, including *Bryum argenteum*, exhibit cytotoxicity against epithelial/cervical (HeLa), ovarian (T47D), and breast (A2780) cancer cell lines. Methanol and water extracts exhibited no such activity. In the same study, tufted thread moss, also known as matted bryum or sidewalk moss (*Bryum caespiticium*) was also evaluated. The researchers found various solvent extracts exhibit cytotoxicity against epithelial/cervical (HeLa), ovarian (T47D), and breast (A2780) cancer cell lines.

Work by Singh et al. (2011) found *Bryum argenteum* and other mosses and lichens were more active against gram-negative bacteria when extracted with chloroform, while those subjected to butanol exhibited greater activity against gram-positive bacteria, especially *Staphylococcus aureus*.

CALLICLADIUM

Beautiful Branch Moss Haldane's Moss Tousled Treasure Moss

Haldane's moss or beautiful branch moss (*Callicladium haldaneanum* syn. *Hypnum haldaneanum* possesses antioxidant activity (Smolinska-Kondla et al. 2022). In horticulture it is referred to as tousled treasure moss. This beautifully colored moss is prized for its use in terrariums.

CALLIERGONELLA

Pointed Spear Moss

The genus name may derive from the Greek *kallos*, "fine" or "beautiful," and *ergon*, "work," alluding to its elegant appearance and pretty workmanship. Pointed spear moss, *Calliergonella cuspidata*, is one of our most common and easily identified species. Some early common names include waxed-moustache moss, rolled umbrella moss, and dagger feather moss.

Calliergonella cuspidata contains phenols and exhibits antioxidant activity (Pejin and Bogdanovic-Pristov 2012). Work by Vollár et al. (2018) found chloroform extracts exhibit cytotoxicity against epithelial/cervical (HeLa) and ovarian (T47D) cancer cell lines. They also inhibit *Staphylococcus aureus* in vitro.

Pointed spear moss and nine other mosses out of twenty-three exhibited good antimicrobial activity against *Paenibacillus* larvae isolates that cause American foulbrood diseases in honeybee larvae in a study by Sevim et al. (2017). The other mosses showing benefit were *Calliergonella lindbergi*, *Polytrichum formosum* and *Polytrichum commune*, *Metzgeria conjugata*, *Isothecium alopecuroides*, *Syntrichia calcicola*, *S. montana* (syn. *S. intermedia*), *Tortella densa*, and *Grimmia alpestris*.

CALOHYPNUM

Cypress-leaved Plaitmoss Feather Moss

The genus contains about 210 species, many of them taxonomically difficult to differentiate.

A 70% ethanol extract of *Calohypnum plumiforme* syn. *Hypnum plumaeforme* was given to mice that were fed a high-fat diet. This work by Shin et al. (2016) found the moss reduces blood serum lipid levels as well as insulin and leptin levels. Insulin resistance, or type-2 diabetes, in which insulin continues to be secreted by beta cells in the pancreas, but blood sugar is not efficiently transferred to red blood cells, is a growing concern. Lowering leptin levels is thus beneficial, as elevated numbers are related to the accumulation of body fat and weight gain. Free-radical scavenging ability confirms the highest antioxidant activity in this moss was found in extracts made from deionized water.

Green-leaved plant moss (*Calohypnum plumiforme* syn. *Hypnum plumiforme*) is found worldwide. It contains momilactones A–B and F, acrenol, and 8(14)-podocarpen-13-on-18-oic acid. The latter compound exhibits strong growth promotion of lettuce (Li, Wie et al. 2020).

CALYMPERES

The genus name is derived from the Greek *kalymma*, meaning "covering" or "veil" and *peres*, "going beyond," or peiro "pierce," referring to the fissured calyptra forming a covering that encloses the capsule.

Calymperes erosum moss extracts exhibit antibacterial activity against

Bacillus subtilis, Staphylococcus aureus, Streptococcus pyogenes, and *Escherichia coli* (Oyesiku and Caleb 2015). Previous work by Tedela et al. (2014) found ethanol extracts also inhibit *Klebsiella pneumoniae, Enterococcus faecalis, Bacillus pumilis,* and *Enterobacter cloacea* in decreasing order of sensitivity. *Bacillus pumilis* is a gram-positive soil bacterium that has been harnessed to create commercial fungicides as well as the enzyme keratinase and vanillin (a phenolic aldehyde and the principal constituent of vanilla), which are ingredients in several traditional fermented foods. Several strains are used as probiotics for animals. Ironically, *Bacillus pumilis* is also a pathogen that causes ginger rhizome rot disease (Yuan and Gao 2015).

Enterobacter cloacae is emerging as a global, multidrug-resistant, gram-negative bacteria, resistant to last-resort carbapenems, a class of antibiotics used in cases of severe infections. Pneumonia, urinary tract infections, endocarditis, intra-abdominal skin and soft-tissue infections, and septicemia may present with such infections. Some are acquired in hospitals and have the highest mortality rate of all *Enterobacter* infections. This moss shows efficacy in the exchange of these resistant genes to create a stubborn defense.

Calymperes motleyi is a common moss in parts of Southeast Asia and Australia. In Malaysia it is combined with *Campylopus* and *Sphagnum* species for stuffing mattresses.

Kirisanth et al. (2020) dried and extracted this bryophyte as well as *Marchantia* sp., *Fissidens* sp., *Plagiochila* sp., *Sematophyllum demissum,* and *Hypnum cupressiforme* with three organic solvents. Six out of eighteen showed antibacterial activity for gram-positive bacteria, and one was active for gram-negative species. The ethyl acetate extracts were tested for α-amylase activity and three out of six extracts showed moderate inhibition.

CAMPYLIUM

Dull Starry Feather Moss   Yellow Starry Feather Moss

The moss *Campylium stellatum,* with the descriptive common name yellow starry feather moss, is often found in fens and hummocks. In northern Indiana, floating islands have been formed in ponds with this moss a major part of the mat formation. *Campylium stellatum,* according to Pouliot et al. (2012), would be the top pick to grow in the contaminated Athabasca Oil Sands to create new fen peatlands. The researchers also suggest *Ptychostomum pseudotriquetrum* syn. *Bryum pseudotriquetrum* be trialed.

Campylium protensum, dull starry feather moss, inhibits three gram-positive and two gram-negative bacteria (Bukvicki, Veljic et al. 2012).

CAMPYLOPUS

Crooked Stork Fishhook Moss Swan Moss

Campylopus is a fairly large genus, containing 185 accepted species worldwide, with one-tenth found in North America. The genus name is derived from the Greek *kampylos*, meaning "bent" or "curved," and *pous*, "foot," due to the appearance of cygneous seta (Dixon 1954). The genus is often known as crooked stork, fishhook moss, or swan moss.

In Malaysia this moss is used with *Sphagnum* or *Leucobryum* species for stuffing mattresses and cushions.

The heat-tolerant *Campylopus praemorsus* lives close to the steam vents of a dormant volcano near Pahoa, Hawaii.

Valarezo (2018) gathered, steam-distilled, and identified 94 constituents in six moss species found in Ecuador. Essential oil from the moss *Campylopus richardii* contains 15.1% epi-α-muurolol and 12.5% α-cadinol. Epi-αmuurolol is a moderate inhibitor of *Escherichia coli* DNA gyrase subunit B, penicillin binding protein 2X and penicillin binding protein 3 of *Pseudomonas aeruginosa* (The et al. 2022). Alpha-cadinol is a potential angiotensin converting enzyme (ACE) inhibitor suggestive of benefit in treating hypertension (Tripathi et al. 2023).

CERATODON

Fire Moss Red Roof Moss Seventy-Mile-An-Hour Moss
Purple Fork Moss Red Shank Moss Twin-Stalked Fork Moss

Geographic Range: North America, Europe, Antarctica
Habitats: hot, sunny, inhospitable locations; thrives on rooftops
Practical Uses: remediates burn sites and roadsides
Medicinal Applications: anticancer, antibacterial, antifungal, antioxidant

The genus name is derived from the Greek *keratos*, meaning "horn," and *odon*, "tooth." This is due to the resemblance of the peristome teeth of this moss to a goat's horn (Dixon 1954). There are 5 accepted species worldwide.

Fire moss, red shank moss, or purple fork moss (*Ceratodon purpureus*) is found throughout Europe and North America. Other unusual common names

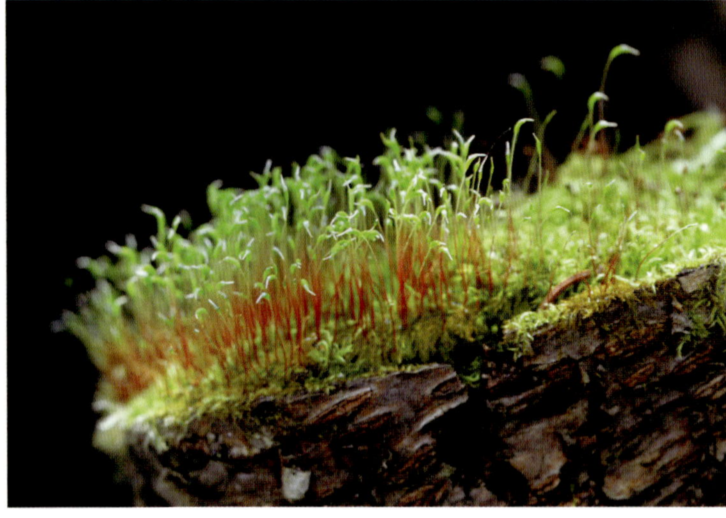

Ceratodon purpureus (Fire Moss)

are red roof moss, seventy-mile-an-hour moss, and twin-stalked fork moss. The sporophytes are not really purple, more red.

Ceratodon purpureus syn. *Dicranum purpureum* goes by the names red shank moss, purple fork moss, fire moss, and purple horn toothed moss. Exudate fractions from this moss were collected and tested for their medicinal activity (Dague et al. 2023). The exudates from the female strain did not exhibit inhibitory activity, but the male moss strain exhibited strong inhibition of several gram-positive bacteria, including *Staphylococcus aureus* and *Enterococcus faecium*. In culture, the exudates increased in antibacterial activity significantly over the four weeks in which the study took place. The authors suggest that the bioactive compounds in this species may give additional options for treating infections caused by antibiotic-resistant gram-positive bacteria.

Unlike some moss species, *Ceratodon purpureus* can handle hot, sunny locations. It is often found along the edges of asphalt parking lots or in cracks in concrete sidewalks.

Frahm (2004) used an extract of this moss to treat fungal infections in horses. This occurred after an equine owner read about Frahm's experiments and made a paste of this moss and *Bryum argenteum*. The fungus disappeared within twenty-four hours, and the rest is history. The patented extract is sold today as a human foot cream to remove odor.

Ceratodon purpureus exhibits significant antioxidant and antibacterial activity (Wolksi et al. 2021; Waterman et al. 2017).

A fungal endophyte living in the tissue of this moss has been identified as *Smardaea* species. Analysis revealed five new isopimarane diterpenes (smardaesidins A–E); and two new 20-nor-isoprimarane diterpenes (smardaesidins F and G); as well as sphaeropsidin A and C–F. Several compounds show significant cytotoxicity. Sphaeropsidin A inhibits the migration of metastatic breast adenocarcinoma (MDA-MB-231) cells at subcytotoxic concentrations (Wang et al. 2011). These constituents shows promise against drug-resistant cancer cells, specifically displaying in vitro activity against melanoma and kidney cancer cell lines.

Studies by Mathieu et al. (2015) found sphaeropsidin A can overcome multi-drug resistance by inducing a marked and rapid cellular shrinkage due to changes in ion homeostasis. Sphaeropsidin A decreases biofilm formation associated with methicillin-resistant *Staphylococcus aureus* and *Pseudomonas aeruginosa* (Roscetto et al. 2020). Sphaeropsidin D has also been discovered in the endophyte as well as in the medicinal mushroom Artist's Conk (*Ganoderma applanatum*), a bracket fungus that binds to receptors associated with anxiety, depression, and pain (Hossen et al. 2021).

Work by Vollár et al. (2018) found various solvent extracts of *Ceratodon purpureus* exhibit cytotoxicity against epithelial/cervical (HeLa), ovarian (T47D), and breast (A2780) cancer cell lines. Methanol extracts were only effective against ovarian cancer cells. Water extracts showed no activity.

Kang et al. (2007) found extracts of this, and other mosses inhibit *Staphylococcus aureus* when enhanced by UV-A light irradiation.

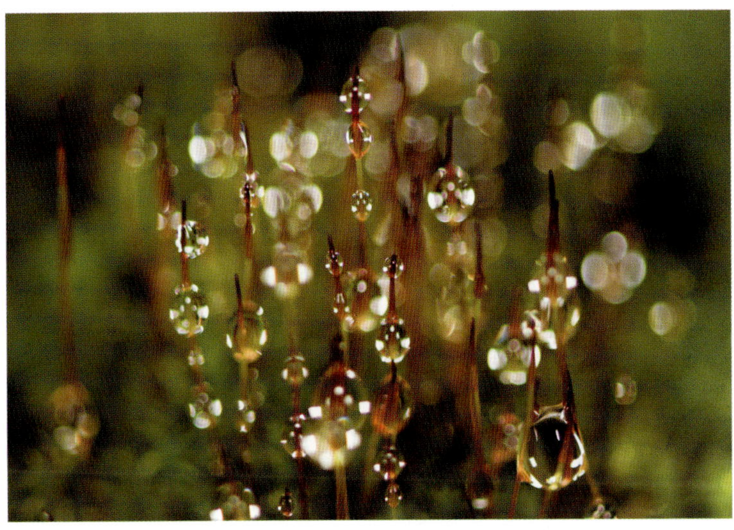

Ceratodon purpureus (Fire Moss)

Homeopathy

In homeopathy, fire moss, *Ceratodon purpureus*, is used for hyperactivity, ADHD, in order to forget the cruelty, to stay on top, to avoid the abyss of boredom, greyness, playing; dancing the madness away.*

The recommended dose is 12C to 30C potency.

CINCLIDOTUS

Lattice Mosses
Net Tooth Moss
Screw Moss
Small Sekra Moss

The genus name derives from *kinklidotos*, meaning "latticed," in reference to the latticed peristome (Dixon 1954).

Smaller lattice moss, fountain lattice moss, or small sekra moss (*Cinclidotus fontinaloides*) loves growing on rocks in streams that change with the seasons. Recent work by Yayintas et al. (2017) found ethanol and water extracts significantly inhibit the bacteria *Escherichia coli*, *Bacillus subtilis*, *Staphylococcus aureus*, and *Pseudomonas aeruginosa*; and the fungus *Candida albicans*; as well as exhibit antioxidant activity. The moss contains various flavonoids, including gallic acid. Methanol extracts of the aquatic moss inhibit the growth of gray mold, *Botrytis cinerea* (Nedeljko et al. 2019), which, like many bacteria and fungi, has developed resistance to fungicides.

CIRRIPHYLLUM

Hair Grass Moss
Hair-Pointed Feather Moss

The genus name may derive from the Latin *cirrus*, "curl," and the Greek *phyllon*, "leaf"; from the Latin *pilus*, meaning "hair," and *ferrum*, referring to the element iron and meaning "strong."

Hair-pointed feather moss or hair grass moss, (*Cirriphyllum piliferum*) is a large and easily identified moss. Work by Vollár et al. (2018) found various solvent extracts exhibit cytotoxicity against epithelial/cervical (HeLa), ovarian (T47D), and breast (A2780) cancer cell lines. Water extracts were only active against epithelial/cervical lines. An extract inhibited *Streptococcus pneumoniae*, the leading cause of community-acquired pneumonia.

*Proving by Jan Scholten, Qjure Homeopathy (website) chapter 3.

CLAOPODIUM

Anomodon Moss | Velvet Tree Apron
Rough Moss | Yellow Yarn

The genus name probably derives from the Greek *klao*, "break," and *podion*, "little foot," alluding to the fragile setae and the pendent appearance of the capsule.

Crispleaf rough moss, *Claopodium crispifolium*, is found on the coast of British Columbia and in southeastern parts of Alberta. Tests conducted for the National Cancer Institute by Spjut et al. (1988) involving 184 mosses identified this species as possessing the strongest antitumor activity.

Studies by Suwanborirux et al. (1990) isolated ansamitocin P-3 from *Claopodium crispifolium*. Subsequent trials found this to be a potent cytotoxic substance against human lung (A-549) and colon (HT29) cancer cell lines. The compound is also found in the mosses *Pseudanomodon attenuates* syn. *Anomodon attenuatus* and *Thamnobryum subseriatum* syn. *Thamnobryum sandei*. It has low solubility, so loading it into photo-responsive liposomes may create a product useful for treating breast cancer (Jin et al. 2023). Spjut et al. (1988) found cytotoxic and antitumor activity against both murine lymphocytic leukemia (P-388) and epidermoid (HL-60) cell cultures. The *Nostoc* genus of blue-green algae was found present on the samples with the highest levels of activity. This suggests *Nostoc* may be the source of bioactivity, or it precipitates allelopathy, the suppression of growth of one plant species due to the release of toxic substances.

Yellow yarn, velvet tree apron, or anomodon moss (*Claopodium rostratum* syn. *Anomodon rostratus*) grows on calcareous rocks and prefers alkaline soil. The word *rostratus*, derived from the Latin, means "beaked" or "curved," in reference to the beaked operculum. Early work by McCleary et al. (1960) found this moss inhibited the growth of the pathogens *Micrococcus flavus*, *M. rubens* syn. *Kocuria rosea*, *Streptococcus pyogenes*, and *Candida albicans*. It is effective against *Kocuria rosea*, a novel bacterium native to the human microbiome that can cause a bloodstream infection from the insertion of a catheter and has become multi-drug-resistant to standard antibiotics like cephalosporin, fluoroquinolone, and macrolide drugs. Cases involving endocarditis and necrotizing fasciitis (flesh-eating disease) are also cited in the literature.

CLIMACIUM

Common Longevity Moss
Glistering Shrub Moss
Ground Pine Moss
Palm Moss
Staircase Moss
Tree Climacium Moss
Tree-Shaped Feather Moss

The genus name is derived from the Greek *klimakion*, meaning "staircase" or "ladder." This alludes to the appearance of the process of the inner peristome, the two halves of which are regularly united by projections between the perforations, giving the appearance of a ladder (Dixon 1954), reflected in one of this plant's common names, staircase moss.

Tree climacium moss, or common longevity moss, (*Climacium dendroides*) resembles little trees. The moss is found all over the Canadian prairies, save for the driest areas of southeastern Alberta and southwestern Saskatchewan. On the West Coast, extending south through the Pacific Northwest and Northern California, it is a common yard weed, but on the prairies it is found in fens and calcareous tundra conditions. Other common names reflect this moss' appearance: glistering shrub moss, palm moss, and tree-shaped feather moss. Compared to most mosses it is a giant and considered an invasive weed in the Pacific Northwest.

In parts of England, the dried moss was artificially colored and used to decorate women's hats.

The moss is used in Traditional Chinese Medicine for rheumatism, bone pain, and as a muscle relaxant (Zhong Hua Ben Cao 1999).

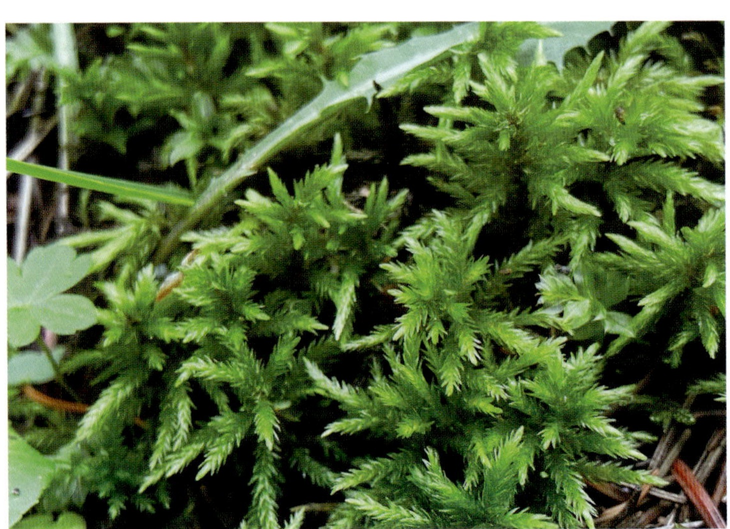

Climacium dendroides (Tree Climacium Moss)
Photo by Graham Steinruck

Research by Nerlo and Kosior (1977) identified the sterol content in *Climacium dendroides* and concluded that it is cytotoxic to one or more hormonal cancer cell lines. Work by Klavina et al. (2015) found ethanol extracts exhibit weak antiproliferative activity against five of the six cancer cell lines tested. The team identified atraric acid, 7,8-dihydroxy-5-methoxycoumarin-7-β sophoroside, as well as 4-O- and 5-O-caffeoylquinic acid. Atraric acid is an androgen receptor antagonist and inhibits prostate cancer cell growth. In vivo studies by Ehsani et al. (2022) found that it suppresses androgen-regulated neo-angiogensis of castration-resistant prostate cancer through angiopoietin 2. Atraric acid is widely used in perfumes due to its pleasant scent; external use ameliorates hyperpigmentation of the skin (Li, Jiang et al. 2022).

Vollár et al. (2018) selected 42 bryophytes from which they made 168 water and organic extracts. They then screened for activity against cervical epithelial adenocarcinoma (HeLa) as well as ovarian (A2780) and invasive ductal breast (T47D) cancer cell lines. Ninety-nine of the organic extracts derived from forty-one species exerted more than 25% inhibition of at least one of the cancer cell lines at 10 μg/mL. Water extracts were not active against the breast cancer cell line. Only 19 samples from 15 taxa showed moderate antibacterial activity, with *Staphylococcus aureus* the most susceptible to this moss.

CRATONEURON

Cowhorn Moss
Fern Feather
Fern-Leaved Hook Moss
Golden Fern Moss
Shaguma Moss
Tufa Moss

The genus name derives from the Greek *kratos*, "strong," and *neuron* "nerve," alluding to the strong leaf costa. The genus is commonly referred to as cowhorn moss or tufa moss. In Japan, it is commonly known as Shaguma moss, referring to a wooden hair-tool.

Fern-leaved hook moss, cowhorn moss, fern feather, and golden fern moss (*Cratoneuron filicinum*) is often found in the northern prairies on calcareous rocks. In India, this moss is traditionally taken internally to treat heart disease (Chandra et al. 2017; Ding et al. 1982). There it is a specific remedy indicated for *malum cardis*, "bad heart" (Alam et al. 2015).

Bukvicki, Veljic et al. (2012) found methanol extracts of *Cratoneuron filicinum* to possess significant antimicrobial activity against both gram-positive and gram-negative bacteria.

CRYPHAEA

Hidden Capsule Moss   Thread Cedar Moss

The genus name is derived from the Greek *kryphos*, meaning, "secret" or "hidden," in reference to the immersed capsule, which is more or less hidden by the perichaetial leaves (Dixon 1954). This is reflected in one of this genus's common names, hidden capsule; it is also called thread cedar moss.

Lateral cryphaea, odd-sided dalton, or lateral daltonia (*Cryphaea heteromalla*), is one of about 26 species found worldwide. This moss is generally found in pollution-free environments, usually at the base of willows or hardwood trees. Two of the common names were given in honor of the British bryologist James Dalton (1764–1843), who was a close friend of the Hooker family and godfather of British botanist and explorer Joseph Dalton Hooker. As well, the bryophyte genus *Daltonia* was dedicated to him in 1818.

Provenzano et al. (2019) investigated three different solvent extractions of *Cryphaea heteromalla*: pure water, 80% ethanol, and 80% methanol. The water extract proved the best solvent with the highest content of bisphenols and highest oxygen radical absorbance capacity. When analyzed, 14 compounds were detected, and five were phenolic derivatives of benzoic, caffeic,

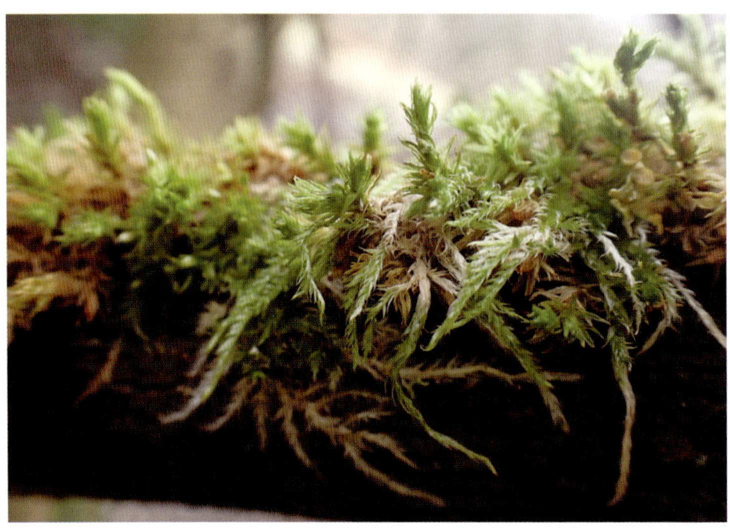

Cryphaea heteromalla (Lateral Cryphaea)

and coumaric acids. When tested against reactive oxygen species (ROS) on murine fibroblast (NIH-3T3) cell lines, the water extract showed protective effects.

An aqueous extract was trialed in a hydrogel film for application as a wound dressing in work by Ditta et al. (2020). The investigation found an absence of cytotoxicity and an ability to reduce oxidative stress, as demonstrated on NIH-3T3 fibroblast cell cultures.

CTENIDIUM

Comb Mosses   Schofield's Ctenidium Moss

The genus name is derived from *ktenos* (comb) and diminuitive suffix *-idion*, alluding to the neat, comblike appearance of the branching.

Chalk comb moss, *Ctenidium molluscum*, is common in Europe and North America. The name refers to the respiratory or gill structure of ocean mollusks. There are numerous varieties: *Ctenidium condensatum* is dense comb moss; *C. fastigiatum* is slender comb moss; *C. robustum* is vinous comb moss; and *C. sylvaticum* is wood comb moss.

Ctenidium molluscum is one of the more popular bryophytes used in traditional nativity scenes in Croatia. A study of farmer's markets in parts of southeastern Europe found it commonly used in Christmas festivities (Bucar et al. 2022). It contains polyphenols and flavonoids that exhibit antioxidant activity (Erturk et al. 2015).

Schofield's ctenidium moss, *Ctenidium schofieldii*, is a species restricted to Haida Gwaii in British Columbia and Adak Island off the coast of Alaska. It is named in honor of Canadian bryologist Wilfred "Wilf" Borden Schofield (1927–2008). Born in Nova Scotia, Schofield later became a full professor of biology at the University of British Columbia. When he first arrived at UBC, the bryophyte collection at the Beaty Biodiversity Museum held 3,000 specimens; today it holds over 260,000. Some authors, including myself, consider him the foremost bryologist in Canada. The bryophytes *Sphagnum wilfii*, *Plagiochila schofieldiana* (an older name for *Plagiochila gracilis*), and *Plagiothecium schofieldii* were also named in his honor.

CYCLODICTYON

Cave Moss

The generic name refers to the rounded, netlike outlines of the laminal cells from the Greek *kūklos*, "circle," and *diktyon*, "net." This large genus contains 83 accepted species, mainly in the Neotropics.

Cyclodictyon species moss was collected from the wall of an ancient water well in southwest Nigeria as part of a 2015 study by Oyesiku and Caleb. Ethanol extracts inhibited various fungi, including *Trichoderma* spp., *Aspergillus niger*, and *Microsporum gypseum*.

CYNODONTIUM

Dog Tooth Moss Loose-Leaved Fork Moss

Dog tooth or loose-leaved fork moss (*Cynodontium laxifolia* syn. *Oreoweisia laxifolia* syn. *Dicranum laxifolium*) contains phospholipids rich in the antimicrobial dicranin, an acetylenic fatty acid (Chowdhuri et al. 2018). Platelet aggregation induced by either thrombin or arachidonic acid was inhibited by 10^{-4} M of dicranin (Guichardant et al. 1992).

DALTONIA

Dalton's Moss Irish Daltonia

The genus name was given in honor of the British bryologist James Dalton (1764–1843), who was a close friend of the botanically oriented Hooker family and godfather of botanist Joseph Dalton Hooker. This bryophyte was dedicated to him in 1818 by William Jackson Hooker and Thomas Taylor in their 1818 book on bryophytes, *Muscologia Britannica*. There are 30 accepted species, mainly tropical.

Dalton's moss, or Irish daltonia, (*Daltonia splachnoides*) is the best-known species. It is rare in Canada, with only three sites, one in the temperate rain forests of Haida Gwaii, British Columbia. This beautiful, small, glossy-yellow to bronze-colored moss is also found in the moist climates of Australia, New Zealand, Great Britain, Central and South America, and the West Indies. It is red listed on the IUCN Red List of Threatened Species in Canada and Europe.

DAWSONIA

Giant Moss Giant Royal Moss

The genus is named in honor of Dawson Turner (1775–1858), a banker, botanist, antiquarian, artist, and good friend of Scottish botanist Robert Brown, who pioneered the use of the microscope in biology. Brown (1811) wrote, "I have named this remarkable genus in honor of my esteemed friend Dawson Turner, Esq., a gentleman eminently distinguished in every part of Cryptogamic botany, and from whom, after he has finished the incomparable work on *Fuci*, in which he is now engaged, we may expect a general history of Mosses." Turner died on June 20, 1858, just ten days after Brown. There are 10 accepted species.

Dawsonia species are some of our tallest bryophytes; they can grow up to two feet tall in parts of Australia. They have adapted to a lack of vascular tissue by transporting water by conduit widening of their hydraulic structure.

Dawsonia species and other mosses are used in Papua, New Guinea, to decorate the body and as ornaments in head gear, particularly *Dawsonia grandis*, which is stripped of leaves, split, and braided into a red rope to decorate bags and baskets. In Malaysia this moss is used along with *Spiridens* and *Pogonatum* species for body decoration and to ward off evil spirits.

Dawsonia longifolia, a synonym of *Dawsonia superba*, is used as a diuretic in India and to encourage hair growth (Chandra et al. 2017; Azuelo et al. 2011).

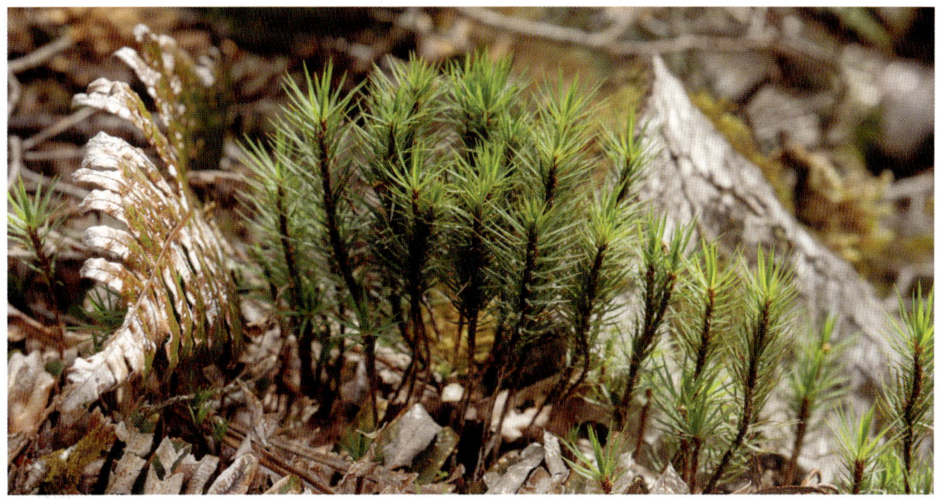

Dawsonia superba (Giant Moss)

GIANT ROYAL MOSS ESSENCE

This Essence prepared from *Dawsonia superba* anchors cosmic light into the fourth layer of DNA. It creates a powerful and magical connection with the Sacred Altars of the West and the places of true emotional well-being.

Giant Royal Moss Essence No. 164 can be found at First Light Flower Essences of New Zealand.

DENDROPOGONELLA

Pastle Amarillo
Tree Beard
Yellow Curtains
Yellow Moss

Only one species, *Dendropogonella rufescens*. The Zapotec name *begachi yaa'xia* means "yellow moss." *Pastle amarillo* is derived from the Náhuatl pachtli (herb that grows and hangs from trees) and the Spanish *amarillo* meaning "yellow." *Cortinas amarillas*, "yellow curtains," is the Spanish name as is *musgo amarillo*, "yellow moss."

Dendropogonella rufescens was traditional tea in southeastern Mexico to relieve the pain and discomfort suffered by new mothers following childbirth. It generally relieves body and bone pain, kidney and lung complaints, diabetic-related conditions, and blindness. The moss tea is also prepared as an appetizer or beverage consumed either warm or cold in Zapotec communities of southeastern Mexico (Hernández-Rodríguez and López-Santiago 2021). It is traditional to smoke this moss with the stalk of *Agave americana* and dry corn to provide relief for bone and muscle pain. The moss is also used for decorations at ceremonies, weddings, and festivals, and in crafts, beds, pillows, and even molded into hats in Central America.

DICRANELLA

Silky Forklet Moss

Dicranella is the diminutive of *Dicranum* (see below). German bryologist Carl Müller (1818–1899) coined the name for three species in this genus that were previously included in the taxon *Dicranum*. During his career he collected a moss herbarium of 12,000 bryophyte species. *Dicranella* resemble *Dicranum* species but are smaller and have scarcely differentiated alar cells.

Dicranella spiralis syn. *Anisothecium spirale*, a moss from the eastern Himalayas, contains high levels of dicranin (Mitra 2017). (The synonym *Anisothecium* derives from the Greek *aniso*, "unequal" or "different," and *thekion*, "little vessel," "container," or "sheath.") The valuable phytochemical dicranin, found in this moss, is an acetylenic fatty acid with anti-fibrotic, anti-inflammatory, and anticancer effects and found in many other moss species. Platelet aggregation induced by either thrombin or arachidonic acid was inhibited by 10^{-4} M of dicranin. This suggests possible benefits in conditions such as thrombophlebitis and other blood clot disorders. (Guichardant et al. 1992).

SILKY FORKLET MOSS ESSENCE

This moss essence prepared from *Dicranella heteromalla* helps those who fear light and freedom in their lives, in particular those who hold shadow issues. Within these dark spaces there is a fear of joy and freedom and the responsibility that comes with it. With such people there is not overall gloom, but rather small, dark spaces that nevertheless seriously affect their lives. Some of these areas may be very guilt laden as a result of old patterns (Bailey 1996).*

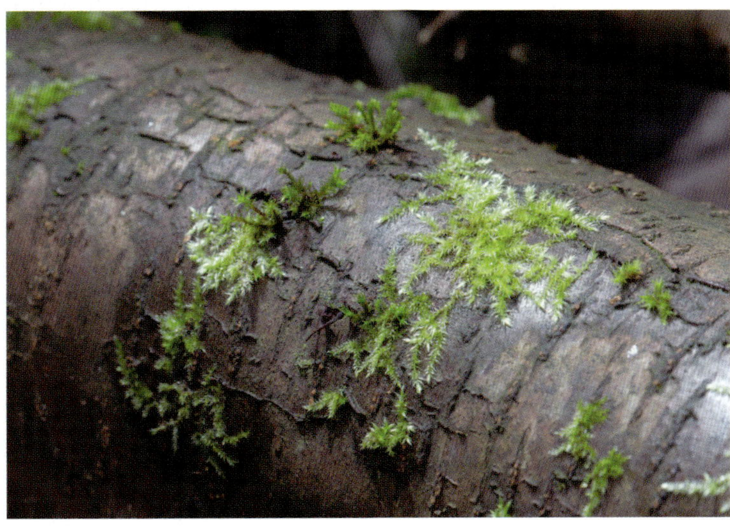

Dicranella heteromalla (Silky Forklet Moss)

*This product is no longer commercially available.

DICRANOLOMA

The genus name is a combination of *Dicranum* and *loma*, meaning "border," alluding to the border of narrow, elongate cells on the leaf margin.

Dicranoloma mosses are commonly found in the Southern Hemisphere (40 species), as distinguished from *Dicranum* mosses, which are common to the Northern Hemisphere. *Dicranoloma braunii* syn. *D. brevisetum* var. *samoanum* was collected and studied for volatile compounds (Koid et al. 2022). The moss contains 32.7% pentanoic acid, 2.2.4-trimethyl-3-carboxyisopropyl isobutyl ester, 10.5% decanal, and minor amounts of limonene, β-elemene, geranylacetone, dodecane, tetradecane, 1-dodecene, and nonanal.

Geranylacetone in particular was found to have trypanostatic activity and could protect livestock against the pathogenic parasite *Trypanosoma congolense* that causes anemia. This may be through the inhibition of sialidase and/or the protection of parasite-induced hepatosplenomegaly (Saad et al. 2019).

DICRANUM

Broken-Leaf Curved-Tail Moss
Broom Fork Moss
Cushion Moss
Electric Eels Moss
Fork Mosses
Footstool Moss
Fragile Fork Moss
Giant Green Moss
Purple Horn Toothed Moss
Rugose Fork Moss
Tail Mosses
Wavy Dicranum

Geographic Range: worldwide

Habitats: acidic soils, tree stumps, shaded forests

Practical Uses: bedding and mattresses, candle wicks, diapers, window displays, insecticides, meat fermentation, moss gardens

Medicinal Applications: antibacterial, anticancer, antifungal, anti-inflammatory, cough suppressant, digestive

The genus name *Dicranum* is derived from the Greek *dikranon*, "two-headed," referring to the two forked teeth around the mouth of the capsule. These teeth control spore dispersal by opening and closing according to changes of humidity. There are 94 accepted species worldwide.

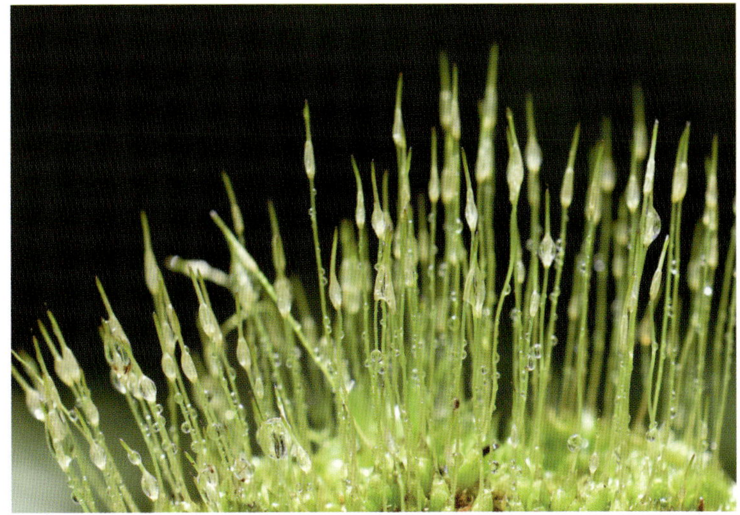

Dicranum sp.

Although many *Dicranum* species have since been reclassified as *Orthodicranum*, Robin Wall Kimmerer, in her book *Gathering Moss: A Natural and Cultural History of Mosses*, describes the relationships between the species with such excellence that I've preserved her original intent here.

> In the *Dicranum* clan, there are family roles that could easily apply to sisters in any big family. [*Dicranum*] *montanum* [now *Orthodicranum montanum*], is the unassuming one; you know the type—nondescript, overlooked with her short curls always in disarray. . . . Moist, shady rocks are the habitat of the glamorous [*Dicranum*] *scoparium*, the one who draws the looks with her long, shiny leaves tossed to one side. . . . [*Dicranum*] *flagellare* [now *Orthodicranum flagellare*], with her trim and straight leaves that resemble a military buzzcut, remains aloof from the others, choosing to live only on logs in an advanced state of decay. She's the conservative one, celibate for the most part, foregoing family in favor of her own personal advancement by cloning. Solitary and intensely green, [*Dicranum*] *viride* has a hidden fragile side, with leaf tips always broken off like bitten fingernails. [*Dicranum*] *polysetum*, on the other hand, is the most prolific mother of the family, an inevitable outcome of her multiple sporophytes. Then there's the long, wavy-leafed [*Dicranum*] *undulatum*, capping the tops of boggy hummocks, and [*Dicranum*] *fulvum* [now *Orthodicranum fulvum*], the black sheep of the family.

Orthodicranum fulvum shows moderate activity against murine lymphoma (P-388) cancer cell lines (Spjut et al. 1986).

Lawn moss, *Dicranum montanum* (now *Orthodicranum montanum*) possesses significant antioxidant activity (Smolinska-Kondla et al. 2022).

Dicranum aquaticum (now *Dichodontium pellucidum*) exhibits inhibition of the necotrophic fungi *Botrytis cinerea* and *Alternaria solani* (Mekuria et al. 2005).

Crisped fork moss, *Dicranum bonjeannii*, also called marsh fork moss and thin-rib curved tailmoss, has been used by traditional peoples in North America for its absorbent properties such as in diapers (Moerman 1998; Thieret 1956). Long-forked moss, *Dicranum elongatum*, and other *Dicranum* species were used by the Cree for lamp wicks (Bland 1971), as in nature there are only a few fibers that produce carbonless wicks that do not burn up like standard cotton.

As a sidenote, the fluff of the flowering plant known as fireweed (*Epilobium angustifolium* syn. *Chamerion angustifolium*) also produces a carbonless wick. It was traditionally woven with mountain goat or sheep hair to produce waterproof clothing (Rogers 2017). *Dicranum elongatum* is known as *maniq* by the Inuit of Baffin Island; it is prepared dry or in a broth for indigestion or to treat sickness that required bed rest. At one time it was used as diaper material for babies. Cushion moss (*Dicranum groenlandicum*) is known to the Chipewyan of northern Canada as *nódhulé* and was used for its long parallel stems that absorb grease and make good wicks (Marles et al. 2000).

Greater forked moss, or giant green moss, *Dicranum majus*, is used in TCM as a cough suppressant (Zhong Hua Ben Cao 1999). It also inhibits nitric oxide production without cytotoxic effects, which suggests an innovative therapeutic pathway for reducing inflammation in new cough syrup products (Marques et al. 2022).

Dicranin, found in *Dicranum scoparium* and *Anisothecium spirale*, exhibits 15-lipoxygenase inhibition, suggestive of antioxidant activity (Borel et al. 1993). Dicranin is considered a chemotaxonomic marker for Dicranaceae members.

In vitro evaluation of *Dicranum scoparium* showed significant decrease in *Klebsiella pneumoniae* and *Escherichia coli* shedding and colonizing. (Karpinksi and Adamczak 2017).

A study by El-Shiekh et al. (2023) suggests the *Dicranum* spp. constituent L4N is a potential substitute for or perhaps an adjunctive with (based on the author's observation) traditional antibiotics.

Rugose fork moss, *Dicranum polysetum*, is a common moss found on the floors of deciduous forests. Other common names for this species are wavy dicranum, wavy-leaf curved-tail moss, and electric eels moss. American foulbrood is a serious disease in honeybee colonies caused by the *Paenibacillus* genus. Ethanol extracts of *Dicranum polysetum* contain 7,8-dihydroxy-5-methoxycoumarin-7-β sophoroside, and minor amounts of atraric acid and 4-hydroxybenzoic acid. These were found to considerably reduce infection in the honeybee larvae, which was clinically halted when the extract was administered in the first twenty-four hours after spore contamination. The extract neither reduces larvae viability and live weight nor affect the production of royal jelly (Karaoglu et al. 2023).

Work by Klavina et al. (2015) examined the antiproliferative activity of *Dicranum polysetum* against six cancer cell lines. Significant inhibition of rat glioma (C6) and mouse melanoma (B16-F10) was noted.

This moss exhibits significant activity against the nonpathogenic *Staphyloccocus carnosus* (Altuner et al. 2014), an important starter culture for meat fermentation.

Broom fork moss, mood moss, or footstool moss, (*Dicranum scoparium*), is widespread in North America and around the world. It makes a great ottoman for the front of benches, hence one of the common names. This moss is frequently used in shop window displays and in moss gardens, and is traditionally used in bedding, mattresses, cushions, and pillows. Its presence is usually a good indicator of acidic soil. Martin (2015) notes it cannot tolerant too much moisture or too much sun, hence it is "moody." However, she says, "Golden sporophytes with almond-shaped capsules light up green colonies like glowing candles."

Moss extracts of *Dicranum scoparium* inhibit *Bacillus cereus*, *B. subtilis*, *B. stearothermophilus*, *Staphylococcus aureus*, and *Escherichia coli* in a study by Borel et al. (1993). The compound dicranin, when isolated, was found to

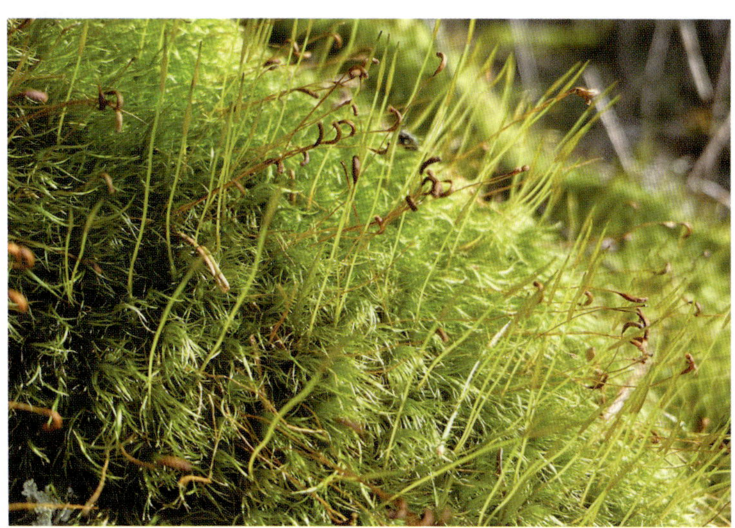

Dicranum scoparium (Broom Fork Moss)
Photo by Drew T. Henderson

be the most active inhibitor against *Streptococcus faecalis* but inactive against *Escherichia coli*. This seems confirmed by a much earlier 1963 study by Pavletic and Stilinovic, who found *Dicranum scoparium* strongly inhibits all bacteria tested, including *Micrococcus luteus* but not *Escherichia coli*.

A 2017 study by Karpinski and Adamczak investigated 12 moss species including *Dicranum scoparium* and found minor inhibition of *Streptococcus pyogenes, Staphylococcus aureus, Escherichia coli, Enterococcus faecalis, and Klebsiella pneumoniae.*

Guichardant et al. (1992) found dicranin, an acetylenic fatty acid extracted from *D. scoparium*, to be an inhibitor of platelet aggregation when induced by either thrombin or arachidonic acid. Seven flavonoids were isolated from this and four other moss species. The flavonoids were apigenin, apigenin-7-O-triglycoside, lucenin-2, luteolin-7-O-neohesperidoside, saponarine, and vitex; and the biflavonoid bartramiaflavone was isolated as well. Some of them showed significant inhibition of the gram-negative bacteria *Enterobacter cloaceae, E. aerogenes*, and *Pseudomonas aeruginosa* (Basile et al. 1999). Moreover, another constituent, luteolin 4'-neohesperidoside (L4N), inhibits four antibiotic-resistant bacteria, including MRSA, *Klebsiella pneumoniae*, the fosA-positive shiga toxin that produces the *Escherichia coli* serogroup O111, and *Bacillus cereus*.

Significant synergistic activity against the gram-negative bacteria *Bacillus cereus*, for example, was noted in cases when the drug-resistant antibiotics gentamicin and vancomycin were combined with *Dicranum scoparium* (El-Shiekh et al. 2023).

In a study of five mosses, including *Dicranum scoparium* the flavonoid apigenin-7-O-triglycoside was found to inhibit the gram-negative bacteria *Pseudomonas aeruginosa* (Basile et al. 1999). Fatty acid derivatives obtained from dichloromethane extracts of *Dicranum scoparium* exhibit antiproliferative effects. Hexane extracts, rich in omega-9 fatty acid, exhibit strong antiproliferative activity against epithelial/cervical (HeLa) cancer cell lines when compared to the topical skin cancer drug fluorouracil (5-FU).

In Turkey, *Dicranum scoparium* is traditionally used as an insecticide against the wheat weevil (*Sitophilus granarius*). Compounds present in this moss species such as myristic, palmitic, and lauric acids exhibit specific insecticidal activity (Abay et al 2015). Novel acetylenic oxylipins derived from *Dicranum scoparium* exhibit antifeedant activity against herbivorous slugs (Rempt and Pohnert 2010).

Fragile fork moss, or broken-leaf curved-tail moss, (*Dicranum tauricum*) is found on old tree stumps in shaded forests. Its common name makes it easy to identify. Simply wet a finger and place it on a moss clump and a few leaflets

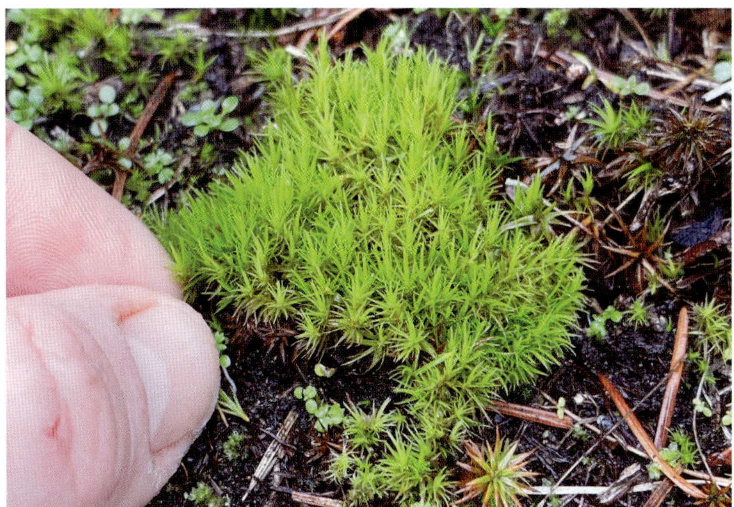

Dicranum tauricum (Fragile Fork Moss)
Photo by Drew T. Henderson

will adhere and pull off. Work by Vollár et al. (2018) found various solvent and water extracts exhibited cytotoxicity against epithelial/cervical (HeLa), ovarian (T47D), and breast (A2780) cancer cell lines, although the water extract exhibited no activity against the breast cancer cell line. The same study found solvent extracts inhibited *Streptococcus pneumoniae* in vitro.

DISTICHOPHYLLUM

Joint-Toothed Mosses

The genus name derives from the Greek *distichos*, meaning "in two rows," and *phyllon*, "leaf," alluding to the apparently distichous (but in fact flattened) leaf arrangement.

The Southern Hemisphere moss *Distichophyllum mittenii* was collected and studied for volatile compounds (Koid et al. 2022). It contains over 32% pentanoic acid; 2,2,4-trimethyl-3-carboxyisopropyl-isobutyl ester; limonene (17.8%); and minor amounts of menthol, tetradecane, 1-dodecene, 1-tetradecene, 1-hexanol, 2-ethyl, decanal, and naphthalene.

DITRICHUM

Gold Thread Moss Hair Mosses

The genus name is derived from the Greek *di*, meaning "two," and *trichos*, "hair," alluding to the divided filiform peristome teeth (Dixon 1954), hence common names such as two hair moss, cow hair moss, gold thread moss, and gold hair moss. Brown ditrichum (*Ditrichum pallidum*) has been used traditionally in India to treat convulsions, especially in children (Harris 2008; Asakawa 2015; Chandra et al. 2017).

ENCALYPTA

Spiral Extinguisher Moss

The genus name derives from the Greek *en*, "within," and *kalyptos*, "cover" or "lid," meaning to cover or conceal, with a veil, a reference to this moss's large calyptra (Dixon 1954). There are 41 accepted species.

Spiral extinguisher moss (*Encalypta streptocarpa*) is cytotoxic to one or more gynecological cancer cell lines. Vollár et al. (2018) selected forty-two bryophytes and then did 168 water and organic extracts. They then screened for activity against cervical/epithelial (HeLa), ovarian (A2780), and invasive ductal breast (T47D) cancer cell lines. Ninety-nine of the extracts derived from 41 species exerted more than 25% inhibition of at least one of the cancer cell lines at 10 μg/mL. Both methanol and water extracts exhibited no cytotoxicity against breast (T47D) cancer cell lines. Only 19 samples out of 15 taxa showed moderate antibacterial activity, with *Staphylococcus aureus* and MRSA the most susceptible.

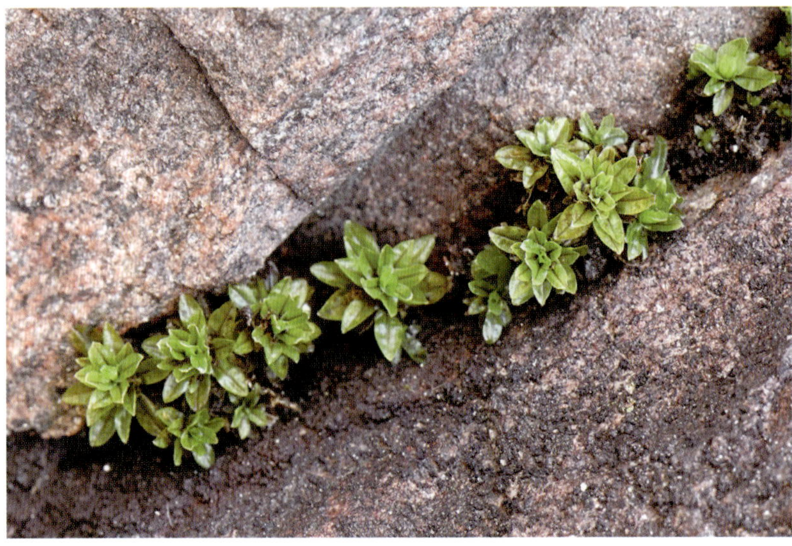

Encalypta streptocarpa (Spiral Extinguisher Moss)

ENTODON

Cord Glade Moss
Cucumber Scented Moss
Flat Glaze Moss
Seductive Entodon Moss
Shiny Sexy Moss
Silk Mosses
Toothpick Moss
Tooth within Moss

Geographic Range: North America, Asia

Habitat: logs and tree trunks; moist shaded areas on rocks; patios and moss lawns

Practical Uses: hydrogen production

Medicinal Applications: anticancer, anti-inflammatory, antimicrobial, anti-ulcer, diuretic, earache, endometriosis, fertility, hepatoprotective, neuroprotective, sedative

The genus name is derived from the Greek *entos*, "inside," and *odon*, "tooth," alluding to the insertion of the outer peristome teeth inside the capsule mouth, as reflected in one of this taxon's common names, tooth within moss.

Flat glaze moss (*Entodon cladorrhizans* syn. *E. compressus*) is used in TCM as a sedative and diuretic (Ding 1982).

Entodon flavescens is used to treat earaches by the Kani in Western Ghats, India (Chandra et al. 2017). The fresh leaf juice is squeezed directly into the

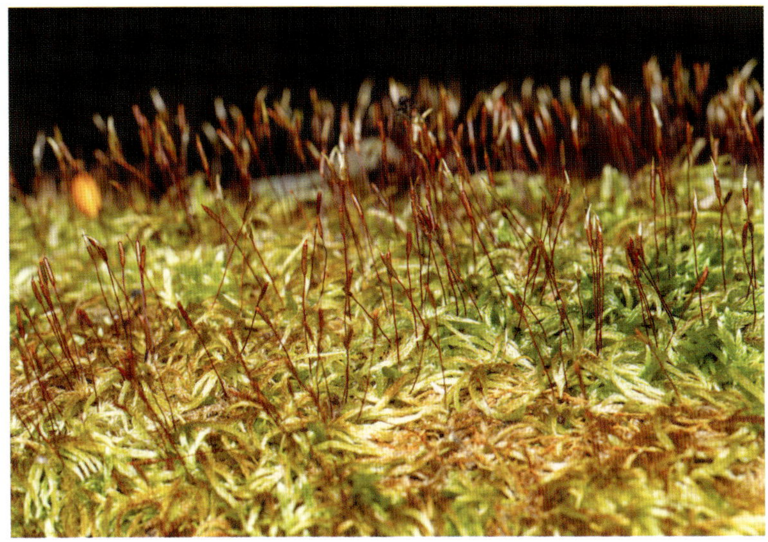

Entodon sp.

ear. When taken orally for colds or for inducing female fertility, another application, the leaf juice is taken with equal parts garlic and black pepper once daily for three days after the menstrual period ends.

Venous catheter insertion and some surgeries can cause bloodstream infections. *Entodon myurus* possesses antibacterial properties against *Klebsiella aerogenes* and *Klebsiella pneumoniae* (Kumar and Chaudhary 2010). *Klebsiella aerogenes* is a gram-negative bacterium generally found in the human gastrointestinal system. It can become a problem due to specific antibiotic treatment, and then it becomes resistant to standard antibiotics. This moss has an interesting practical aspect: it is an outstanding producer of hydrogen, with a short doubling time that allows it to consume various sugars. Unlike the cultivation of strict anaerobes, no special work is needed to remove oxygen from the fermenter. This suggests an alternative method of producing hydrogen, the fossil-free fuel of the future.

Ethanol and methanol extracts of *Entodon nepalensis* were tested against three bacteria: *Escherichia coli*, *Salmonella typhimurium*, and *Bacillus subtilis*. The extracts showed significant zones of inhibition against the former two species. *Bacillus subtilis* showed very low inhibition, even lower than the water extracts of the other two (Alam et al. 2012, "Antibacterial Activity").

Entodon luridus syn. *E. okamurae* was examined for its compounds by Zhang et al. (2003). The species synonym is named in honor of Shûtai Okamura (1877–1947), a Japanese bryologist noted for his identification of over 80 species. The moss compounds found in the study are dryocrassol, chrysophanol, physcion, 10-nonacosamnol, n-hexadecanol, phthalic acid isodibutyl ester, curcumol, β-sitosterol, daucosterol, and entokamurol. Four of them possess significant anticancer activity. Chrysophanol in particular is widely studied and shows anticancer, hepatoprotective, neuroprotective, anti-inflammatory, anti-ulcer, and antimicrobial properties. Over 700 abstracts on this compound are listed in PubMed. Chrysophanol has been trialed in vitro against various cancers, including oral squamous, colorectal, lymphoblastic leukemia, lung, and glioma. Standard chemotherapy drugs such as the chemical compound cisplatin are nephrotoxic. Work by Ma et al. (2021) suggests chrysophanol may inhibit and suppress acute kidney injury when administered pre-treatment.

Physcion, another compound isolated in this moss, induces pro-apoptotic effects on cervical cancer cell lines (Trybus et al. 2021). There are numerous other studies on its health benefits.

Curcumol, also found in this moss, reduces oxidative stress and inhibits cancer, microbial infections, neurodegeneration, and inflammation. It induces apoptosis in numerous cancer cell lines (Wei et al. 2019). Endometriosis is a debilitating and increasingly common disease. Curcumol inhibits the proliferation of ectopic endometrial stromal cells, promotes cell apoptosis, and weakens cell migration. It reduces expression of bcl-2-like protein 4 and caspase-3 protein and increases expression of Bcl2 (Wang, Nie et al. 2022), thus attenuating endometriosis.

Another compound found in this moss, daucosterol, induces autophagic-dependent apoptosis in prostate cancer via JNK activation (Gao et al. 2019).

Cucumber-scented moss, the visceral common name of *Entodon plicatus*, is easy to identify olfactorily, as the common name suggests. This moss's extracts inhibit *Bacillus cereus* but exhibit weaker activity against *Bacillus subtilis* (Singh et al. 2016).

Entodon flavescens syn. *E. rubicundus* ethanol extracts were tested on five gram-positive and six gram-negative bacteria, and eight fungi. Activity of seven out of fifteen mosses studied, including this one, was found against all nineteen species in a study by Singh et al. (2007).

Shiny sexy moss or seductive entodon moss, a few of the alluring common names of *Entodon seductrix*, is native to North America. These names sound much more interesting than some of the other common names: round-stemmed entodon moss, toothpick moss, and cord glade moss. *Entodon seductrix* gets superbly shiny according to Martin (2015): "As if coated in a metallic paint, it

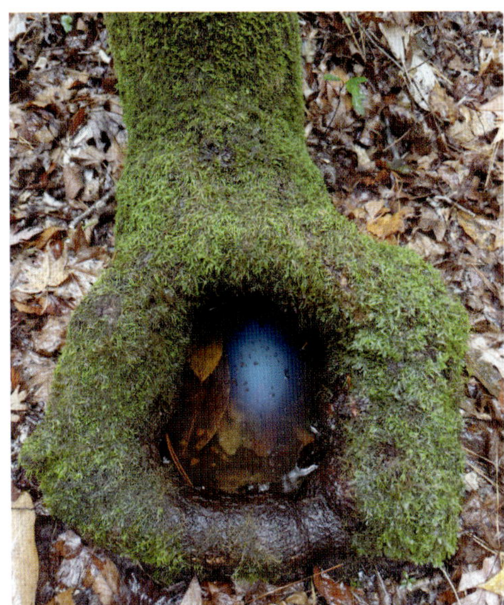

Entodon seductrix (Seductive Entodon Moss)
Photo by Alan Rockefeller

shimmers with an iridescent quality, whether green, golden or brownish." I can find no specific medicinal properties, but in time someone will produce a moss essence that invokes support for issues around human gender, sexuality, and binary patterns.

EUCLADIUM

Whorled Tufa Moss

The genus name derives from the Greek *eu*, "good" or "well," and *klados*, "branch," alluding to the well-developed whorls of the stem leaves.

Whorled tufa moss (*Eucladium verticillatum*) is generally found on rocks around water springs. It contains diphenylamine, used in agriculture as a fungicide and livestock dewormer. This compound's presence in the anti-inflammatory drugs diclofenac and tolfenamic acid (both NSAIDS) may present cytotoxicity. In a 2019 study it was found that diphenylamine derivatives selectively kill leukemic cells over normal cells by arresting the cells in the G_1 phase of the cell cycle (Janovec et al.). Human leukemic (L1210) cells were more sensitive to the inhibitory action of diphenylamine than embryonic kidney (HEK293T) cells.

EURHYNCHIUM

Blunt-Leaved Beaked Moss   Striated Feather Mosses

The genus name *Eurhynchium* derives from the Greek *eu*, meaning "well" or "good," and *rhynchion*, "beak," alluding to the long beak of the operculum (Dixon 1954). Hence one of the common names, beaked moss.

The related mosses, blunt-leaved beak moss, *Eurhynchium angustirete*, and common striated feather moss, *Eurhynchium striatum*, were distilled and examined for their antimicrobial activity by Tosun et al. (2015). The main compound in the former is eicosane (28.6%), and in the latter, 3-octanone (48.1%). Essential oils from both species showed antitubercular activity against *Mycobacterium smegmatis*, a nonpathogenic species used as a model for researching tuberculosis. Eicosane shows both in vitro and in vivo anti-biofilm activity against *Candida albicans*. A reduction in the biomass and thickness of the biofilm, as well as significant reduction in adhesion and colonization of yeast cells, was noted (Shafreen et al. 2022).

Eurhynchium angustirete essential oil was investigated by Yücel and Erata (2021). It contains the chemical constituents trans-pinocarveol (23%)

and myrtenal (14.1%), which inhibits *Escherichia coli*, *Staphylococcus aureus*, *Enterococcus faecalis*, *Pseudomonas aeruginosa*, and *Streptococcus mutans*.

The related elegant feather moss, *Eurhynchium pulchellum*, was distilled as an essential oil by Kahriman et al. (2009). The main constituent is n-nonanal (36.2%). Another study by Özdemir et al. (2009) found minor constituents include decane (8.1%), n-decanal (4.6%), α-muurolene (4.9%), n-undecanal (5.1%), n-pentadecanal (12%), and hexahydrofarnesyl acetone (10%). Alpha-muurolene exhibits antifungal activity against *Cladosporium cucumerinum*, which is especially problematic for producers of cucumbers grown organically in greenhouses.

EXSERTOTHECA

Exsertotheca genus, in the Neckeraceae family, contains just three species.

Early inhabitants of what is now Switzerland used *Exsertotheca crispa* syn. *Neckera crispa* for upper body clothing, leggings, aprons, twisted thongs, and hair decorations (Oschner 1975).

Crisped neckera moss (*Exsertotheca crispa* syn. *Neckera crispa*) shows antifungal activity against *Trichoderma viride*, *Penicillium ochrachloron*, *P. funiculosum*, and *Aspergillus flavus* (Bukvicki, Veljic et al. 2012). It also exhibits significant inhibition of *Staphylococcus aureus*, *Micrococcus flavus*, *Bacillus cereus*, *Escherichia coli*, and *Salmonella typhimurium*. As a sidenote, *Penicillium funiculosum* has been cultured from the rinds of Marzolino, an Italian fresh pecorina cheese.

FISSIDENS

Fern Mosses
Flat Fork Moss
Great Yew Moss
Phoenix Moss
Plume Moss
Pocket Mosses

Geographic Range: North and South America, Europe, Asia

Habitat: damp soil; shady spots near fast-running brooks or waterfalls

Practical Uses: aquariums, hair tonic

Medicinal Applications: antibacterial, antifungal, antidiabetic, antioxidant, bladder issues, digestion, diuretic, dysentery, galactagogue, hair growth, jaundice, leukorrhea, malaria, mouth ulcers, pulmonary tuberculosis, vulnerary

Fissidens is derived from the Latin *fissus*, meaning "split," and *dens*, "tooth," alluding to the split peristome teeth. There are 478 accepted species worldwide, many of them tropical and subtropical species. They are commonly referred to as fern mosses.

Maidenhair pocket moss, *Fissidens adianthoides*, is found in North and South America, Europe, Asia, and elsewhere. It enjoys shady spots near running water and is often found on damp soil, hence the other common names: marsh fern moss, great yew moss, and plume moss. Common names given by early Anglo-Saxons describe its soft, pubic hairlike nature. The Nitinaht of Vancouver Island use it to staunch bleeding wounds. In China and India it is used to improve hair growth and is considered an effective diuretic.

Fissidens bryoides shows antifungal activity against the pathogen *Agrobacterium tumefaciens* (Deora and Bhati 2007), which causes crown gall in members of the rose family, including apples, pears, cherries, and raspberries.

Asakawa (2015) identified compounds in the moss that may help promote hair growth.

In the Southern Hemisphere, *Fissidens crispulus* was collected and studied for volatile compounds (Koid et al. 2022). The essential oil contains pentanoic acid; 2,2,4-trimethyl-3-carboxyisopropyl; isobutyl ester (16.9%); tetradecamethyl-cyclohjeptasiloxane (15.7%); naphthalene (13.2%); 1-tetracedene (11.5%); limonene (10.3%); and minor amounts of methyl salicylate, decanal, tetradecane, 1-hexanol, and 2-ethyl.

Large-leafed pocket moss, *Fissidens grandifrons*, is the largest of the family

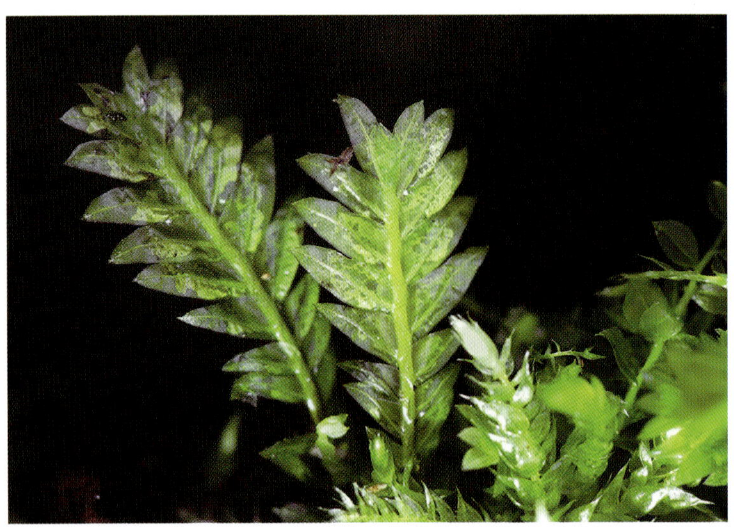

Fissidens adianthoides (Maidenhair Pocket Moss)

Fissidentaceae. It grows submerged in waterfalls and fast-running brooks. It is hepaprotective in ethanol-intoxicated rats (Meka et al. 2022). This species is not to be confused with *Fissidens grandifolia*, which possesses antioxidant and antidiabetic activity (Hieu et al. 2020).

Fissidens crenulatus was used traditionally in India for bladder issues, pulmonary tuberculosis, dysentery, and as galactagogue (increasing breast milk production). TCM uses *Fissidens nobilis* mosses to stimulate hair growth and the decoction of the cooled tea as a diuretic (Harris 2008). *Fissidens nobilis* is traditionally used for jaundice as well (Asakawa 2015).

Plume moss, pocket moss, or flat fork moss (*Fissidens dubius*) has each new leaf fitting into the pocket on the base of a previous leaf unlike other moss genera. This helps conserve water accumulation.

Fissidens flaccidus is traditionally used in India for mouth ulcers, leukorrhea, malaria, and flatulence in cattle.

Fissidens pellucidus syn. *F. flexinervis* is used by the Chácabo of Bolivia for digestive problems (Boom et al. 1996).

Fissidens laxitextus is used to heal skin burns and is noted for its diuretic activity and the treatment of jaundice in the eastern Himalayas (Alam et al. 2015). In India, *Fissidens nobilis* is used for hair growth; the dried moss is burned and then rubbed into the scalp.

Phoenix moss, *Fissidens nobilis*, has been used traditionally as a diuretic and health-restoring tonic; it is also used for infections and externally for swellings, and as a hair treatment (Azuelo et al. 2011). Due to its bright green color this aquatic species is prized for freshwater aquariums.

In China and Bolivia, *Fissidens* species, possibly purple-stalked pocket moss, *Fissidens osmundoides*, is used as an antibacterial gargle for sore and swollen throat (Glime 2017).

FLATBERGIUM

Silky Flatbergium

Flatbergium sericeum syn. *Sphagnum sericeum* has been used to treat eye disease (Azuelo et al. 2011; Chandra et al. 2017). It was originally described as a *Sphagnum* species, but further genetic work gave it a new designation.

Flatbergium sericeum is used in Traditional Chinese Medicine and in the Philippines for acne, insect bites, scabies, acne, hemorrhoids, and eye disease (Ding 1982).

FONTINALIS

Brook Mosses Fireproof Spring Moss Watermosses

Geographic Range: North and South Americas, Iceland, Eurasia

Habitat: attached to submerged rocks and logs

Practical Uses: aquariums, bryoremediation

Medicinal Applications: antianxiety, antibacterial, antidepressant, antidiabetic, antioxidant, antiparasitic, antiplatelet, antipyretic, detoxification, hypotensive

The genus name *Fontinalis* is derived from the Latin for "belonging to springs or water" (Dixon 1954). There are 17 accepted species. The Nlaka'pamux of British Columbia, formerly known as the Thompson River Salish, know it as *n/q*^{w}*zem=étk*^{w}*u* "water moss." In other parts of the world, *Fontinalis dalecarlica* is called common watermoss or brook moss, while *Fontinalis hypnoides* is feather-branched watermoss. Brook mosses, a general term for *Fontinalis* species, are common. This moss stabilizes weirs in streams and is sold as a freshwater aquarium plant.

Fontanilis species hyperaccumulate cadmium and absorb up to 43% of phenols in a water environment. It is a bioaccumulator of uranium and iron as well and is used as a bioindicator of excessive ethylene glycol in water, hence

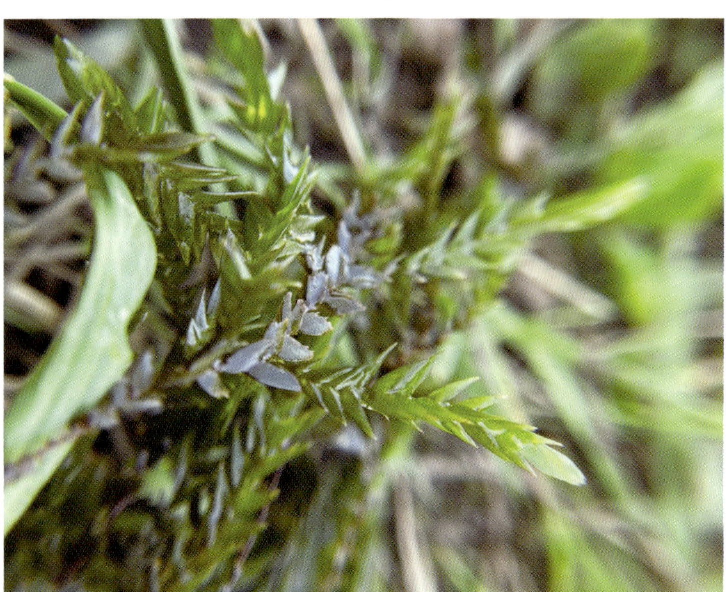

Fontinalis antipyretica (Fireproof Spring Moss) Photo by Graham Steinruck

generally speaking, *Fontinalis* species are good monitors of water pollution.

Fireproof spring moss, *Fontinalis antipyretica*, was given its curious species name by Linnaeus based on its ability to reduce fever (maybe). Some authors suggest the name was derived from its use as chimney insulation (probably not a good idea) or to plug empty spaces between bricks in walls (a better idea). TCM uses this moss for its antipyretic properties (Wu and Jia 2003; Harris 2008). It was traditionally boiled with beer and used as a footbath to relieve chest fever, microbial infections, and to detoxify (Drobnik and Stebel 2021). *Fontinalis antipyretica* methanol extracts show activity against the fungi *Aspergillus niger, A. flavus, A. fumigatus, Trichoderma viride, Penicillium funiculosum*, and *P. ochrochloron* (Veljic et al. 2009). Methanol extracts showed the strongest activity against the bacteria *Escherichia coli, Salmonella enteritidis, Shigella epidermidis, Bacillus subtilis*, and *Micrococcus flavus*.

Work by Savaroglu, Iscen et al. (2011) found organic solvent extracts of *Fontinalis antipyretica* inhibit the fungi *Aspergillus parasiticus* and *A. fumigatus*. The former pathogen causes aspergillus ear rot in corn crops and in agricultural storage facilities. It is also one of the major causes of human hepatocellular carcinoma in developing countries. Aflatoxin B_1, produced by *Aspergillus parasiticus* and *A. fumigatus*, is classified as a group 1 human carcinogen by the International Agency for Research on Cancer and is a common contaminant in many foods.

Alpine watermoss, *Fontinalis squamosa*, unlike most liverworts and other mosses, contains nitrogen metabolites, fontinalin, and two harmane alkaloids, harmane and harmaline, which possess a wide range of activities, including antianxiety, antidepressant, antiplatelet, antidiabetic, acetylcholinesterase and myeloperoxidase inhibition, antioxidant, antiparasitic, and hypotensive. Harmine and harmaline compounds also alleviate morphine withdrawal syndrome (Alijanpour et al. 2021).

Harmine and harmaline are β-carbonlines with selective and reversible inhibition of monoamine oxidase (MAO-A), an enzyme encoded in the MAOA gene that has been associated with a variety of psychiatric disorders, including antisocial behavior. Ayahuasca, the well-known entheogenic combination of two plants from South America, is based on a plant rich in DMT combined with an MAO inhibitor. This prevents degradation in the stomach, allowing the herbs to influence the brain. I spent time in Peru (1982–83) and was introduced to the ayahuasca herbal combination as well as to the mescaline-rich San Pedro cacti by several curanderos.

FUNARIA

Bonfire Moss
Charcoal Peddler
Cinderella Moss
Cord Mosses
Fire Moss
Golden Bulbed Moss
Predictor Moss
Water-Measuring Cord Moss

Geographic Range: worldwide from arctic to tropical regions

Habitat: common in disturbed areas

Practical Uses: gardens, removing lead from water, teaching life cycle of mosses in schools

Medicinal Applications: alopecia, antibacterial, anticancer, antifungal, anti-inflammatory, antiparasitic, antipyretic, bronchitis, bruises, cardiovascular, expectorant, hematemesis (vomiting of blood), hemostasis, jaundice, pneumonia, tuberculosis

The genus name *Funaria* is derived from the Latin *funis*, "rope," and *aris*, "resembling." This is in reference to the seta of *Funaria hygrometrica*, which twists in a spiral when the moss is old or dry (Dixon 1954).

Bonfire moss or common cord moss (*Funaria hygrometrica*) is found almost everywhere and has been used worldwide as a folk remedy for external use for wounds and skin problems, and internally for hypertension and other cardiovascular concerns. Like *Bryum argenteum*, it is frequently classified as a weed moss. It is fond of old campfire sites or forests that have burned, when the nutrients become available. It's a short-lived moss, living only two to three years, before it is replaced with herbaceous plants, then shrubs, and finally trees.

Being that it is so widely known, this moss has acquired numerous common names: charcoal peddler, Cinderella moss, golden bulbed moss, twisted-cord moss, fire moss, predictor moss, and water-measuring cord moss, to name a few. "Twisted cord refers to the setae (stem of the sporophyte) of older mosses, which are contorted and twisted together. Martin (2015) notes it must be tolerant of large doses of fertilizer, as it is commonly used on the soil of potted plants in greenhouses.

In Traditional Chinese Medicine, *Funaria hygrometrica* is used for hemostasis, pulmonary tuberculosis, hematemesis (vomiting of blood), bruises, and athlete's foot and other fungal infections (Asakawa 2015). In the western

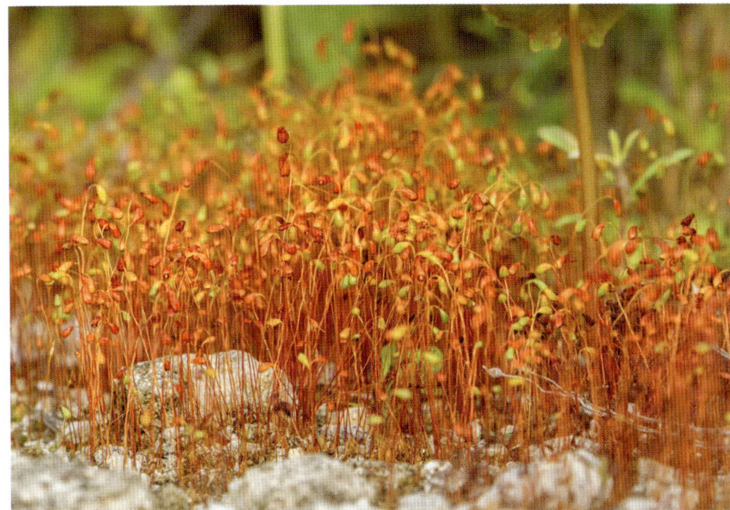

Funaria hygrometrica (Bonfire Moss)

Himalayas it is used for pulmonary tuberculosis, jaundice, hematemesis, and nosebleeds (Alam et al. 2015). Other ethnobryology uses include alopecia (hair loss), bronchitis, pneumonia, morning vomiting of excess mucus, and fever.

Moss extracts of *Funaria hygrometrica* inhibit *Bacillus subtilis*, *Pseudomonas aeruginosa*, *Staphylococcus aureus*, and *Escherichia fergusonii* (Savaroglu, Ilhan et al. 2011). The latter bacterium, named for William W. Ferguson, an American microbiologist, is closely related to its more famous cousin *Escherichia coli*. Some strains that infect open wounds can caused bacteraemia or urinary tract infections. These bacteria are highly resistant to ampicillin, and in some cases, gentamicin and chloroamphenicol as well.

Funaria hygrometrica is anti-inflammatory and relieves pain. Work by Asif et al. (2023) identified numerous constituents, including chitobiose, chlorovulone III, gamma-tocotrienol, emmotin, cassine, hexacosanedioic acid, neophytadiene, fumaric acid, neophytadiene, hexadecenoic acid, phytol, and stigmasterol. The closely related chlorovulone II exhibits cytotoxicity against human prostate (PC-3) and human colon (HT20) cancer cell lines (Shen et al. 2004). Chitobiose is an effective antioxidant, but it also promotes growth of the spirochete *Borrelia burgdorferi*, associated with Lyme disease. A chloroform extract of the moss was tested in vivo and found to exhibit central analgesic activity and anti-inflammatory relief in a rat paw study. Acute inflammatory mediators such as TNF-α, IL-6, and IL-4 were reduced, and IL-10 was upregulated in a treated group, compared to a control group.

In a study on the flowering plant *Senna racemosa*, cassine, also found in

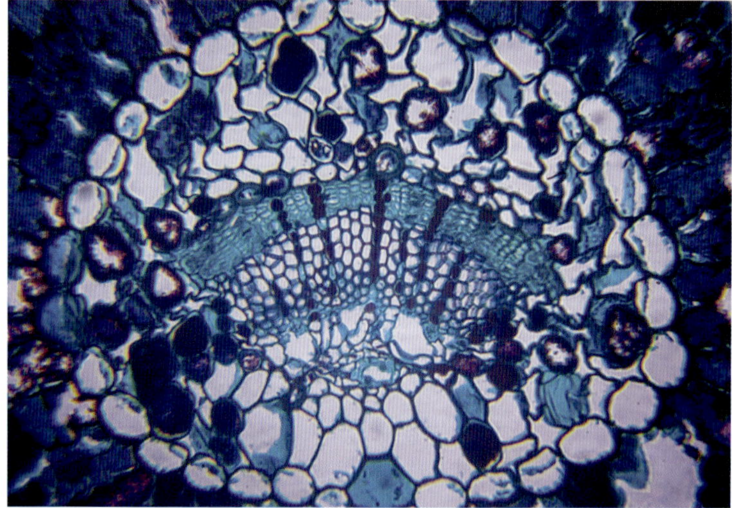

Funaria microstoma (Small Cord Moss) under a microscope

Funaria hygrometrica, shows activity against *Staphylococcus aureus*, *Bacillus subtilis*, and *Candida albicans* (Sansores-Peraza et al. 2000). Cassine also shows activity against *Giardia intestinalis*, a protozoal pathogen (Moo-Puc et al. 2007). Also known as beaver fever, giardia causes diarrhea and is the fifth most common source of intestinal distress in Canada.

Work by Vollár et al. (2018) found various solvent and water extracts of *Funaria hygrometrica* exhibit cytotoxicity against epithelial/cervical (HeLa), ovarian (T47D), and breast (A2780) cancer cell lines.

GAROVAGLIA

Garovaglia genus mosses have been placed in the Ptychomniaceae family. The genus name honors Santo Garovaglio (1805–1885), a professor of botany in Lombardy, Italy, who was instrumental in establishing the Laboratorio di Botanica Crittogamica at the University of Pavia.

Garovaglia elegans volatiles were collected by headspace (a technique for sampling and examining the volatiles associated with a solid or liquid sample); they include 1-tetradecene, 2-ethyl-1-hexanol, decanal, pentanoic acid, 2,2,4-trimethyl-3-carboxyisopropyl, isobutyl ester, limonene, and naphthalene (Koid et al. 2022).

GEMMABRYUM

Bicolored Bryum
Crowned Thread Moss
Handbell Moss
Tufted Bryum Moss

Gemma is derived from Latin meaning "gem," or "jewel." Crowned thread moss (*Gemmabryum coronatum* syn. *Bryum coronatum*) contains secondary metabolites with anti-inflammatory activity (Ayinke et al. 2015). Ethanol extracts show relatively low activity against four bacteria (Tedela et al. 2014).

GRIMMIA

Blunt-Beak Moss
Grey Cushion Moss
Hoary Tile Moss
Montana Grimmia
Ostrich Moss
Pulvinate Dry Rock Moss
Scarce Hedgehog Moss
Toothless Grimmia Moss

The genus name honors Johann Friedrich Carl Grimm (1737–1821), a German botanist and physician who became the personal physician to the duke of Saxe-Gotha-Alternburg and was commissioned to study diseases prevalent in Ronneburg, a town noted for its mineral springs. He translated and published four volumes of the medical works of Hippocrates. Grimm corresponded with Linnaeus and was bestowed the genus name by his contemporary, German botanist Jakob Friedrich Ehrhart, who originally identified and named the moss.

The *Grimmia* genus, found worldwide, is very difficult to identify as to species. In fact, Geneva Sayre (1911–1992), an American bryologist worked on a North American monograph for many years and noted, "It contains an ambigua, a varia, a decipiens, a controversa, a revisa, and at least two anomalas." Now that over 800 species have been recorded over time, this logjam is slowly being resolved. The number of accepted species is now closer to 108.

Species of *Grimmia* are used in China for unspecified (at least unknown to me) medical purposes.

Grimmia alpestris and nine other mosses out of twenty-three exhibited good antimicrobial activity against *Paenibacillus* larvae isolates that cause American foulbrood diseases in honeybee larvae (Sevim et al. 2017). The other mosses showing antibacterial activity are *Polytrichum formosum*, *Polytrichum commune*, *Calliergonella cuspidata*, *C. lindbergi*, *Metzgeria conjugata*, *Isothecium alopecuroides*, *Syntrichia calcicola*, *S. intermedia*, and *Tortella densa*.

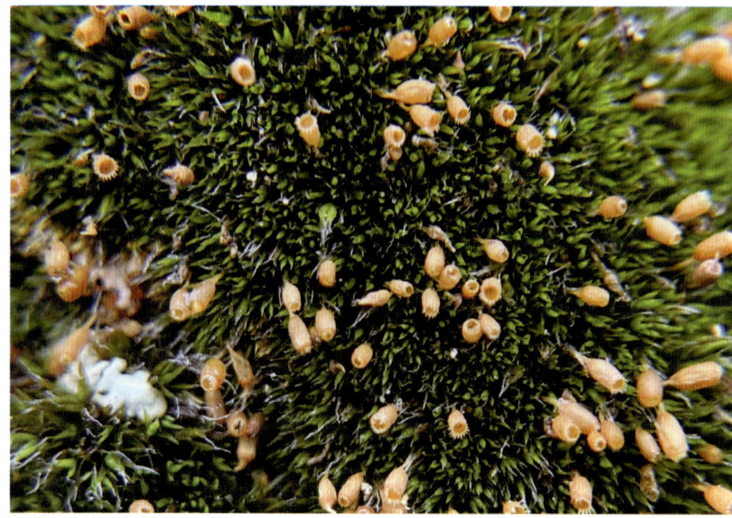

Grimmia sp.
Photo by
Graham Steinruck

Toothless grimmia moss, or scarce hedgehog moss, *Grimmia anodon*, is resistant to drought and found in Southern Alberta, southern British Columbia; and across the Western United States. It is rare and endangered in Great Britain, usually growing on rocks. Solvent extracts were found to inhibit *Bacillus subtilis*, *B. cereus*, *Salmonella* sp., *Staphylococcus aureus*, *Pseudomonas aeruginosa*, and *Escherichia coli* (Elibol et al. 2011).

Montana grimmia, *Grimmia montana*, contains 54 genera of bacterial endophytes. Their benefit to the host, or to medical research, is yet to be determined (Liu et al. 2014).

Grey cushion moss, blunt-beak moss, or pulvinate dry rock moss (*Grimmia pulvinata* syn. *Dryptodon pulvinatus*) is found on stones and walls in temperate climates worldwide. Other common names are ostrich moss and hoary tile moss. It has been used for biomonitoring of airborne metals in cemeteries near Paris and Lyon, France. In Paris, some moss contained up to 84% antimony (but mostly 20% to 60%), while in Lyon, 5% vanadium was noted (Leguy et al. 2022).

Grimmia pulvinata syn. *Dryptodon pulvinatus* exhibits significant antioxidant, antibacterial, and cytotoxic activity (Wolski et al. 2021). At higher concentrations the extracts exert the strongest negative effect on mouse fibroblast cell line L929 associated with the development of novel anticancer treatments. Also, a 2017 study by Karpinski and Adamczak found significant inhibition of *Streptococcus pyogenes*, *Staphylococcus aureus*, *Escherichia coli*, *Enterococcus faecalis*, and *Klebsiella pneumoniae*.

HAMATOCAULIS

Slender Green Feather Moss Varnished Hook Moss

Like all mammals, including humans, mosses are territorial. They like to maintain and spread their sphere of influence and repel competitive mosses. Slender green feather moss, or varnished hook moss (*Hamatocaulis vernicosus* syn. *Drepanocladus vernicosus*) is a great example.

Vicherová et al. (2020) investigated the reaction of *Hamatocaulis vernicosus* to volatile organic compounds of its common competitor, *Sphagnum flexuosum*. When exposed, the shoots of *Hamatocaulis vernicosus* elongated and emitted six times higher amounts of a stress-signaling compound related to β-cyclocitral. Notably, an analog of β-cyclocitral and curcumin shows strong cytotoxic activity and apoptosis in hepatic (HCC, HepG2, and Huh-7) cancer cell lines. Moreover, a beneficial combination with sorafenib, a kidney, liver, and thyroid cancer drug, significantly increased synergistic cytotoxicity in hepatic cells (Han et al. 2023).

A phenethyl alcohol core substituted with a β-cyclocitral derivative exhibited activity against *Mycobacterium smegmatis*. Work by Crusco et al. (2019) revealed β-cyclocitral significantly impacts amino acid, nitrogen, nucleotides, and the folate-dependent one-carbon metabolism of the mycobacterium.

HAPLOCLADIUM

Five-Pointed Leaf Little Feather Moss Tiny-Leaved Haplocladium Moss

Similar to many other mosses, this moss employs a strategy to abate drought stress.

Five-pointed leaf little feather moss (*Haplocladium microphyllum* subsp. *capillatum*) is traditionally used to treat pneumonia, tonsilitis, and fever (Ding 1982; Chandra 2017).

In TCM the moss is known as *jian ye xiao yu xian*. As a cool, bitter, pungent moss it helps remove toxic heat from the lungs, kidneys, bladder, and breasts. Urethritis, cystitis, mastitis, bronchitis, and other inflamed organ systems are treated. It has also been successful in cases of tinnitus.

In the Himalayas tiny-leaved hypocladium, *Haplocladium microphyllum*, is used to treat bronchitis (Kumar et al. 2007), as well as tonsillitis and pneumonia (Chandra et al. 2017).

Haplocladium microphyllum syn. *H. capillatum* has been traditionally used in parts of India for tonsillitis, bronchitis, tympanitis (eardrum) and inner ear infections and inflammation, as well as erysipelas (a bacterial infection of the skin), mammary gland infections, postpartum infections, and cystitis (Chandra et al. 2017; Ding 1982; Pant 1998).

HAPLODONTIUM

One of the rarest mosses in the entire Northern Hemisphere is found in two locales in western Alberta, Canada. *Haplodontium macrocarpum* syn. *Mielichhoferia macrocarpa* is found on wet, seeping, calcareous formations at the back of waterfalls.

Natalie Cleavitt, a PhD student at the University of Alberta, drew attention to it in the late 1990s when a mine was planning a road that would have wiped out this rare population. With only ten localities in the entire world, the fight for retaining biodiversity came front and center. Dr. René Belland, a moss expert from the University of Alberta who is also associated with the University of Alberta Gardens near Edmonton, found a small cluster of these rare mosses in the summer of 2007 near Jasper. René and I worked together for a short time on an Alberta Native Plant Adopt-a-Plant Alberta initiative for which I was hired as a volunteer coordinator in 2006.

HEDWIGIA

Dreadlock Moss
Hedwig's Fringe Leaf Moss
Hoarmosses
Medussa Moss
Old Rock Moss
Tiger Tail Moss
White-Tipped Moss

Geographic Range: worldwide

Habitat: temperate forest floors

Practical Uses: landscapes, moss gardening, green walls, gravel paths

Medicinal Applications: antibacterial, anticancer, antidiabetic, anti-neuroinflammatory

The genus is named in honor of German botanist Johannes (or Johann) Hedwig (1730–1799), considered by many to be the father of bryology. He was born in Brasov, Transylvania, the son of a shoemaker. He became fascinated with mosses at an early age and received his medical degree from the University of Leipzig in

1759. The next twenty years saw him practice as a physician. He published his first work, the two-volume *Fundamentum historiae naturalis muscorum frondosorum*, in 1782. His main work, *Species Muscorum frondosorum*, was published a few years after his death. The peer-reviewed journal *Nova Hedwigia* is named in his honor. The Hedwig Medal is today given by the International Association of Bryologists to scientists for their contributions to bryology. Hedwig, incidently, is also the name of the owl in the Harry Potter books. Twelve accepted species.

White-tipped moss, ciliate hoarmoss, fringed hoarmoss, dusky hoarmoss, Medussa moss, dreadlock moss, tiger tail moss, old rock moss, and Hedwig's fringe leaf moss are some of the common names of *Hedwigia ciliata*. It is commonly found on temperate forest floors. Seven flavonoids were isolated from this and four other moss species (Basile et al. 1999). The flavonoids are apigenin, apigenin-7-0-triglycoside, lucenin-2, luteolin-7-0-neohesperidoside-4'-O-sophoroside, saponarine, vitex, and the biflavonoid bartramiaflavone. Some flavonoids show significant inhibition of *Enterobacter cloacae*, *E. aerogenes*, and *Pseudomonas aeruginosa*, all gram-negative bacteria. Lucenin-2 and bartramiaflavone inhibit *Pseudomonas aeruginosa*.

Luteolin 4'-neohesperidoside (L4N) inhibits four antibiotic-resistant bacteria, including MRSA, *Klebsiella pneumoniae*, the fosA-positive shiga toxin producing the *Escherichia coli* serogroup (STEC 0111), and *Bacillus cereus*. Significant synergistic activity was noted in cases of use with gentamycin against gram-negative bacteria. *Bacillus cereus*, for example, was highly inhibited by a combination of vancomycin with L4N, despite the pathogen

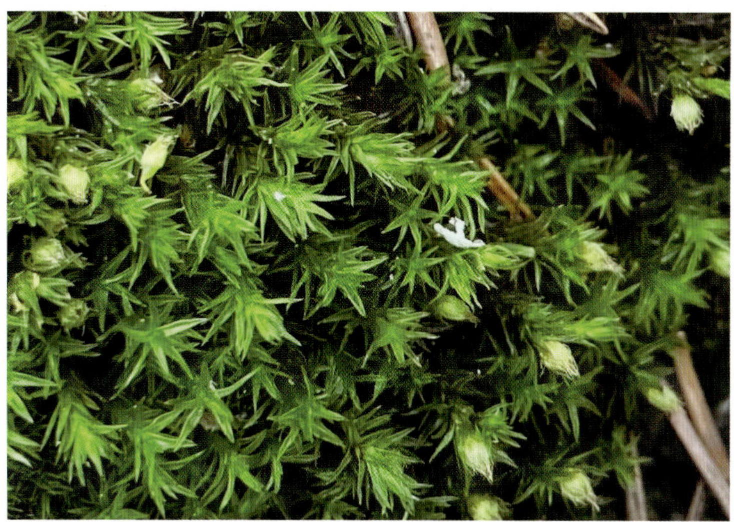

Hedwigia ciliata (White-tipped Moss)
Photo by Graham Steinruck

being vancomycin-resistant. In vivo evaluation showed significant decrease in *Klebsiella pneumoniae* and STEC shedding and colonizing. Renal and pulmonary lesions in lab animals were remarkably reduced, with significant decreases in bacteria-infected tissue (El-Shiekh et al. 2023).

Their study suggests L4N as a potential substitute for or perhaps an adjunctive with (author observation) traditional antibiotics. A 96% ethanol extract of *Hedwigia ciliata* yielded more than 50% antiproliferative activity against the human breast adenocarcinoma (MDA-MB-230) cell line. It also exhibited significant anti-neuroinflammatory activity, significantly reducing nitric oxide production. Acetylcholinesterase inhibition was 60% for acetyl acetate extracts and 80% for tyrosinase based on a 70% ethanol extract. The extracts also exhibit significant antidiabetic effects by mediating α-glucosidase inhibition (80% for ethyl acetate) (Mandic et al. 2021).

HOMALIA

Blunt Feather Moss

The genus name *Homalia* is derived from the Greek *homalos*, meaning "flattened," "even," or "level," from the appearance of the expanded or complanate leaves (Dixon 1954).

The original name of this genus, *Omalia*, which lacked the aspirated *H*, was coined by Swiss-German bryologist Samuel Elisée Bridel-Brideri (1761–1828) and was later corrected by German bryologist Wilhelm Schimper (1804–1878).

Blunt feather moss (*Homalia trichomanoides*) contains 3-β-methoxyserrat-14-en-21β-op, atranorin, methyl 2,4-dihydroxy-3,6-dimethylbenzoate, and trichomanin. Work by Wang, Yu et al. (2005) found that three of these compounds are active against *Candida albicans*.

HOMALOTHECIUM

Nuttall's Homalothecium Moss Smoky Feather Moss Silky Wall Feather Moss

The essential oil of smoky feather moss, *Homalothecium lutescens*, contains nonanal (36.8%) and tricosane (6.5%) (Ücüncü et al. 2010). Extracts are used in Turkey as insecticidal agents against the wheat weevil (*Sitophilus granarius*). Work by Vollár et al. (2018) found various solvent and water extracts exhibit cytotoxicity against epithelial/cervical (HeLa), ovarian (T47D) and breast

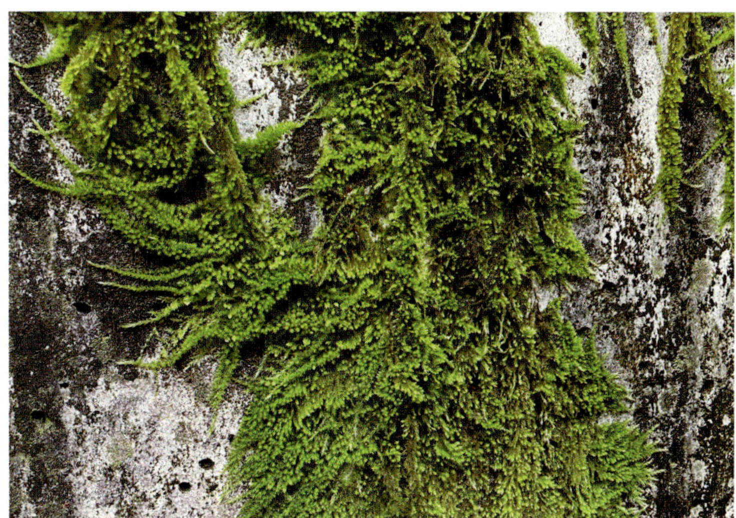

Homalothecium nuttallii (Nuttall's Homalothecium Moss)
Photo by Graham Steinruck

(A2780) cancer cell lines. Methanol extracts exhibited no cytotoxicity. *Homalothecium philippeanum* was tested in the same study. All extracts showed cytotoxicity against all cancer cell lines, except for water extracts, which only inhibited breast cancer cell lines.

Silky wall feather moss, *Homalothecium sericeum*, is found in North America and elsewhere. Özerkan et al. (2022) evaluated ethyl extracts of this and four other mosses on 5-fluorouracil-resistant colorectal cancer lines (HCT116 and HT29). All bryophytes tested exhibit cytotoxicity.

In England this moss was traditionally used to treat whooping cough (Belcher and Swale 1998).

Various extracts of *Homalothecium sericeum* were tested for antibacterial and antiproliferative activity by Oztopcu-Vatan et al. (2011). Acetone extracts exhibit inhibition of *Pseudomonas aeruginosa* and antiproliferative activity against rat glioma (C6) cancer cell line.

Work by Colak et al. (2011) found methanol extracts of *Homalothecium sericeum* inhibit *Bacillus subtilis*, *B. cereus*, *Saccharomyces cerevisiae*, *Pseudomonas aeruginosa*, and *Escherichiacoli*. Ethanol extracts of the moss were combined with ruthenium nanoparticles and tested against human colon (HCT116) cancer cell lines. Cell death of this cancer line was induced, as was the death of multidrug resistant protein ABCG2, suggesting its use in multidrug-resistant pharmacology (Samir et al. 2023).

Unspecified *Homalothecium* syn. *Camptothecium* species inhibit the polio virus (Witthauer et al. 1976).

HYDROGONIUM

Joint-Toothed Moss

The genus name may derive from the Greek *hydro*, meaning "water," and either *gonia*, "angle," or *gonos* or *gono*, "seed." Not sure. Many species reproduce asexually by gemmae on stalks in leaf axils. There are 16 accepted species.

Hydrogonium arcuatum syn. *H. gracilentum* syn. *H. gangeticum* inhibits methicillin-resistant *Staphylococcus aureus* (MRSA) and *Escherichia coli* (Kandpal et al 2016). Ethanol extracts exhibit significant activity against the gram-negative bacteria *Dickeya dadantii*, a soft rot pathogenic bacterium that affects potato and other crops, and acetone extracts were effective against *Pseudomonas aeruginosa*, a gram-negative bacterium that can affect plants and animals, including humans.

There is another side to *Dickeya dadantii*, however. The enzyme asparaginase derived from this bacterium shows significant glutaminase activity, depleting glutamine. This is a useful strategy in patients suffering acute lymphoblastic leukemia, acute myeloid leukemia, and lymphoblastic lymphoma (Emadi et al. 2018; Gao et al. 2022).

Water and ethanol extracts of *Hydrogonium arcuatum* syn. *Barbula gracilenta* syn. *Hydrogonium gracilentum*, were found to inhibit methicillin-resistant *Staphylococcus aureus* (MRSA) (Kandpal et al. 2016). The moss is known as *you-ye shi-hui xian* in TCM.

Ethanol extracts of *Hydrogonium javanicum* syn. *Barbula javanica* and *Barbula arcuata*, *Hydrogonium arcuatum syn. Barbula arcuata* were among 7 out of 15 mosses tested on five gram-positive and six gram-negative bacteria and eight fungi.

Earlier work by Gupta and Singh (1971) found *Hydrogonium* (then named *Barbula*) species inhibited some bacteria by up to 36%. Work by Vollár et al. (2018) found various solvent and water extracts exhibit cytotoxicity against epithelial/cervical (HeLa), ovarian (T47D); and breast cancer (A2780) cell lines. The extracts were found to be active against all 19 bacteria species (Singh et al. 2007).

HYGROAMBLYSTEGIUM

Feather Mosses Swamp Feather Moss

Fountain feather moss or swamp feather moss, *Hygroamblystegium tenax*, is easily identified and common—it has a very sharp, pointed leaf.

Work by Vollár et al. (2018) found various solvent and water extracts exhibit cytotoxicity against epithelial/cervical (HeLa) and ovarian (T47D) cancer cell lines.

HYLOCOMIADELPHUS

Big Shaggy Moss

Big Shaggy Moss is a large terrestrial pale green to golden-brown moss, and easy to identify. It prefers sheltered, north-facing grassy slopes and open woodland.

Big shaggy moss, *Hylocomiadelphus triquetrus* syn. *Rhytidiadelphus triquetrus*, is a northern moss that also goes by the name rough gooseneck moss and the cartoonish name electrified cat's tail moss. The Nlaka'pamux of British Columbia know this moss as *tek q^w^ zém*, meaning "short moss" (Turner et al. 1990). The eastern Iroquois (Haudenosaunee Confederacy) use the moss externally to treat pain (Herrick 1995).

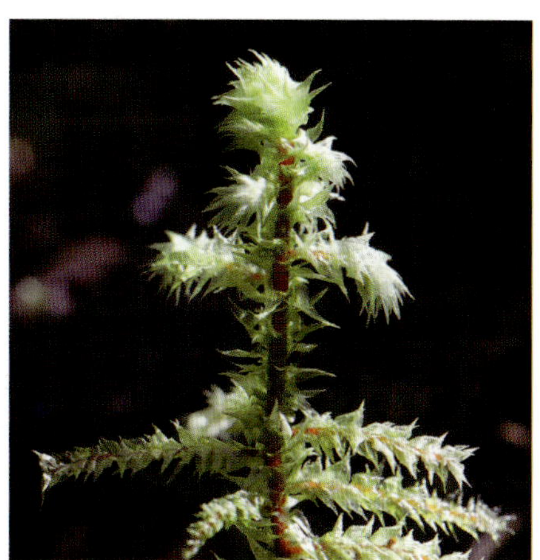

Hylocomiadelphus triquetrus (Big Shaggy Moss)

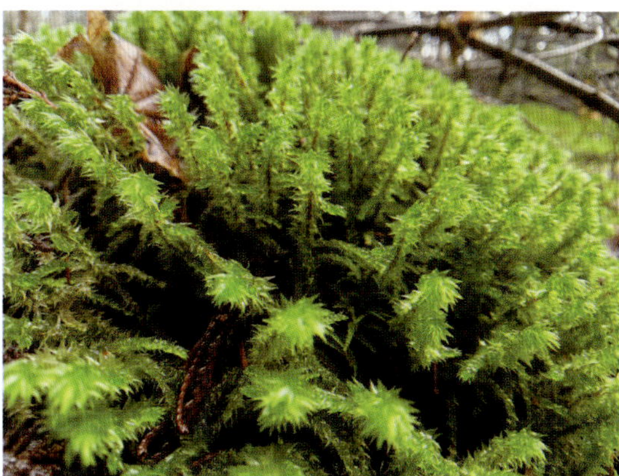

Hylocomiadelphus triquetrus (Big Shaggy Moss)
Photo by Drew T. Henderson

Hylocomiadelphus triquetrus contains palmitic, 4-hydroxy benzoic, salicylic, gallic, caffeic, and gensitic acid (Yaghuglu et al. 2017). Most importantly, various extracts showed significant antiproliferative activity against cervical (HeLa) and rat glioma (C6) cancer cell lines.

GOOSENECK MOSS ESSENCE

This essence, also called frightened cattail moss essence, from *Hylocomiadelphus triquetrus* syn. *Rhytidiadelphus triquetrus*, is a restorer. It clears deep blocks and trauma not known on the surface. It restores at the core and cellular level, bringing deep shifting and new freedom. It can create profound changes within a person.* This description is from Canadian Forest Essences.

HYLOCOMIUM

Glittering Wood Moss
Mountain Fern Moss
Splendid Feather Moss
Stair-Step Moss

Geographic Range: Europe, North America, Asia

Habitat: moist coniferous forest settings

Practical Uses: insulation, bryoremediation

Medicinal Applications: antibacterial, anticancer, antifungal, anti-inflammatory, vulnerary

The genus name may derive from the Greek *hylokomos*, meaning "a lover of moisture" or "forest dweller," alluding to the habitat of the two *Hylocomium* species (Dixon 1954).

Splendid feather moss, glittering wood moss, or stair-step moss (*Hylocomium splendens*), a northern moss, is also known as splendid feather moss, stair-step moss, and mountain fern moss. It is found in coniferous forests with poor soil, often growing with *Pleurozium schreberi*, red-stemmed feather moss. It is probably the most common moss of the boreal forests and is often used to insulate log cabins in the north. The common name stair-step moss comes from the stair-step annual growth pattern that is easy to recognize.

*This product is no longer commercially available.

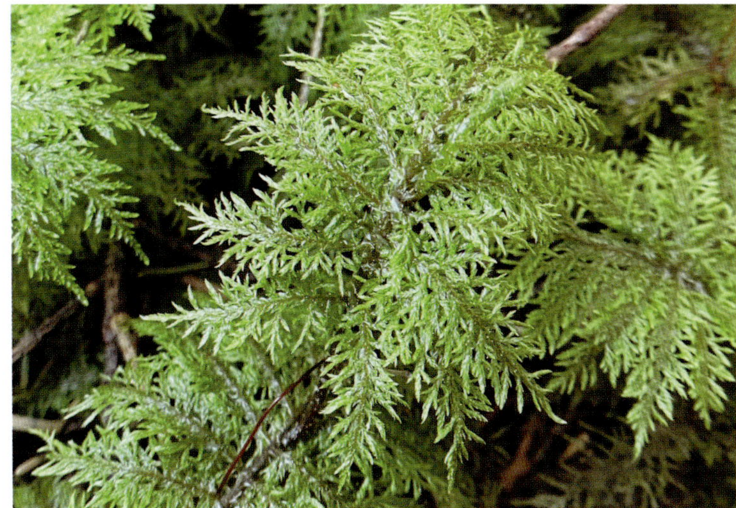

Hylocomium splendens (Splendid Feather Moss)
Photo by Drew T. Henderson

The Nlaka'pamux in British Columbia know this moss as */qʷ zém*, meaning "long moss." One resident mentioned it is steeped in hot water, "as hot as you can stand it," and when cool it is used as a vulnerary, specifically as a poultice on sores (Turner et al. 1990). The Wsánec, on the Saanich peninsula of Vancouver Island, know all mosses as *keji*. They used them for bedding, floors, and cleaning fish (Turner and Hebda 2012).

In northern climates this moss has been used as wall insulation and as seals around doors and windows. When I built a log cabin in the mid-1970s, I used this moss and *Pleurozium schreberi* as chinking between the logs. This was then slathered over with lime. Both mosses likely secrete species-specific chemo-attractants when limited by nitrogen access. In turn, this guides cyanobacteria to them, by which they gain nitrogen. This signaling is regulated by the nitrogen demands of the moss and serves as a control of nitrogen input in boreal forests (Bay et al. 2013).

Another practical use of this moss is in India, where traditionally, women use it as a cushion to carry water vessels on their heads.

Like many bryophytes, this moss accumulates fatty acids to maintain cell fluidity in a harsh environment. It accumulates long-chain polyunsaturated fatty acids (l-PUFAs) such as arachidonic acid (AA) and eicosapentaenoic acid (EPA), which help keep cell fluidity in cold or freezing temperatures. Work by Lu et al. (2023) examined the lipid composition of 39 species in Iceland and found the AA and EPA of six mosses, including *Hylocomium splendens*, were abundantly distributed in the phospholipids (mainly PC and PE) and glycerolipids (MGDG and DGDG). This moss accumulates high concentrations of PUFA-containing triacylglycerols. Ethanol extracts contain 7,8-dihydroxy-5-methoxycoumarin-7-β sophoroside; 3-methoxy-4-hydroxybenzoic; and abscisic, atraric, and sphagnic acids.

As a result of its absorptive capabilities this moss is commonly used in bryometers, which are really just bags of mosses hung to monitor pollution. Most species, including this one, are injured in 10 to 40 hours by 0.8 ppm of sulfur dioxide. I wonder how well a bryometer would do downwind of one of the oil sands projects in Northern Alberta? Probably no better than the lichen project initiated some 40 years ago, where they all died. I've written about this in my *Medicinal Lichens: Traditional Knowledge and Modern Pharmacology* (2025). Due to its water absorption rate of 55%, this moss is bagged to assess heavy metal concentrations in Finland. Studies have found that *Hylocomium splendens* possesses significant murine lymphatic leukemia (P-388) cytotoxicity (Kimb et al. 2007).

Kang et al. (2007) found that an 80% methanol extract shows significant activity against gram-positive bacteria, while ethyl acetate fractions show even stronger activity. The research team found this and the other mosses studied, *Bartramia pomiformis*, *Ceratodon purpureus*, and *Neckera douglasii*, to all be active against *Staphylococcus* species when exposed to UVA irradiation.

Hylocomium splendens is also antifungal; in a 2005 study it was shown to inhibit *Botrytis cinerea* and *Alternaria solani* (Mekuria et al. 2005).

This moss is still used today in Italy as a poultice for skin sores (dei Cas et al. 2015).

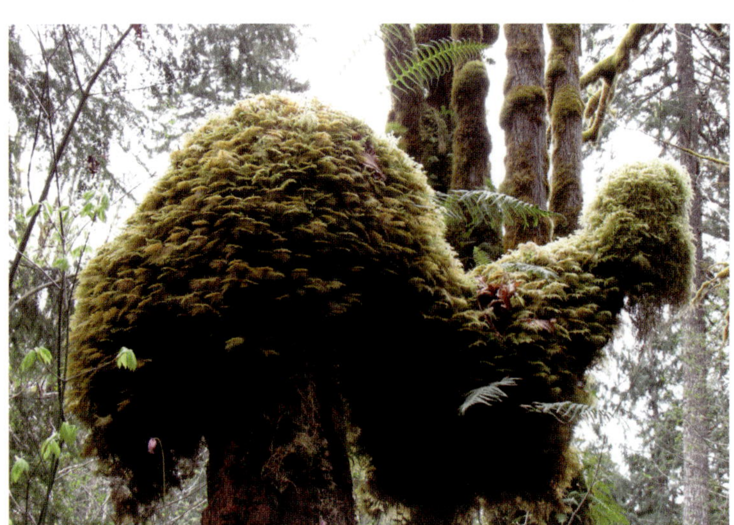

Hylocomium splendens (Stair-Step Moss)
Photo by Drew T. Henderson

The essential oil derived from *Hylocomium splendens* contains 58 compounds rich in β-pinene (11.6%) and α-pinene (8.9%). The oil shows activity against the bacteria *Escherichia coli*, *Staphylococcus aureus*, *Enterococcus faecalis*, *Bacillus cereus*, *Mycobacterium smegmatis*, as well as the fungi *Candida albicans* and *Yersinia pseudotuberculosis* (Cansu et al. 2013).

Yersinia pseudotuberculosis in particular can move from the small intestine through Peyer's patches (an important part of gut-associated lymphoid tissue usually found in humans in the lowest portion of the small intestine) and lymphatic vessels to infect the mesenteric lymph nodes. The result is mesenteric lymphadenitis, a swelling of the lymph nodes in the mesentery that can present in the formation of pyogranulomas, painful nodules that frequently present in dogs. The gram-negative bacteria can spread through the food chain.

Yersinia pseudotuberculosis is relatively rare in humans, but it can present as strawberry tongue. It is called Izumi fever in Japan and is known elsewhere as Far East scarlet-like fever. These infections are more common in Europe than in Asia, and when they do occur in humans they are found more frequently in children rather than adults. Infections can mimic appendicitis and can result in *Erythema nodosum*, an inflammatory condition presenting as reddish-blue bumps on the shins, thighs, arms, and elsewhere. It is remotely related to *Yersinia pestis*, the bacteria that caused the Great Plague (Black Death) of 1665–66. Spread by fleas and rodents, it is rare but still appears occasionally in North America.

GOLDEN FOREST MOSS ESSENCE

Golden forest moss essence, from *Hylocomium* species, anchors cosmic light into the eighth layer of DNA. It creates a powerful, magical linkage and connection with the Sacred Altars of the Infinite and the places of true emotional well-being.

First Light Flower Essence of New Zealand produces No. 168, Golden Forest Moss.

HYMENOSTYLIUM

Hook Beak Tufa Moss

Hook beak tufa moss, the descriptive common name of *Hymenostylium recurvirostrum*, favors magnesite-rich soil. In Cornwall, England, it is found on former tin and copper mine sites. Magnesium carbonate (magnesite) is a mineral supplement sometimes suggested for stomach hyperacidity; it is found in the antacid drug Gaviscon and other over-the-counter medications. In clinical practice I found that over 80% of clients taking Tums, Rolaids, and other proton pump inhibitors suffered from low stomach acid. The consequences of incomplete protein digestion and lack of mineral uptake are profound.

Homeopathy

The related magnesia carbonica (carbonate of magnesia) remedy relieves gastrointestinal catarrh. It is frequently indicated in children when the whole body smells sour and is disposed to boils. It also is indicated in women who suffer from a sore throat before menses or who later in life suffer from uterine and menopause-related disorders. Patients easily startle, with diminished hearing and a tearing pain in shoulders as if dislocated. Symptoms are worse from warmth of bed or changes of temperature, better from warm air and walking outdoors in open air.

The recommended dose is 3C to 30C potency.*

HYOPHILA

Feather Moss
Ground Mosses
Log Moss
Pott Moss
Rain Moss
Rolled-Leaf Wet Ground Moss
Water Moss

The genus name derives from the Greek *hyo*, "water" or "rain," and *philia*, "fondness" or "loving," alluding to its love of being close to or in water. Common names for the genus reflect these characteristics: water moss, rain moss, Pott moss (Pottiaceae), and wet ground moss. There are about 85 species.

In India, *Hyophila involuta* syn. *H. attenuata* is traditionally used as a tea for coughs and colds (Lubaina et al. 2014). It is combined with a pinch of black pepper for these complaints as well as for neck pain. The leaf juice is used to treat earache, fungal infections of the skin, neurasthenia, and to increase sexual potency.

Rolled-leaf wet ground moss (*Hyophila involuta*) is found on wet rocks alongside streams. It has been used traditionally for symptoms associated with colds, coughs, and sore throat. The leaf decoction, along with a pinch of black pepper, is taken daily (Chandra et al. 2017; Harris 2008).

*Case study by William Boericke M.D. in the 9th ed. Pocket Manual of *Homeopathic Materia Medica & Repertory* (1927)

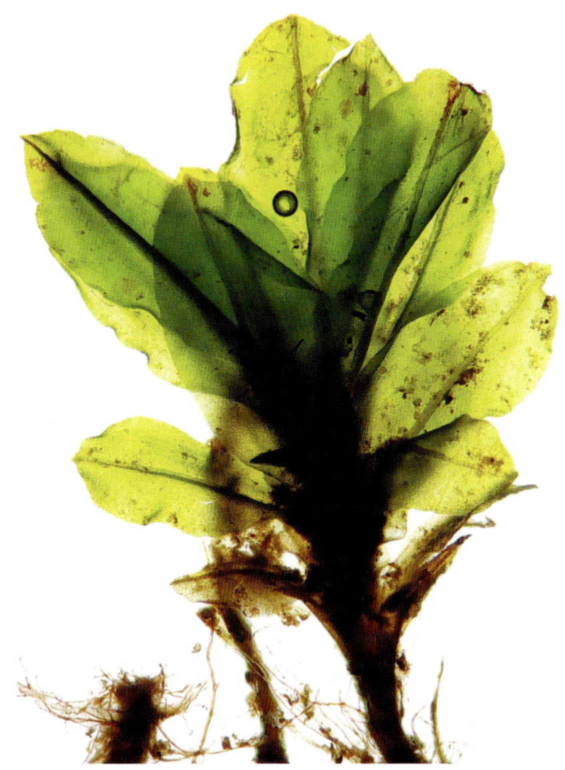

Hyophila involuta (Rolled Leaf Wet Ground Moss)

This moss shows promise as an antifungal. Work by Subhisha and Subranomiam (2007) tested in vitro and in vivo activity against *Aspergillus niger*, *A. fumigatus*, and *Candida albicans*. The alcohol extract exhibited the most significant inhibition, and *A. fumigatus* was the most sensitive fungus. An active chloroform fraction from the alcohol extract protected all the immune-suppressed mice, while all untreated mice died. The fraction did not show any short-term toxicity.

Both acetone and ethanol extracts contain cardiac glycosides (Makinde et al. 2015). Work by this research team found the extract active against *Staphylococcus aureus* and *Aspergillus niger*.

A study by Singh et al. (2016) found methanol extracts inhibit various gram-positive *Bacillus* spp. more strongly than gram-negative *Escherichia coli*.

Hyophila spathulata ethanol and methanol extracts show significant antifungal activity against *Aspergillus niger*, *Fusarium solani*, and *Trichoderma viride*, with better results than the standard antifungal medication Fluconazole (Bishnoi et al. 2015).

HYPNUM

Coiled-Leaf Claw Moss
Cypress-Leaved Plait-Moss
Feather Moss
Green-Leaved Plant Moss
Natural Sheet Moss
Pillow Moss
Rose Moss

Geographic Range: worldwide

Habitat: moist shady environments on tree trunks; rotting logs; aquatic environments

Practical Uses: bryoremediation, herbicide, moss gardens, pillows

Medicinal Applications: antibacterial, anticancer, antifungal, antimicrobial, antioxidant, antiviral, diabetes, heavy metal chelation, neuroprotective

There are about 80 *Hypnum* species found around the world. The genus name may derive from the Greek *hypnon*, meaning "moss" or referring to some other cryptogamic plant (Dixon 1954). Or it may derive from the Greek *hypnos*, meaning "sleep," as in hypnotize, referring to its use as a filler for pillows, hence one of the common names, pillow moss. Such pillows, being insect-repellant and rot-resistant, not only make for excellent bedding material, but they also supposedly induce a special trancelike sleep. In traditional India, this moss, as well as *Hylocomium* and *Trachypodopsis* species, are stuffed into cloth sacks to make the *sirona*, a head cushion used when hauling water (Pant and Tewari 1989). Another prosaic use of this moss is in France, where it is used in window displays, particularly in nativity scenes. Various species are commonly used in moss gardens today.

Cypress-leaved plait moss, or feather moss, (*Hypnum cupressiforme*) is a common ground covering in much of western Alberta, from north to south. Extracts have been reported to possess antimicrobial and antiviral activity.

In nineteenth-century Europe, *Hypnum cupressiforme* was used to treat pertussis (whooping cough); recent studies in Korea indicate that aromadendrin-derived flavonoids may play a role (Lee et al. 2024).

Studies by Bargagli et al. (2020) have shown *Hypnum cupressiforme* to be a most efficient accumulator of trace elements. It accumulates up to three times concentrations of zinc, copper, and cadmium. This makes it an excellent determinant of heavy metal contamination from power plants, refineries, and chemical processors (Nordström 2019). Mosses in general, and feather moss in particular, are quite suitable as bryo-monitors.

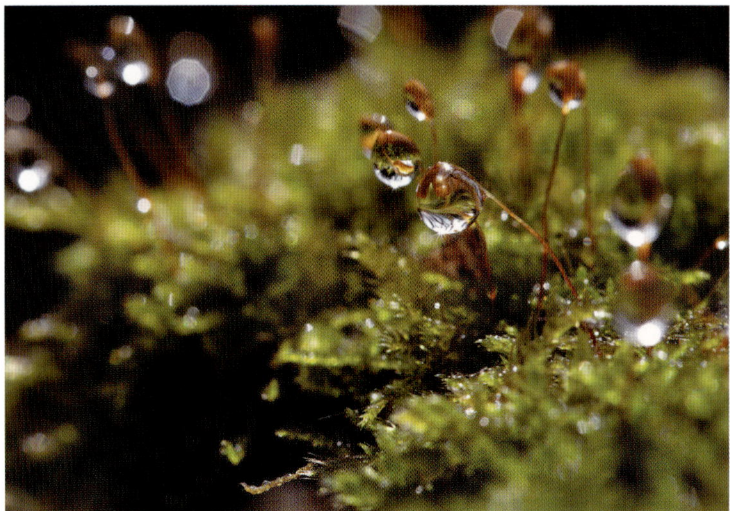

Hypnum cupressiforme (Cypress-Leaved Plait Moss)

This moss possesses antioxidant, antibacterial, and antifungal activities. Methanol extracts exhibit activity against the fungi *Aspergillus niger, A. flavus, A. fumigatus, Trichoderma viride, Penicillium funiculosum, and P. ochrochloron* (Veljic et al. 2009). Bacteria tested include *Escherichia coli, Salmonella enteritidis, Shigella epidermidis, Bacillus subtilis*, and *Micrococcus flavus*. In addition, water extracts show activity against *Candida albicans* and *Saccharomyces cerevisiae*. *Penicillium ochrochloron* is responsible for a green mold disease on some medicinal herb crops. On the other hand, it contains chitinase, which inhibits the growth of the cotton bollworm, *Helicoverpa armigera* (Patil and Jadhav 2015).

Savaroglu, Ilhan et al. (2011) found extracts inhibit *Bacillus subtilis, Pseudomonas aeruginos*a, and *Staphylococcus aureus*.

Work by Colak et al. (2011) found methanol extracts inhibit the bacteria *Bacillus cereus* and *Salmonella* species, and the fungus *Saccharomyces cerevisiae*. Chloroform extracts inhibit *Bacillus cereus, B. subtilis, Salmonella* sp., *S. cerevisiae*, and *Pseudomonas aeruginosa*.

The secondary metabolites inhibit inflammatory, oxidative, and acetylcholinesterase, suggesting neuroprotective potential. Moss harvested in summer contains the highest level of metabolites (Lunic et al. 2022). An earlier study (Lunic et al. 2020) found that the main compounds are kaempferol, p-hydroxybenzoic, protocatechuic, p-coumaric, gallic and caffeic acids; as well as numerous flavonoids, including hypnogenol B1, hypnum bioflavonoid A, hypnum acid methyl ether, and hyaluronic acid. Significant antiproliferative activity was found against breast cancer (MDA-MB-231) cell lines.

Hypnum cupressiforme inhibits acute lymphoblastic leukemia (CCRF/CEM) cancer cell lines (Huneck 1983).

Work by Kirisanth et al. (2020) looked at six different air-dried bryophytes, including *Hypnum cupressiforme,* which were cold-extracted with three different organic solvents. They were then screened against three bacterial and one fungal strain. Six of 18 extracts expressed activity against gram-positive bacteria, and two extracts against the fungal strain. Ethyl acetate extracts showed α-amylase inhibition in half of the mosses, ranging from 8% to 30%.

The essential oil of *Hypnum cupressiforme* was analyzed by (Ücüncü et al. 2010). It was found to be rich in nonterpenoid components as aldehydes, and in terpenoid components as sesquiterpene hydrocarbons. A maximum essential oil concentration of *Hypnum cupressiforme* was then tested for antimicrobial activity against the bacteria *Escherichia coli, Yersinia pseudotuberculosis, Pseudomonas aeruginosa, Staphylococcus aureus, Enterococcus faecalis,* and *Bacillus cereus,* and the fungi *Candida albicans* and *Saccharomyces cerevisiae.* The results show antimicrobial activity only against the fungi.

Natural sheet moss (*Hypnum imponens*) also goes by the names feather moss and log moss. Extracts were found to inhibit *Bacillus subtilis, Pseudomonas aeruginosa,* and *Staphylococcus aureus* (Savaroglu, Ilhan et al. 2011).

Momilactones may be useful for crop-friendly herbicides as well as for antifungal and antibacterial agents; some possess cytotoxicity against various cancer cell lines as well (Zhao et al. 2018). Momilactone B inhibits ketosis in vitro. A primary target for treating the metabolic state of ketosis, an abnormal increase of ketones in the body, is angiopoietin-like-3, which modulates lipoprotein metabolism by inhibiting the lipoprotein lipase that breaks down stored fat to produce triglycerides (Kang et al. 2017). Ketogenic diets encourage the body to burn fat as fuel.

Momilactone B also causes cell arrest and apoptosis in human monocytic leukemia (U937) cancer cell lines (Park et al. 2014) and induces apoptosis on human lymphoma T cells (Lee, Chung et al. 2008). In addition, the compound exhibits cytotoxicity against human colon (HT-29 and SW620) cancer cell lines (Kim et al. 2007). Work by Joung et al. (2008) found that momilactone B accelerates hypoxia-induced chemoprevention, that is, it acts therapeutically against human breast cancer cell lines via apoptosis. Moreover, momilactones A and B are cytotoxic in promyelocytic leukemia (HL-60) and multiple myeloma cancer cell lines. The compounds negligibly affect the noncancerous cell line MeT-5A, often used as a control cell line in various scientific investigations

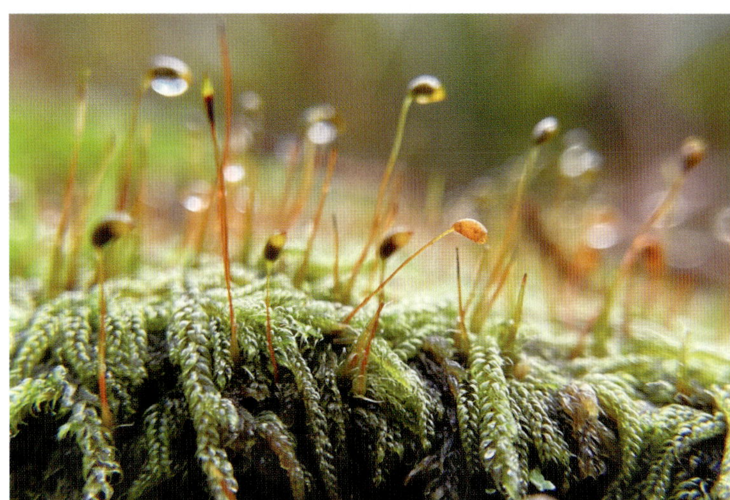

Hypnum cirinale (Coiled-Leaf Claw Moss)
Photo by Graham Steinruck

(Anh et al. 2022). Both compounds exhibit potent inhibitory effect on pancreatic α-amylase, α-glucosidase, and trypsin, suggesting beneficial outcomes for diabetes in terms of blood sugar dysregulation (Quan et al. 2019).

The presence of the compound acrenol in this moss suggests cytotoxicity against the human ovary (A2780) cancer cell line as well as against phytopathogenic fungi, as revealed in a 2005 study about lianas, woody vines that populate tropical rain forests, which also contain this compound (Adou et al. 2005).

The fungal endophyte *Xylaria* sp. was isolated from a *Hypnum* moss species by Wei et al. (2015). Xylaguaianols A–D (oxygenated guaiane-type sesquiterpenes), iso-cadinane-type sesquiterpene isocadinanol A, and an α-pyrone 9-hydroxyxyarone, along with five known sesquiterpenes and four known cytochalasins, were isolated from a culture broth. Cytochalasin D showed significant cytotoxicity against all five cancer cell lines tested. Cytochalasins C and Q exhibited moderate, but selective cytotoxicity. In another study (Huang et al. 2012), cytochalasin D was found to inhibit colorectal (CT26) tumor cell proliferation and induce apoptosis and suppression of angiogenesis. I could go on, as there are over 5,000 citations for this compound in PubMed.

IMBRIBRYUM

Thread Moss

The genus name *Imbribryum* derives from the Greek *imbrex*, meaning "roof tile," and *bryon*, "moss," alluding to the plant's overlapping leaves.

Imbribryum species inhibit the bacterium *Pseudomonas aeruginosa* (Lashin et al. 2015; Abdel-Shafi et al. 2017). A mixture of a methanol extract of the moss and tetracycline showed a synergistic effect. A scanning electron microscope allowed for observation, and it indicated a sheath surrounded the bacteria, with signs of an irregular wrinkled outer surface, adhesion, and aggregation of damaged cells.

ISOPTERYGIUM

Isopterygium Moss

The genus name is derived from the Greek *isos*, meaning "equal," and *pteron*, "wing," alluding to the complanate leaves. There are about 170 species worldwide.

The Chácobo of Bolivia use *Isopterygium tenerum* externally for rheumatic pain (Boom 1996).

ISOTHECIUM

Lesser Striated Feather Moss   Mousetail Mosses

In Greek, *iso* means "equal," and *thecium* derives from *thecio*, meaning "sack," "container," or "capsule," referring to a vessel that holds spores.

Large mousetail moss (*Isothecium alopecuroides*) is antibacterial, with activity against *Bacillus subtilis*, *Candida albicans*, *Escherichia coli*, *Listeria monocytogenes*, *Salmonella enteritidis*, *Shigella flexneri*, *Staphylococcus aureus*,

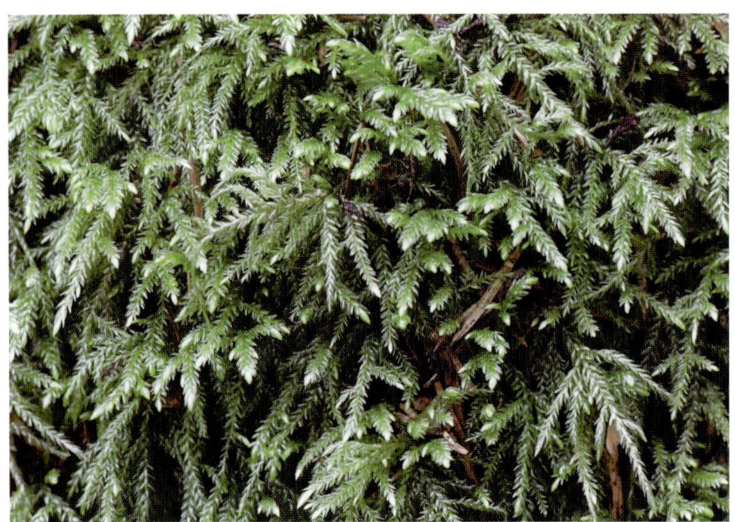

Isothecium alopecuroides (Large Mousetail Moss)

and *Yersinia enterocolitica* (Altuner and Cetin 2018). The latter bacteria cause acute bowel disease, reactive arthritis, erythema nodosum (an inflammatory condition causing painful lumps on legs, arms, and elsewhere), and uveitis (a form of eye inflammation). Research suggests it may also play a role in Crohn's disease (Fang et al. 2023).

In a 2017 study, large mousetail moss and nine other mosses were found to exhibit antimicrobial activity against *Paenibacillus* larvae isolates that cause American foulbrood diseases in honeybee larvae (Sevim et al. 2017). The other mosses that showed benefit were *Polytrichum formosum* and *P. commune*, *Calliergonella cuspidata*, *C. lindbergi*, *Metzgeria conjugata*, *Syntrichia calcicola*, *S. montana*, *Tortella densa*, and *Grimmia alpestris*.

The essential oil of *Isothecium alopecuroides* was analyzed by Yücel and Erata (2021), and the main compounds were found to be biformene (9.9%), α-pinene (9.1%), and bornyl acetate (8.4%). The oil is antibacterial and was found to inhibit *Escherichia coli*, *Staphylococcus aureus*, *Enterococcus faecalis*, *Pseudomonas aeruginosa*, and *Streptococcus mutans*.

Yayintas (2019) found that blunt mousetail moss, *Isothecium myurum*, inhibits *Bacillus subtilis* (Yayintas, 2019).

The Asian-Pacific moss *Isothecium subdiversiforme* (the old name for *Isotheciastrum subdiversiforme*) contains maytansinoids 1, 3, and 4, as well as 15-methoxyansamitocin P-3. All these compounds are potent tumor cytotoxins (Sakai et al. 1988).

Another compound found in this moss, trewiasine, is cytotoxic against ascitic tumor 180 (associated with hypercalcemia, when calcium levels in the blood become too high), lymphoma (U937), murine cervical (U14) carcinoma, hepatocellular carcinoma, and Lewis lung carcinoma (Yue et al. 1992). Trewiasine also possesses agricultural benefits as it exhibits significant activity against the European corn borer, *Ostrinia nubilalis*.

KINDBERGIA

Common Feather Moss

The Hesquiat of Vancouver Island used *Kindbergia oregana* syn. *Eurhynchium oreganum* moss for skin wounds and handwashing (Turner and Efrat 1982).

Common feather moss, *Kindbergia praelonga*, contains phenolic acids and derivatives, including 4-O-caffeoylquinic, 5-O-caffeoylquinic, caffeic, p-coumaric, ferulic and ellagic acids, as well as caffeic and p-coumaric

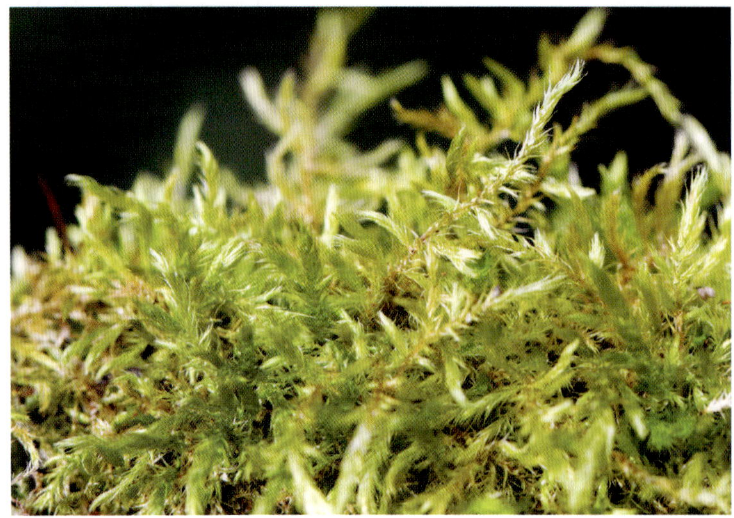

Kindbergia praelonga (Common Feather Moss)

derivatives. It contains three flavonoids: apigenin-7-O-glucoside, luteolin, apigenin, and an unidentified flavanone (Jockovic et al. 2008). According to the authors of the study, many of these compounds have interesting biological activity, including antimicrobial, antifungal, cytotoxic, antitumor, vasopressin antagonist, cardiotonic, tumor effecting, insect antifeedant, insecticidal, molluscicidal, pesticidal, and plant growth regulatory, to name a few.

LEMBOPHYLLUM

Joint-Toothed Moss Feather Moss

The genus name *Lembophyllum* derives from the Greek *lembos*, "skiff," and *phyllon*, "leaf," alluding to this moss's boat-shaped leaves.

Lembophyllum clandestinum is a moss traditionally used in New Zealand as an absorbent diaper or sanitary napkin. It was trialed for venereal disease, but conclusions were doubtful as to its efficacy. Calder et al. (1986) found no antibiotic activity from extracts against *Escherichia coli* or *Staphylococcus aureus*.

LEPTOBRYUM

Golden Thread Moss Long-Necked Bryum

The genus name derives from the Greek *leptos*, meaning "slender," and *bryum*, alluding to the genus *Bryum* and the erect, wide-spreading leaf shape.

Long-necked bryum, *Leptobryum pyriforme*, is found in a variety of habitats, from rotten wood to disturbed sites, even invading greenhouses. The species name *pyriforme* refers to this moss's pear-shaped capsules.

Cell cultures of this moss have shown the ability to synthesize EPA and other fatty acids.

GOLDEN THREAD MOSS ESSENCE

Golden thread moss essence, derived from *Leptobryum pyriforme*, addresses core issues, thereby bringing about freedom and strength to fulfill oneself. It is the anchor to your source; it cuts through fear and illusion and revivifies your deepest goals.* This description is from Canadian Forest Essences.

LEPTODICTYUM

Knapwort   Kneiff's Feather Moss   Streamside Leptodictyum Moss

The Greek *leptos* means "narrow" or "slender," and *diction* means "net," alluding to the areolation of the leaves. There is only one species.

Kneiff's feather moss, knapwort, or streamside leptodictyum moss (*Leptodictyum riparium*) is found worldwide except in the Pacific islands and Australia. It is found in the lakes and rivers of Minnesota and was once found in a Canadian mining lake. It can live in acidic lakes and old volcanic crater lakes with an acidic pH of 1.6.

In the western Himalayan regions of India and in Traditional Chinese Medicine the moss is used for its fever-reducing activity as well as for hepatic (jaundice) and urinary tract issues (Alam et al. 2015). Bile salts in the urine or blood require treatment with this moss (Harris 2008; Pant 1998; Ding 1982).

Extracts from *Leptodictyum riparium* inhibited eight bacteria tested by Castaldo-Cobianchi et al. (1988), including *Pseudomonas aeruginosa*, the bacterium responsible for serious opportunist infections. Acetone extracts were tested on the blood of three human volunteers and results showed that this moss possesses antioxidant activity (Basile et al. 2011).

Leptodictyum spp. contain high levels of phosphates, making this moss suitable for freshwater aquariums.

---

*This product is no longer commercially available.

LEPTODONTIUM

Thin-Teethed Moss

The genus name is derived from the Greek *leptos*, "slender," and *odontos*, "tooth," alluding to the peristome consisting of 32 narrow teeth, hence the common name of the genus, thin-teethed moss. There are 39 species, two in North America.

Valarezo (2018) gathered, steam-distilled, and identified 94 constituents in 6 mosses found in Ecuador. *Leptodontium vitculosoides* contains as its two main components, β-selinene (13.5%) and α-selinene (10.5%).

This moss exhibits antioxidant activity (Téllez-Rocha et al. 2021). It contains phospholipids rich in dicranin (Chowdhuri et al. 2018), an acetylenic fatty acid with anti-fibrotic, anti-inflammatory, and anticancer effects. Platelet aggregation induced by either thrombin or arachidonic acid was inhibited by 10^{-4} M of dicranin (Guichardant et al. 1992).

LEPTOSTOMUM

Pincushion Moss

The Greek *leptos* means "slender" or "delicate," and *stoma* means "mouth," alluding to the appearance of the rudimentary peristome.

Pincushion moss, *Leptostomum inclinans*, is found on tree trunks and sometimes on soil or rocks in Australia and New Zealand. Work by Calder et al. (1986) found ethanol extracts strongly active against *Staphylococcus aureus*.

LESKEA

Many-Fruited Leskea Marsh Feather Moss

Many-fruited leskea or marsh feather moss (*Leskea polycarpa*) is often found alongside streams covered with stream silt but also found in drier areas alongside rural dirt roads. There are about 112 species found worldwide.

Work by Vollár et al. (2018) found various solvent extracts exhibit cytotoxicity against epithelial/cervical (HeLa), ovarian (T47D), and breast (A2780) cancer cell lines.

LEUCOBRYUM

Cloud Moss
Cushion Mosses
Hooked Moss
Pincushion Mosses
White Mosses

Geographic Range: Eastern North America and Europe

Habitat: dry and thin soil or rocks in open upland woodlands; pine bark

Practical Uses: detergents, fabric softener, perfume

Medicinal Applications: antibiotic, anticancer, anticonvulsant, antidepressant, antidiabetic, antihypertensive, anti-inflammatory, antimicrobial, antineurodegenerative, antipsychotic, antitubercular, antiviral, vulnerary

The Greek *leukos* means "white," and bryon "moss," alluding to the white or very pale green color of this moss. Martin (2015) explains: "In this species, hyaline and chlorphyllous cells are interwoven. As top layers dry out, they lose their color. Upon rehydration, *Leucobryum* soaks up water like a sponge." This is one of the few mosses that grow on pine bark. Eighty accepted species.

Leucobryum species are absorptive and antibiotic and have traditionally been used to treat serious wounds (Nordström 2019).

Extracts of hooked moss or spiked white moss (*Leucobryum aduncum*) inhibit the growth of *Staphylococcus aureus* and *Escherichia coli*. The compounds 1-nonadecene, 5-eicosene, and cyclotetracosane were derived from nonpolar extracts (Makajanma et al. 2020). Two of this moss' constituents, 1-nonadecene and cyclotetracosane, also found in an extract of the perennial herb *Wurfbainia villosa* var. *xanthioides*, were found to reduce gastric acid production and exhibit cytotoxicity on human gastric cancer cell lines (Lee et al. 2007).

Bowring's pincushion moss (*Leucobryum bowringii*) exhibits antibacterial activity according to Manoj et al. (2016). Methanol extracts strongly inhibit various pathogens, including *Salmonella typhimurium*, *Staphylococcus aureus*, *Klebsiella pneumoniae*, *Escherichia coli*, *Bacillus cereus*, *B. subtilis*, *Proteus vulgaris*, and *Pseudomonas aeruginosa*. Earlier work by Manoj et al. (2012) found that methanol extracts inhibit growth, migration, and invasion of human breast (MCF-7) cancer cell lines as well.

In parts of India, an external paste is prepared from the leaf tips of *Leucobryum bowringii* in a cup of silver date palm (*Phoenix sylvestris*) to treat

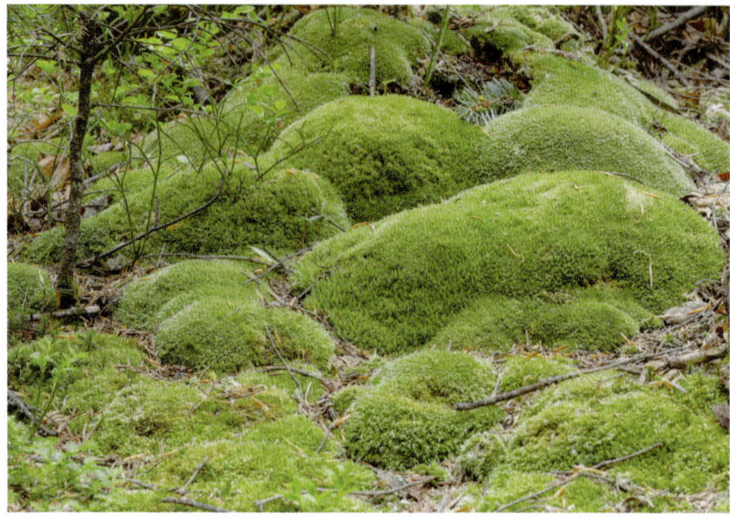

Leucobryum glaucum (Large White Moss)

pain (Lubaina et al. 2014; Chandra et al. 2017). The *yama-goke*, or *araha shiraga-goke*, moss is found at the base of Japanese cedar trees. It is widely used as a base for bonsai trees.

The essential oil from *Leucobryum glaucum*, large white moss contains 47 compounds, the two most plentiful being thujopsadiene (35.5%) and β-curcumene (25.4%), cedrol (7.6%) and isolongifolene (5%) were also isolated (Celik 2020). The oil showed no activity against gram-negative bacteria, however, *Mycobacterium smegmatis* exhibited the largest zone of inhibition.

A 70% ethanol extract of *Leucobryum juniperoideum*, smaller white moss, was given to mice fed a high fat diet by Shin et al. (2016). The research team found that the moss reduces blood serum lipid and insulin and leptin levels. Insulin resistance, or type-2 diabetes, in which insulin continues to be secreted by beta cells in the pancreas, but blood sugar is not efficiently transferred to red blood cells, is a growing concern today. Lowering leptin levels is beneficial, as elevated numbers are related to the accumulation of body fat and weight gain.

Essential oil derived from large white moss, or cloud moss, *Leucobryum martianum*, that was collected in the Brazilian rainforest contains naphthalene (72.51%), phthalic acid derivative (7.09%), hexadecanoic acid (5.08%), and minor amounts of safrole (0.43%), maaliol, and galaxolide (Rezende-Moraes 2023). The latter compound is musky and has been synthesized for perfume, fabric softener, and detergents. It is, however, an androgen disruptor that has a toxic effect on the development of the male reproductive organs (Li, Wang et al. 2023). Naphthalene is cytotoxic and has applications in various anticancer,

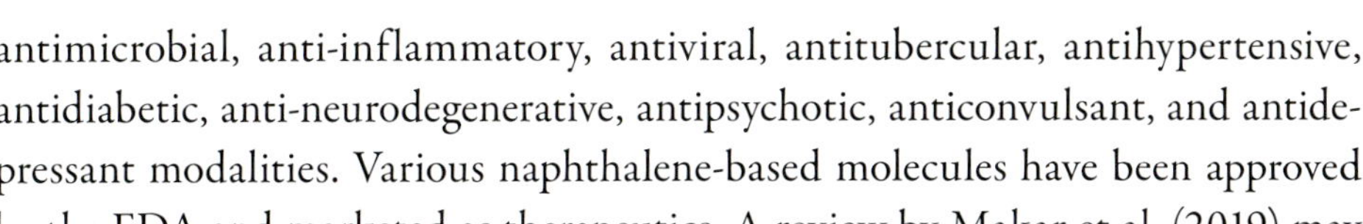

antimicrobial, anti-inflammatory, antiviral, antitubercular, antihypertensive, antidiabetic, anti-neurodegenerative, antipsychotic, anticonvulsant, and antidepressant modalities. Various naphthalene-based molecules have been approved by the FDA and marketed as therapeutics. A review by Makar et al. (2019) may be useful to those interested.

GREEN WOODLAND MOSS ESSENCE

This essence from *Leucobryum* spp. anchors cosmic light into the third layer of DNA. It creates a powerful and magical linkage and connection with the Sacred Altars of the West and the places of true emotional well-being.

It is available through First Light Flower Essence of New Zealand as No. 163, Green Woodland Moss.

LEUCODON

Squirrel-Tail Moss

The genus name derives from the Greek *leukos*, meaning "white," and *odon*, "tooth," referring to the pale peristome teeth. Thirty-eight species worldwide.

Essential oil derived from squirrel-tail moss, *Leucodon sciuroides*, contains nonanal (26.8%) and heptanal (13.7%) (Cansu et al. 2013). The inhibition of *Candida albicans* fungi was noted.

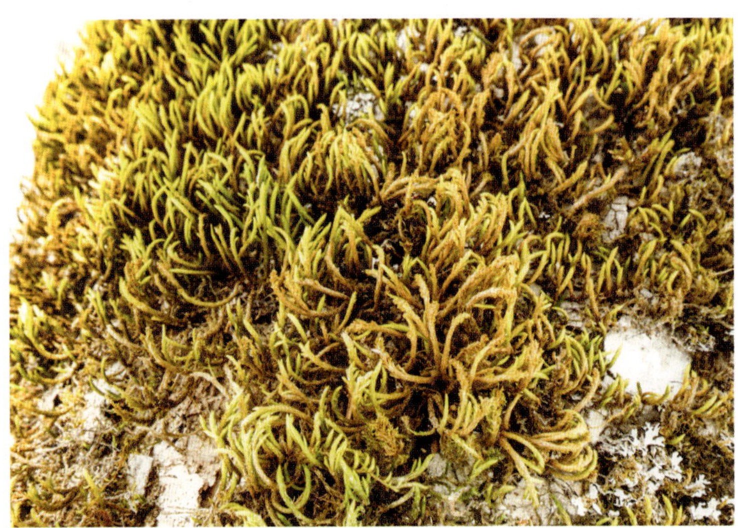

Leucodon sp.

Work by Vollár et al. (2018) found various solvent extracts exhibit cytotoxicity against epithelial/cervical (HeLa), ovarian (T47D), and breast (A2780) cancer cell lines. Water extracts were inactive.

Ethanol extracts were found to inhibit *Salmonella* species, *Candida albicans*, *Staphylococcus aureus*, and *Pseudomonas aeruginosa*, while chloroform extracts inhibited *Escherichia coli* (Colak et al. 2011).

Traditional Chinese Medicine makes use of *Leucodon secundus* mosses to stop bleeding and to relieve pain, as well as to treat headache and stomachache (Zhong Hua Ben Cao 1999; Harris 2008).

LEUCOLEPSIS

Menzies' Tree Moss

The genus name derives from the Greek *leukos*, meaning "white," and *lepsis*, "scale," alluding to the stem leaves.

Menzies' tree moss (*Leucolepsis acanthoneuron*) exhibits modest activity against *Bacillus subtilis* (Russell 2010).

LEWINSKYA

Bristle Mosses

Rock bristle moss, or Sturm's bristle moss (*Lewinskya rupestris* syn. *Orthotrichum rupestre*), prefers to grow on igneous rock formations. Solvent extracts inhibit various bacterial growth, including *Bacillus subtilis*, *B. cereus*, *Staphylococcus aureus*, and *Escherichia coli* (Elibol et al. 2011).

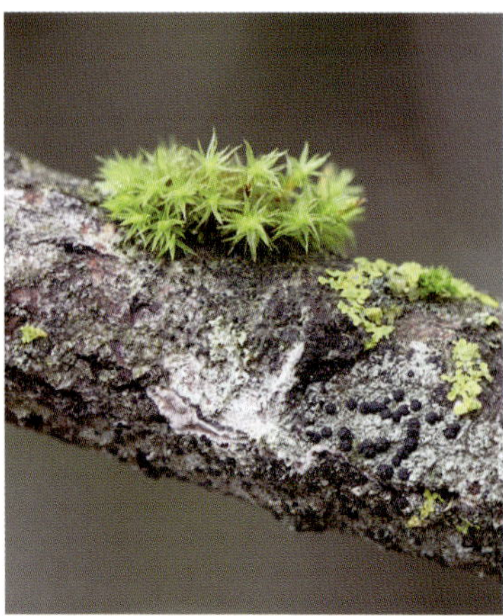

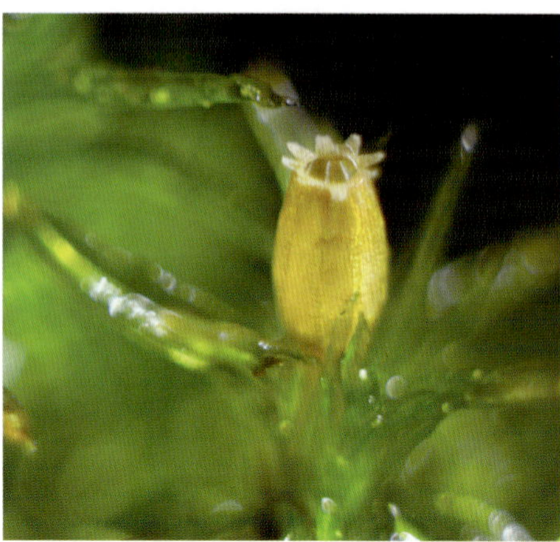

Lewinskya speciosum (Showy Bristle Moss)

MICROCALPE

Microcalpe subsimplex moss is widespread throughout central and northern South America; the Caribbean; in isolated part of southeastern United States; and a few countries in West Africa.

Microcalpe subsimplex syn. *Sematophyllum subsimplex* gathered in the Brazilian Amazon was steam-distilled and the essential oil analyzed by Rezende-Moraes et al. (2023). It contains naphthalene (26.62%), phthalic acid derivative (13.98%), curcuphenol (7.74%), hexadecanoic acid (7.51%), n-nonanal (5.41%), and minor amounts of methyl linoleate, (2E)-octenal and octenol, and galaxolide (0.66%). The latter compound has a musky scent, and the synthetic chemical is widely used in perfumes, fabric softeners, and detergents. It is also an environmental androgen that exerts toxicological effects on the development of male reproductive organs (Li, Wang et al. 2023).

MACROMITRIUM

Raincoat Moss Umbrella Moss

The genus name *Macromitrium* derives from the Greek *makros*, "long," and *mitra*, "cap," alluding to this moss's obviously long calyptra. *Macromitrium* species are called raincoat moss or umbrella moss in some parts of the world.

Valarezo (2018) gathered, steam-distilled, and identified 94 constituents in 6 mosses found in Ecuador. The three main compounds in *Macromitrium perreflexum* mosses are selina-3, 11-dien-6-α-ol (19.7%), and curcuphenol (10.6%). Curcuphenol inhibits cell proliferation, DNA replication, and induces cell death (apoptosis) in human colon (Caco-2) cancer cell lines. Apoptosis is associated with the stimulation of caspase-3 activity (Rodrigo et al. 2010).

Mucormycosis is a serious infection of the sinuses, eyes, and even the brain, which can occur one to two weeks, sometimes longer, after contracting COVID-19. It is caused by various fungi, with 70% of cases due to *Rhizopus oryzae*. Symptoms include one-sided headache, nasal and sinus congestion, and black lesions on the nasal bridge or upper inside of mouth. Fever, lethargy, slurred speech, partial paralysis, and death can occur if left untreated. Work by Pokharkar et al. (2022) found (+) curcuphenol to be a promising compound due to its broad-spectrum target potential for inhibiting the pathogen.

It should be noted that curcuphenol is found in turmeric and curcumins.

MIELICHHOFERIA

Copper Moss

Copper moss (*Mielichhoferia mielichhoferiana* and *M. elongata*) has been widely used by prospectors as a determinate for heavy metal deposits. Substrate copper levels of 30–770 ppm have been found for some copper moss species.

MERCEYOPSIS

Tongue-Leaf Copper Moss

Tongue-leaf copper moss, *Merceyopsis cataractae* syn. *Scopelophila cataractae* enjoys living on copper-rich soil. The species derives from the Latin *cataracta* meaning "waterfall" and the Ancient Greek *katarrhaktēs* "down-rushing," or katarassō "to dash down."

Once believed to be quite rare, it's found throughout the world in temperate climates. It is not so much a bryo-indicator of copper-rich soil, but rather prone to invading older contaminated mine sites. One analysis of this moss found growing near Swansea, Wales, found 1.54 ppm of copper and 1.4 ppm of zinc.

METEORIELLA

The genus name is derived from the Greek *meteoron*, "high in the sky," alluding to its dangling epiphytic habit.

Meteoriella soluta is used in China as an anti-inflammatory, for relief of pain, and for gastrointestinal and respiratory bleeding (Ding 1982).

MNIUM

Horn Calcareous Moss
Red Penny Moss
Stream Moss
Thyme Mosses

The genus name *Mnium* means "moss" in Greek. Nineteen species are noted.

Two species of *Mnium*, *M. cuspidatum* and *M. medium* are rich in arachidonic acid, used to treat fatty acid deficiencies associated with lack of alpha-linolenic and linolenic acid as well as to treat eczema in dogs and hogs. It also inhibits lipoxygenase, an enzyme that mediates the occurrence of inflammation.

Many species of the genus have been moved to the *Plagiomnium* genus.

Various *Mnium* species are used in the Philippines as a poultice for burns, bruises, and wounds (Azuelo et al. 2011).

In India, stream moss or bordered thyme moss, as *Mnium marginatum* is commonly called, is traditionally applied to cuts, wounds, burn infections, and other skin disorders. Work by Singh et al. (2007) found *Mnium marginatum* active against five gram-positive and six gram-negative bacteria, as well as eight fungi species. The 15 mosses studied by this team were found to contain various ferulic and m- and p-coumaric acids. Later work by Singh et al. (2011) identified this moss as having the highest inhibition of *Staphylococcus aureus* out of the many species tested.

Essential oil obtained by hydro-distillation of *Mnium hornum*, commonly called lipstick thyme moss, horn calcareous moss, or swan's neck thyme moss, contains the highly beneficial sesquiterpenes (+)-10-epi-muurola-4,11-diene and 10,11-dihyroxy-α-cuparenone, as well as (+)-dauca-8,11-diene (Saritas et al. 2001).

Red penny moss, or dotted thyme moss, (*Rhizomnium punctatum* syn. *Mnium punctatum*), is used by several Indigenous peoples of the central and northern coasts of British Columbia for painful swellings (Compton 1993). Several groups use the fresh leaves as a poultice for burns.

Starry thyme moss, *Mnium stellare*, exhibits antibacterial activity against *Bacillus subtilis*, *Staphylococcus aureus*, *S. carnosus*, *S. epidermidis*, and *Salmonella typhimurium* (Singh et al. 2011; Canli et al. 2015). The latter bacterium is a major cause of food-borne illness, with an estimated one million Americans affected annually, resulting in four hundred deaths, mainly in immune-compromised persons. Drug-resistant salmonella is a growing concern.

NECKERA

Feather Mosses   Neckera Mosses

The genus *Neckera* is named in honor of Noël Martin Joseph de Necker (1729–1793), an eighteenth-century Belgian physician, botanist, and bryologist. He was the personal physician to the court of the Electoral Palatinate in Mannheim, a constituent state of the Holy Roman Empire. Dr. Necker wrote several books on mosses and one on fungi. He was born on Christmas day, hence his first name. The genus contains about 50 species worldwide.

Neckera mosses, due to their absorptive and antibacterial properties, were historically prized for their use in outdoor privies.

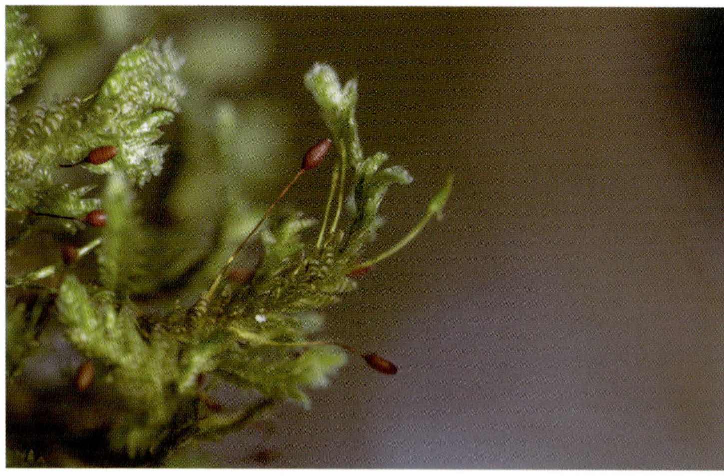

Neckera pumila (Dwarf Neckera)

Kang et al. (2007) found that extracts of Douglas neckera, *Neckera douglasii*, were active against *Staphylococcus aureus* when enhanced by UV-A light irradiation. This species is named in honor of the nineteenth-century Scottish explorer David Douglas. His survey of western North America led to several species named in his honor, including the Douglas fir, well-known to many botanists.

NECKEROPSIS

The tropical *Neckeropsis undulata* syn. *Pilotrichum undulatum*, found growing in the Brazilian Amazon, was collected and distilled by Miranda et al. (2021). Ten compounds were identified with respect to their medicinal value, with the major ones being 1-oct-3-ol (35.7%), α-muurolol (21.4%), naphthalene (11.3%), and *n*-hexanal (10%).

NIPHOTRICHUM

Fringe Mosses

Niphotrichum is derived from the Greek, roughly translating as "snow hair" in reference to its hoary appearance.

Hoary fringe moss (*Niphotrichum canescens* syn. *Racomitrium canescens*) is called *tek* q^{w} *zém* (meaning "rock moss" and "mossy rock moss") by the Nlaka'pamux of British Columbia (Turner et al. 1990). It is found on gravel and sandy sites in higher elevations. The Inuit of North America and Greenland collect this moss and make a type of porridge (Nordström 2019).

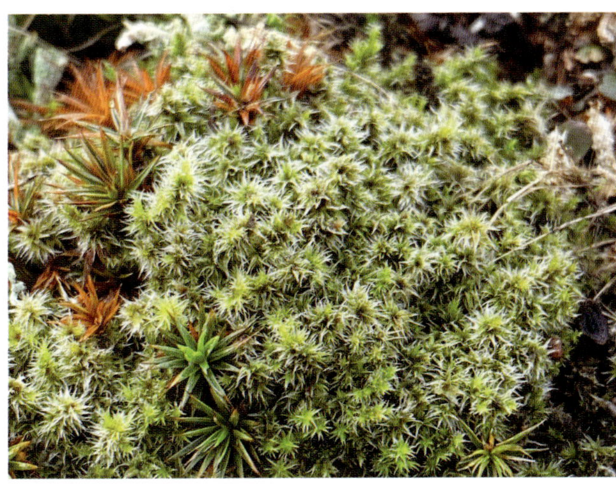

Niphotrichum canescens (Fringe Moss)
Photo by
Drew T. Henderson

It is also used for fill gaps in cabin walls and as lamp wicks by Labrador Inuit. It is especially popular in Japan for landscaping miniature gardens.

A study by Kim et al. (2021) compared the anti-inflammatory effect of methanol extract of this moss and the liverwort *Marchantia polymorpha*. The extract significantly decreased LPS-induced nitric oxide production in human keratinocyte (HaCaT) cells in both, but the liverwort exhibited more effective inhibition.

The essential oil contains mainly estragole (58.86%) and d-limonene (7.2%) (Hong et al. 2021). Estragole is found in tarragon, basil, and other essential oils. It is toxic in large amounts taken internally, but an effective anti-inflammatory when used externally. It should be noted that despite the urging of several large Multi-Level Marketing essential oil companies, essential oils should not be ingested. Essential oils of lemon or peppermint are not a problem, but as little as 5 ml of eucalyptus essential oil swallowed by a baby is toxic and can result in death. My wife Laurie and I have owned a small essential oil company, Scents of Wonder, for over 35 years and taught aromatherapy courses for most of that time frame.

OCTOBLEPHARUM

Bun Moss
Common Octoblepharum Moss
Dwarf Larch Moss
Missionary Moss
White Moss

The genus name derives from the Greek *okto*, "eight," and *blepharis*, "eyelash," alluding to this moss's eight-toothed peristome. Twenty accepted species.

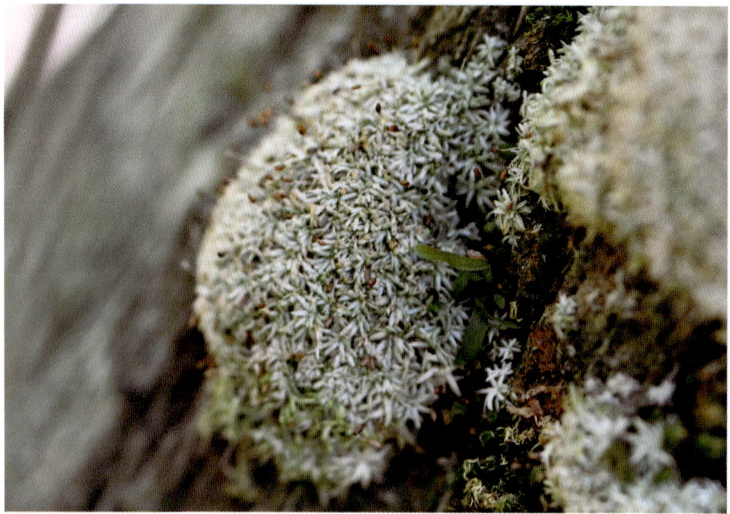

Octoblepharum albidum (Bun Moss)
Photo by Alan Rockefeller

Bun moss, white moss, or common octoblepharum moss (*Octoblepharum albidum*), is used externally by the Seminole of Florida for fever and body pain (Sturtevant 1954; Chandra et al. 2017). Other common names include dwarf larch moss, and for some unknown reason it is also named missionary moss.

The Chácobo of Bolivia use this moss as an antipyretic and to relieve headache (Boom 1996).

Octoblepharum albidum contains daucosterol and friedelin. Daucosterol shows benefit in various cancers, and it also protects neurons from oxygen and glucose deprivation, suggesting an efficient and inexpensive neuroprotectant (Jiang et al. 2015). Work by Naidu et al. (2020) found extracts inhibit the growth and survival of ovarian (PA1), cervical (C-33A), and lung (NCI-H358) cancer cell lines. Daucosterol linoleate, derived from sweet potato, induces apoptosis and prevents metastasis in breast (MCF-7) cancer cell lines (Han, Jiang et al. 2018). A mouse study by Jang et al. (2019) found that daucosterol significantly alleviates colitis.

Friedelin, a triterpenoid chemical compound, reverses scopolamine-induced neuropathy, suggesting a possible benefit in Alzheimer's disease (Sandu et al. 2022). It is also a novel inhibitor of prostate cancer (Joshi, Bhandare et al. 2022) and ameliorates ulcerative colitis by inhibiting inflammation and regulation of autophagy (Shi et al. 2021). Thus it appears that the two main constituents of this *Octoblepharum* species, daucosterol and friedelin, possess anticancer activity, neuronal benefit, and alleviate colitis and ulcerative colitis.

Octoblepharum albidum metabolites show antimicrobial inhibition as well. Manoj et al. (2016) examined the antibacterial potential of methanol extracts, which strongly inhibit pathogens, including *Salmonella typhimurium*, *Staphylococcus aureus*, *Klebsiella pneumoniae*, *Escherichia coli*, *Bacillus cereus*, *B. subtilis*, *Proteus vulgaris*, and *Pseudomonas aeruginosa*. Ethanol extracts inhibited only the latter bacterium (Vidal et al. 2012).

Both fatty acids and essential oils have been produced and analyzed (Alves et al. 2022). Hexadecanoic (palmitic) acid comprises nearly 44% of fatty acids. The main compound in the essential oil is E-isoeugenol (7.09%), followed by 1-octen-3-ol (5.87%), 3-octanone (2.76%), 2-methoxy-4-methyl-phenol (1.91%), and 1-octen-3-yl acetate (1.33%). These compounds are reported in the scientific literature to be possible insecticides that could be used in agricultural formulations.

OLIGOTRICHUM

Balding Moss
Hercynian Haircap Moss
Incurved Hair Moss
Rock Bristle-Moss

The genus name derives from the Greek *oligo*, meaning "few," and *trichos*, "hair" (Dixon 1954). This alludes to the sparse hairs on the calyptra, hence one of the common names, balding moss. Twenty-four accepted species.

Hercynian haircap moss or incurved hair moss (*Oligotrichum hercynicum*) is found on the west side of the Continental Divide and along the coastlines of British Columbia and Washington State, usually at higher elevations. Solvent extracts inhibit the fungi *Fusarium bulbigenum* and *Pyricularia oryzae* (Furuyama et al. 2021). The latter causes rice blast, a pathogenic destruction of rice crops. There is also an upside: Dihydropyriculol, a major secondary metabolite of *Pyricularia oryzae*, inhibits the growth of the bacteria *Streptomyces griseus*. And *Streptomyces griseus* strains are well-known producers of antibiotics such as streptomycin and other such commercially significant secondary metabolites and are a normal part of human microflora. But there is a downside as well: *Streptomyces griseus* strains have been found to cause infection of the sacroiliac joint in a 26-year-old woman (Song et al. 2021). Perhaps even more sinister is the presence of the fungus toxins in the air of water-damaged schools and day care centers. Valinomycin-producing *Streptomyces griseus* strains can cause a loss of sperm motility as well (Andersson et al. 1998).

Early work by McCleary et al. (1960) found the moss, *Oligotrichum hercynicum*, inhibits the growth of *Micrococcus flavus*, *M. rubens*, *Streptococcus pyogenes*, and *Candida albicans*.

Rock bristle-moss (*Oligotrichum rupestre*) is found worldwide on noncalcareous boulders and rock cliffs.

OREAS

Golden Oreas Moss

The genus name is derived from the Greek *oread*, referring to the primeval gods or daimones (spirits) of the mountains, the progeny of Gaia according to Greek mythology. The Greeks rarely personified a mountain, but each one was said to have its own local nymph, an Oread. Golden oreas moss, *Oreas martiana*, is found at high mountain elevations around the world. It is considered rare or critically imperiled in North America, but found in Alberta, British Columbia, Alaska, and Colorado.

This golden-colored moss has been traditionally used to treat wounds, as a hemostatic, and as an anodyne to stop pain and to treat nervous exhaustion and epilepsy (Asakawa 2007). In China it was used traditionally for menorrhagia, prolonged bleeding associated with menstruation (Chandra et al. 2017).

ORTHODICRANUM

Fork Moss Lawn Moss

Many *Dicranum* species have been recategorized to this genus, but for the ease of discussion, they are discussed in the *Dicranum* section.

ORTHOSTICHELLA

The genus name is derived from the Latin *ortho*, meaning "straight," and *stichos*, "row," referring to the moss's straight leaves, while *ella* is from the Latin giving the name a diminutive meaning. The species name *rigida* is obvious. *Orthostichella rigida* is found in tropical regions of Mexico and South America and parts of Africa. Nine species are recognized.

Work by Rodrigues et al. (2020) examined ethanol extracts for antimicrobial activity. Susceptible species are the bacteria *Staphylococcus aureus*, *Escherichia coli*, *Salmonella enteritidis*, and *Listeria monocytogenes*; and the fungi *Candida albicans* and *Cryptococcus neoformans*. The latter fungus is often found in bird excrement, causing cryptococcosis infections in human lungs. Fungal meningitis and encephalitis, especially in AIDS patients, is often caused by this opportunistic pathogen, which causes death in 10% to 30% of patients. Cryptococcal meningitis is increasingly common in immunocompromised persons, resulting in a death rate of up to 90%. After invading the lungs, it enters the bloodstream and then finds its way across the blood-brain barrier. The anticancer drug vandetanib, an oral receptor tyrosine kinase inhibitor used in some cases of thyroid cancer, may be helpful.

ORTHOSTICHOPSIS

Orthostichopsis tortipilis is common throughout South America and Cuba. In Ecuador it is used to relieve cuts, snake bites, and stomach pain (Kohn 1992).

ORTHOTRICHUM

Bristle Mosses

The genus name derives from the Greek *orthos*, "upright" or "straight," and *trichos*, "hair," alluding to the more or less erect hairs on the capsules of most species.

Work by Karpinski and Adamczak (2017) found that *Orthotrichum anomalum* (anomalous bristle moss or red-shafted hood moss) exhibits significant inhibition of *Streptococcus pyogenes, Staphylococcus aureus, Escherichia coli, Enterococcus faecalis, and Klebsiella pneumoniae.*

Vollár et al. (2018) found various solvent and water extracts of *Orthotrichum diaphanum* (white-tipped bristle moss) exhibit cytotoxicity against epithelial/cervical (HeLa), ovarian (T47D), and breast (A2780) cancer cell lines.

OXYRRHYNCHIUM

Feather Mosses

The genus names derives from the Greek *oxys*, "acute," and *rynchos*, "nose," alluding to the beaked operculum. Swartz's feather moss or emerald feather moss (*Oxyrrhynchium hians* syn. *Eurhynchium hians* syn. *O. swartzii*) is diverse and somewhat difficult to identify with four distinct lineages.

Work by Vollár et al. (2018) found various n-hexane and chloroform extracts exhibit cytotoxicity against epithelial/cervical (HeLa), ovarian (T47D), and breast (A2780) cancer cell lines. Extracts also inhibited both *Staphylococcus aureus* and other methicillin-resistant bacterial strains.

Ethanol extracts of the moss *Oxyrrhynchium vagans* syn. *Rhynchostegium vagans* exhibit in vitro inhibition of the fungi *Aspergillus flavus* var. *columnaris* and *A. parasiticus* var. *globosus*, and the gram-negative bacteria *Escherichia coli*, *Erwinia chrysanthemi*, and *Salmonella enterica* (Negi and Chaturvedi 2016). Asparaginase has been used to treat acute lymphoblastic leukemia for the past 50 years, with some success. The FDA has approved two preparations, one from *Escherichia coli* and the other from *E. chrysanthemi*. Up to 30% of patients are hypersensitive to the former, and thus the latter chemotherapy regimen is used. The ethanol extract was found to be superior to the antibiotic chloramphenicol and the fungicide fluconazole.

PALUSTRIELLA

Hookmosses

The genus name comes from the Latin *palustris*, "marshy," and *ella*, a diminutive that refers to the habitat, which is usually near moving water or calcareous wetlands. Bristly hookmoss and claw-leaved hookmoss, as *Palustriella falcata* syn. *Cratoneuron commutatum* is used in Traditional Chinese Medicine to reduce fever and to detoxify (Harris 2008).

Work by Ilhan et al. (2006) found acetone extracts of *Palustriella commutata* inhibit *Bacillus subtilis*, *B. cereus*, *B. mycoides*, and *Micrococcus luteus*, all gram-positive bacteria, as well as *Klebsiella pneumoniae*, *Yersinia enterocolitica*, *Pseudomonas aeruginosa*, *Escherichia coli*, and *Enterobacter aerogenes*, all gram-negative bacteria. Acetone extracts also inhibit methicillin-resistant *Staphylococcus aureus* (MRSA). An acetone extract was more potent against *Bacillus mycoides* than the standard drugs penicillin and cefotaxime. *Bacillus mycoides* can cause disease in fish, including necrotic lesions in commercial channel catfish raised in Alabama.

Yayintas et al. (2017) found ethanol and water extracts of *Palustriella commutata* significantly inhibit *Escherichia coli*, *Bacillus subtilis*, *Staphylococcus aureus, Pseudomonas aeruginosa*, and *Candida albicans*, and exhibit antioxidant activity as well.

Palustriella commutata is utilized in TCM to treat cardiovascular conditions and bacterial infections.

PAPILLARIA

Nipplewort

The genus name is from the Latin *papula*, "nipple," alluding to the leaf cell papillae. Martin (2015) notes, "Naturalists, wilderness adventurers, and mossers can apply a tincture of *Papillaria* and *Thuidium* species as an insect repellent."

Papillaria crocea, an epiphyte in moist forests, concentrates cadmium, chromium, lead, and zinc, and may be useful for biomonitoring trace mineral contamination (Bing et al. 2016). The species name derives from the Latin *crocum*, meaning "yellow" or "golden" colored, which in turn led to the word *crocus*, from which the expensive and medicinal saffron is collected.

PARALEUCOBRYUM

Long Leaf Fork Moss   Notch Leaf Moss

The genus name comes from the Greek *para*, "near," and the genus *Leucobryum*, indicating a resemblance. Long leaf fork moss or notch leaf moss (*Paraleucobryum longifolium*) shows the highest activity against three human gynecological cancer cells lines.

Vollár et al. (2018) selected 42 bryophytes, including *Paraleucobryum longifolium*, and did 168 water and organic extracts. The researchers then screened for activity against cervical/epithelial adenocarcinoma (HeLa), ovarian (A2780), and invasive ductal breast (T47D) cancer cell lines.

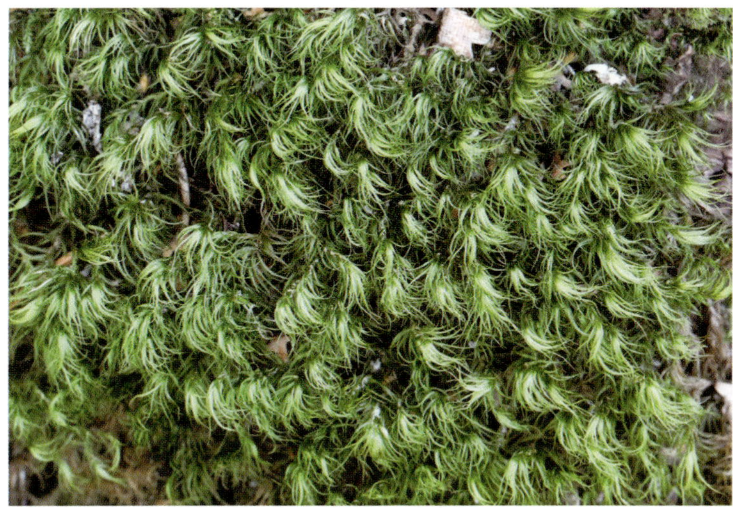

Paraleucobryum longifolium (Long Leaf Fork Moss)

Ninety-nine of the extracts derived from 41 species exerted more than 25% inhibition of at least one of the cancer cell lines at 10 μg/mL, and chloroform extracts exhibited significant inhibition as well. The highest activity (78.54% inhibition of adenocarcinoma) was observed in the case of *Paraleucobryum longifolium*. Moreover, this particular extract was active on all the cell lines. Only 19 samples of 15 taxa showed moderate antibacterial activity, with *Staphylococcus aureus* and *Streptococcus pyogenes* being the most susceptible. The latter bacterium is the cause of strep throat, impetigo, and more serious conditions such as necrotizing fasciitis (flesh-eating disease), which can cause up to 24,000 death-threatening conditions, including cellulitis, toxic shock syndrome, and rheumatic fever. The latter infection caused a heart defect in my father as a young child, leading to his passing at an early age.

Leucobryns A–E were isolated from *Paraleucobryum longifolium* (Csupor et al. 2020). Notably, leucobryns A and B exhibited weak antiproliferative activity against several human cancer cell lines.

PHILONOTIS

Apple Mosses River Moss Spring Bartram Moss Swamp Moss

The genus name derives from the Greek *philo*, "loving," and *notis*, "moisture," hence the names river moss and swamp moss. About 170-180 species to date.

Philonotis angusta moss tea was given to women in India following childbirth.

Fountain apple moss, aquatic apple moss or spring bartram moss (*Philonotis fontana*) is prepared as a tea in southern India to reduce fever and as a gargle for adenopharyngitis, an inflammation of the tonsils and pharynx (Alam et al. 2015; Chandra et al. 2017). This moss was used by the Gasuite of Utah to alleviate burn pain by crushing into a paste and applied as a poultice. It is used to cover bruises and wounds, or used as a padding under splints to set broken limbs. In the Himalayas, it is burned into ash and mixed with fat and honey for cuts, burns, and wounds. It is antipyretic and antidotal for cases of boils. It has traditionally been used as a diuretic in China for urinary obstructions (Harris 2008; Pant 1998).

Unspecified *Philonotis* species have been crushed and the paste applied to burns and bone fractures by Indigenous groups in North America (Saxena 2004).

PHYLLOGONIUM

Broom Moss

The moss *Phyllogonium viride* syn. *P. fulgens* var. *viride* is found on trees in tropical regions of South America. The essential oil is comprised mainly of β-bazzanene (20.3%), β-caryophyllene (17.06%), β-chamigrene (14%), and germacrene B (11.72%). Cytotoxic testing on breast (MCF-7) and colorectal (HCT-116) cancer cell lines did not induce toxicity (Klegin et al. 2021).

PHYSCOMITRIUM

Bladder Mosses Earthmosses Urn Mosses

Geographic Range: North America, Central America, South America, Europe, Asia, Africa, Australia

Habitat: exposed soil of alluvial mud and riverbanks at sea level to low elevations

Practical Uses: cosmetics industry

Medicinal Applications: antibacterial, antifungal, neurodegenerative diseases, hemostasis, kidney disease, malaria

The genus name derives from the Greek *physa*, "bladder," and *mitrion*, "little cap," probably alluding to the urn-like shape of operculum. This may not be a very accurate reference to the calyptra, according to Dixon (1954). The genus *Physcomitrella* is now considered a synonym of the currently accepted *Physcomitrium*. There are about 80 urn mosses identifed to date.

Moss samples of *Physcomitrium patens* were collected from the wild as well as cultured and then extracted with DMSO to test activity against a range of fungi by Sabovljevic et al. (2011). Activity was noted against *Aspergillus versicolor*, *A. fumigatus*, *Penicillium funiculosum*, *P. ochrochloron*, and *Trichoderma viride*. The bryophytes grown in culture had greater antifungal activity than those collected from the wild.

Defective genes in complement-regulating proteins are responsible for a number of kidney diseases, including C3 glomerular issues and atypical hemolytic uremic syndrome, later in life causing increased levels of macular degeneration. Most of these mutations affect the glycoprotein complement factor H, the main regulator. Biologically active factor H has the potential to treat these diseases, but no therapeutic factor H is presently available.

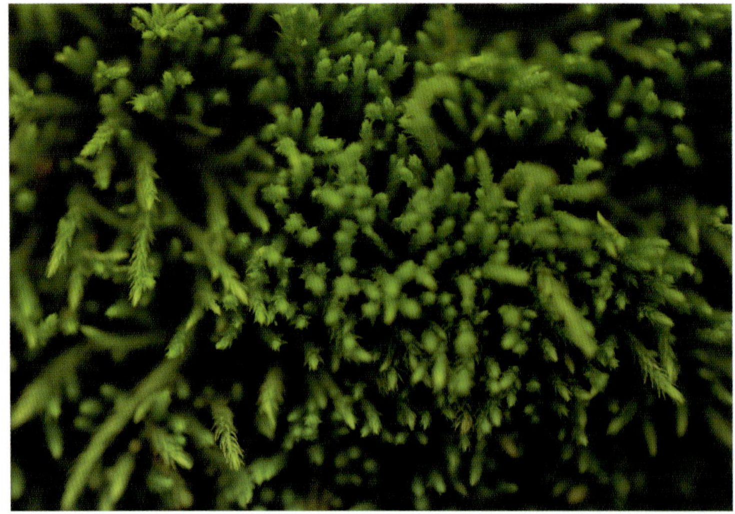

Physcomitrium patens (Spreading Earthmoss)

In a July 23, 2010, article appearing in the journal *Science Daily*, plant biotechnologist Dr. Eva Decker of the University of Freiburg explains: "With the complement factor H we have produced a protein in moss that otherwise occurs only in blood and is important for the immune system. Not enough of this protein in older people is the main cause of blindness for 50 million people worldwide. This age-related macular degeneration is a problem, particularly in industrialized countries."

Michelfelder et al. (2017) found a way to produce an improved recombinant human factor H derived from *Physcomitrium patens* after a multistep purification process. The moss-derived factor H reduced C3 deposition and increased serum C3 levels. It also showed full in vitro complement regulation similar to plasma-derived factor H, and it efficiently blocked LPS-induced alternative pathway activation and hemolysis induced by sera from patients with atypical hemolytic uremic syndrome.

In October 2017, the German company Greenovation Biotech successfully completed a phase 1 study of moss-aGal, a recombinant form of human α-galactosidase used in the treatment of Fabry disease, an inherited condition that can affect the kidneys, heart, brain, and skin, which can in turn lead to organ failure. Six patients were involved in the study and given a single infusion, with an observed drop in urine of the fatty acid globotriaosylceramide (Gb3). The accumulation of Gb3 in cells, tissues, and biological fluids can lead to ventricular hypertrophy, renal insufficiency, and stroke. (Michelfelder et al. 2017).

Fabry disease is a rare lysosomal storage disease due to an inborn deficiency of the α-galactosidase enzyme (aGal). A lysosomal enzyme, aGal breaks down Gb3, and in Fabry disease the absence of aGal causes a continuous accumulation of Gb3 in the cells. *Physcomitrium patens* contains the expression of full-length recombinant factor.

In a 2019 study, *Physomitrium patens* was treated with the stress hormone methyl jasmonate. In turn it released antimicrobial activity. And when protease activity was inhibited during treatment, it resulted in an immune regulatory response (Fesenko et al).

MossCellTec, a skin-care product made by the Mibelle Biochemistry Group, a German company, developed a protoneme culture of this moss and developed an extract for the cosmetics industry. The active compound maintains cell nucleus health in a completely novel antiaging manner. The cell nucleus contains the cell's DNA and is involved in regulating essential cellular processes. Studies have shown MossCellTec No. 1 activates the lamin A gene responsible for the nuclear envelope structure and the nuclear transport gene RanBP17. Both genes are downregulated in aged keratinocytes. Both in vitro and in vivo studies confirm that this extract supports the skin's adaptation to climatic stresses (Wandry et al. 2018). The diterpene ceruchinol in cultivated moss exhibits molecular docking of CAR, AKR1D1, and 17β-HSD1, suggesting potential benefit for cosmetic use (Munoz et al. 2024).

Physomitrium patens contains nine orthologs of the fatty acid amide hydrolase (FAAH) (Haq and Kilaru 2020).

In humans, anandamide, an endocannabinoid ligand, mediates various neurological and physiological processes that are terminated by FAAH. Research shows FAAH is a critical regulator of the endogenous levels of anandamine, suggesting possible avenues of benefit in human pathology. As scientists note, "FAAH inhibitors may be next generation therapeutic drugs of potential value for the treatment of pathologies in the central nervous system and in the periphery" (Maccarrone 2006).

Alzheimer's disease is a growing health concern whose cause is unknown. It is characterized by brain hypometabolism, decreased sugar availability, and ultimately neuron destruction. A hypothesis by Zakirova et al. (2019) involves creating a manner of supplying brain neurons with a fuel supply to help survival, or at least to alleviate symptoms. The team demonstrated that spreading earthmoss cells can be safely co-cultured with human fibroblasts in vitro, showing potential for providing human cells with energy and vital biomolecules to alleviate this disease.

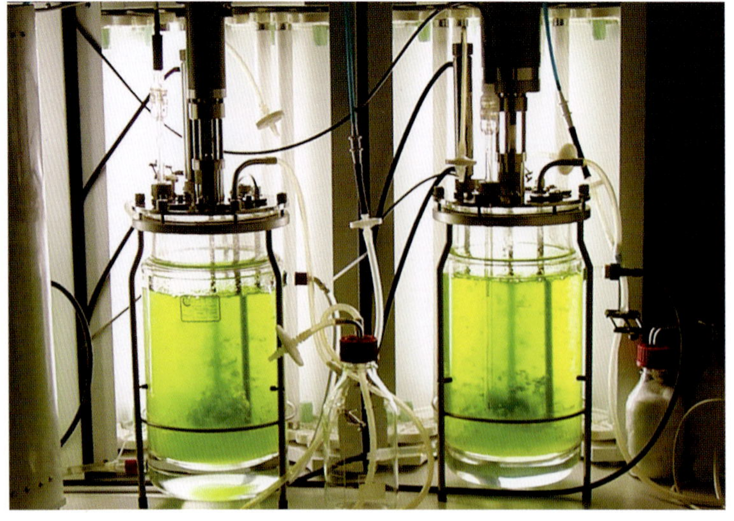

A moss bioreactor, used for production of *Physcomitrium patens* protonemata
Photo by Annette Hohe

An exudate of *Physcomitrium patens* exhibits high levels of antibacterial activity that increased significantly in liquid culture over four weeks in a study by Valeeva et al. (2022). Only gram-positive bacteria were inhibited.

Bryophyte ecologist Janice Glime (2017) shared an amusing story about ingesting a bioreactor liquid culture. A group of about 50 botanists at a party were invited to sample a drink called Psycho Psycho, which contained a teaspoon of protonemata, the early haploid stage in life cycle of *Physcomitrium patens*. The taste was considered quite interesting, and all participants survived. Which reminds me of a bryophyte joke:

What do you call a man with moss on his head?

Pete.

The cultured moss success has led to several novel innovations. Genetically engineered moss can produce patchoulol and α- and β-santalene, both in demand by the fragrance industry. As a long-time proponent of essential oils, I have strong feelings about this, as sandalwood (*Santalum album*) trees are nearly extinct due to overharvesting, and this compound is used to manufacture and sell an adulterated oil. On the other hand, this technology may be useful in the development of a compound that helps alleviate symptoms associated with malaria, from which nearly half the world's population is in real and constant danger of infection. In 2015 over 212 million cases of malaria were reported, along with 429,000 estimated deaths. By inserting five genes involved in the biosynthesis of artemisinin, the effective compound can be more affordable in lower income countries (Ikram et al. 2017).

PLAGIOMNIUM

Baby-Tooth Moss
Magnificent Moss
Saber-Tooth Moss
Sharp-Leaved Moss
Surveyor's Moss
Thread Mosses
Thyme Mosses

Geographic Range: worldwide

Habitat: old-growth boreal forests

Practical Uses: hemostat, terrariums, and small container gardens

Medicinal Applications: antibacterial, anticancer, antifungal, antihemorrhagic, hemostatic, vulnerary

The genus name derives from the Greek *plagios*, "oblique," and *mnion*, "moss," alluding to the presence of plagiotropic stolons in most species, making thread moss one of this genus's common names. Thirty-four accepted species to date.

Sharp-leaved thyme moss (*Plagiomnium acutum*) is found worldwide in old-growth boreal forests. The moss is used commercially in terrariums and small container gardens.

It has been used in Traditional Chinese Medicine for thousands of years, although without human clinical trials to show its history of efficacy. In ethnic use it is considered a hemostatic agent for the nose, gums, and teeth, for spitting and coughing up blood; it is also used as a tea for blood in the urine or stools, as well as for uterine bleeding (Azuelo 2011; Suire et al. 2000).

According to Li, Wang et al. (2022), the essential oil was found to contain 74 constituents, with diterpenes (26.5%), sesquiterpenes (23.89%), and alcohols (21.81%) being the major compounds identified. These include α- and β-cedrene, α acoradiene, and (+)-dolabella-3,7-dien-18-ol, the latter two compounds also found in liverworts. The essential oil shows significant cell growth inhibition of hepatic (HepG2) and lung (A549) cancer cell lines by blocking G1 phase and inducing apoptosis. One of the oil compounds, dolabella-3,7-dien-18-ol, represents over 25% of the oil constituents and is most active against the two cancer cell lines tested.

Many-fruited thyme moss (*Plagiomnium affine* syn. *Mnium affine*) with its constituent flavonoid apigenin, is responsible for inhibiting *Pseudomonas aeruginosa*, a gram-negative bacterium that can cause disease in plants and animals (Basile et al. 1999). It is found in old growth boreal forests. This moss contains up to 6% water-soluble trans-aconitic acid (TAA), a fundamental metabolite and antimicrobial agent (Tachibana and Meeuse 1960).

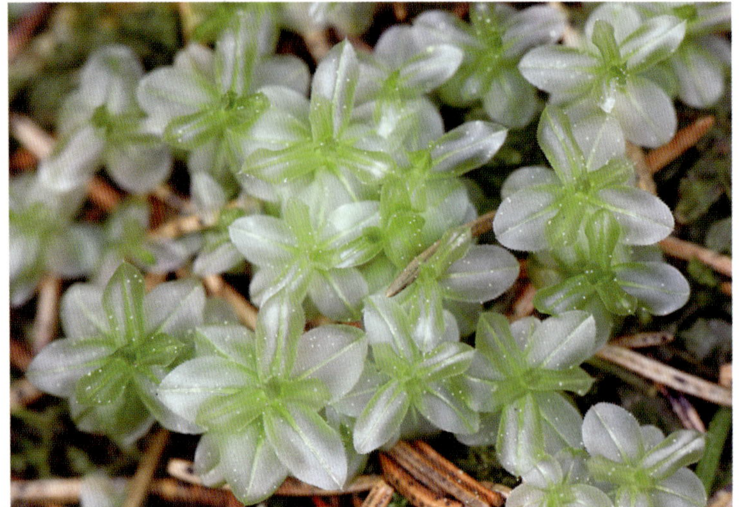

Plagiomnium affine (Many-Fruited Thyme Moss)

Trans-aconitic acid exhibits significant anti-edema activity (de Faria Garcia et al. 2010). Diesters (any compound containing two ester groups) of TAA show benefit in lipopolysaccharide-induced inflammation in the knee joints of mice, suggesting a possible benefit in the management of rheumatoid arthritis according to de Oliveira, do Valle Moreira et al. (2018). This seems confirmed in other work by de Oliveira, Augusto et al. (2018), which found encapsulation of TAA in mucoadhesive microspheres that were given orally to mice provided a sustained release of anti-inflammatory activity in LPS-induced acute arthritis. TAA is an inhibitor of the enzyme aconitase; it specifically inhibits the growth of *Leishmania donovani* parasites. In a hamster model, TAA significantly reduced the parasitic burden in the liver (Misra et al. 1989). In acute toxicity tests there were no deaths in the lab animals, even at a dose level of two grams per kilogram weight per day.

The moss *Plagiomnium cuspidatum* syn. *M. cuspidatum*, when extracted by ethanol, inhibits the growth of *Micrococcus luteus* syn. *Micrococcus flavus* (McCleary et al. 1960). This bacterium rarely affects humans, but in immune-compromised persons can cause endocarditis. As a sidenote, black elderberry extract also exhibits strong activity against this bacterium (Przybylska-Balcerek et al. 2021).

Cow dung was examined and found to contain a strain of *Micrococcus luteus*. When exposed to high-density polyethylene it showed spectacular bacterial colonization and degradation of this sturdy plastic (Sivasankari and Vinotha 2014). This suggests a possible use in bioremediation of this common plastic, which is polluting our entire planet (Gupta et al. 2022). Most milk jugs, detergents, shampoo, and juice bottles are made from high-density polyethylene. Though the plastic is considered "safe," it has been shown to leach estrogenic chemicals dangerous to fetuses and juveniles.

Micrococcus luteus was traditionally used in eastern and western Himalayan regions of India for nosebleeds and hematostasis (Alam et al. 2015).

Many-fruited thread moss or saber-tooth moss (*Plagiomnium ciliare*) appears to have flowers, which is a botanical impossibility. With a hand lens you will initially see what appears to be green blossoms but are actually leaves of the male plant. Martin (2015) explains: "The males form splash platforms at the top (apex) that indeed look like fairy florets . . . You can see dark balls ready to splash out when a giant raindrop hits the cup."

Baby-tooth moss or woodsy thyme moss (*Plagiomnium cuspidatum*) actively inhibits all three human cancer cell lines tested by Vollár et al. (2018)—cervicial/epithelial (HeLa), ovary (A2780), and invasive ductal breast (T470). Early work by McCleary et al. (1960) found inhibition of bacteria and fungi. However, some of the extracts were somewhat unstable or can vary in composition according to the season.

The flavonoid saponarin, an important constituent of *Plagiomnium cuspidatum*, is responsible for inhibiting *Pseudomonas aeruginosa* (Basile et al. 1999). This moss also showed significant inhibition of *Staphylococcus epidermidis, Bacillus subtilis, Streptococcus pyogenes, S. pneumoniae*, and *S. agalactiae*.

The latter bacterium is also known as group B streptococcus. It is common in the gastrointestinal tract and vagina in healthy adults, but it can be problematic in newborns or in adults with chronic medical conditions. It can also be a problem in milk cows, causing mastitis, hence the species name *agalactiae*, which means "of no milk." It can be a pathogenic issue in antibiotic-fed fish farms as well.

Marsh thyme moss or magnificent moss (*Plagiomnium ellipticum*) is a northern moss that accumulates fatty acids to help cell walls retain fluidity in cold weather. Like many other bryophytes it accumulates long-chain polyunsaturated fatty acids (l-PUFAs) such as arachidonic acid (AA) and eicosapentaenoic acid (EPA). Lu et al. (2023) examined the lipid composition of 39 bryophyte species in Iceland and found the AA and EPA of six mosses, including *Plagiomnium. ellipticum*, were abundantly distributed in the phospholipids and glycerolipids. In a 2022 study, ether extracts of this moss showed a high flavonoid content and a high content of 2,2'-azino-bis (3-ethylbenzothiazoline-6-sulfonic acid) antioxidant level in water. It also exhibited a high tyrosinase enzyme activity (Önder et al.).

Indigenous healers of British Columbia use *Plagiomnium insigne* for medicine. Two forms are recognized, and those growing under Douglas fir trees (*Pseudotsuga menziesii*) are considered less effective than the moss growing under spruce trees. Members of the Wuikinuxc Nation, also known as the Oweekeno, call this moss tiny, tiny little trees. It is traditionally used as a poultice for breast abscesses, boils, and swellings (Harris 2008). In the Philippines it is used for infections and swellings (Azeulo 2011).

Four *Plagiomnium* species, including *P. affine*, *P. cuspidatum*, *P. rostratum*, and *P. undulatum*, exhibit anticancer activity. Work by Vollár et al. (2018) found various solvent extracts exhibit cytotoxicity against epithelial/cervical (HeLa), ovarian (T47D), and breast (A2780) cancer cell lines, while water extracts exhibit minimal activity. In the same study, *Plagiomnium affine* showed inhibition of *Bacillus subtilis* and *Streptococcus pneumoniae*.

Surveyor's moss (*Plagiomnium undulatum*) grows on and indicates buried foundations (Saritas et al. 2001) found that the essential oil of mosses collected in Germany and Austria contains (+)-dauca-8,11-diene; 3,4,5-trimethyl-5-pentyl-5H-furan-2-one; and 3,4-dimethyl-5-pentyl-5H-furan-2-one (butenolides). Other compounds include n-heptanal, α-pinene, camphene, 3-octanone, β-pinene, 2-pentylfuran, delta-3-carene, limonene, E-2-octenal, pinocarvone, borneol, β-cyclocitral, bornyl acetate, geosmin, β-cedrene, β-bisabolene, manool, abietatriene, α-cadinol, and various minor compounds.

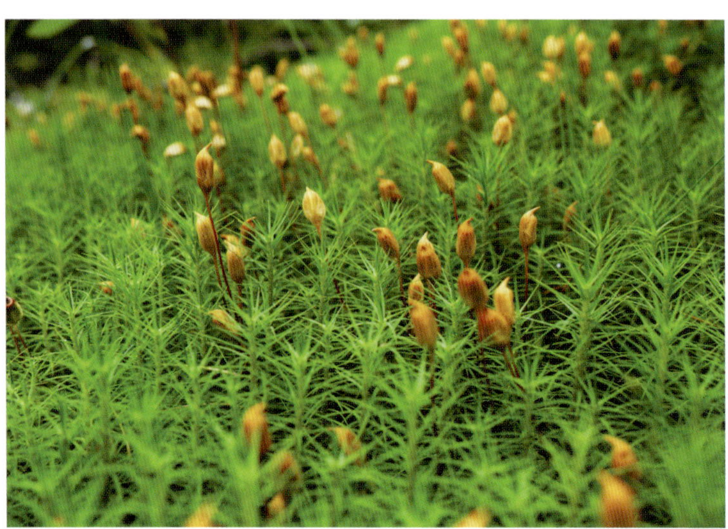

Plagiomnium undulatum (Hart's Tongue Thyme Moss)

The diterpene manool induces cytotoxicity in human cervical adenocarcinoma (HeLa) and human glioblastoma (U343) cell lines (de Oliveira et al. 2016). Manool is an interesting compound. Work by Nicolella et al. (2022) found it to be cytotoxic against murine melanoma (B16F10) cancer cell lines. When combined with cisplatin, an 86.7% reduction of tumor mass was noted. The treatment did not alter the activity of caspase 3 cleaved pathway. Follow-up work by Nicollela et al. (2023) found manool to be cytotoxic to human melanoma cancer cell lines B16F10 and A375.

Manool elicits vascular relaxation and reduced blood pressure in hypertensive rat aorta (Monteiro et al. 2020).

In a study of *Plagiomnium undulatum* and several other mosses Kahriman et al. (2009) identified gamma-elemene (24.1%) as the main constituent in the essential oil. Minor compounds include delta-cadinene (11.7%), α-cadinol (9.5%), tau-muurolol (7.3%), n-nonanal (6.1%), and minor amounts of viridiflorene, chiloscyphone, pentacosane, gamma muurolene, and allo-aromadendrene (Özdemir et al. 2009). Later work by Karpinski and Adamczak (2017) found *Plagiomnium undulatum* significantly inhibits *Streptococcus pyogenes*, *Staphylococcus aureus*, *Escherichia coli*, *Enterococcus faecalis*, and *Klebsiella pneumoniae*.

Plagiomnium venustum moss exhibits anticancer activity against murine lymphoma (P-388) cancer cell lines.

PLAGIOPUS

Oeder's Apple Moss

The genus name derives from the Greek *plagios*, meaning "oblique," and *pous*, foot, describing the curved seta.

Oeder's apple moss (*Plagiopus oederianus* syn. *Plagiopus oederi*) possesses sedative compounds. It is commonly found on moist, calcareous cliffs in the eastern Rockies and is used in the western Himalayas for epilepsy, apoplexy, and heart disease (Alam et al. 2015; Pant 1998; Ding 1982).

PLAGIOTHECIUM

Common Cotton Moss Dented Mosses Hokkaido Ball Moss

The genus name derives from the Greek *plagios*, "oblique," and *theke*, "case" or "little vessel," in reference to the usually oblique, angled capsule. The genus is often called cotton moss or silk moss, and in Japan it is called Hokkaido ball moss.

Dented silk moss or dented hydnum moss (*Plagiothecium denticulatum*) is widespread and found on swampy soil and in grassy fens at the base of trees or on fallen logs. Extracts show antifungal action against *Botrytis allii*, *Rhizoctonia solani*, *Trametes versicolor*, and *Fusarium bulbigenum* (Wolters et al. 1964).

A new species, *Plagiothecium talbotii*, was recently identified on Attu Island in Alaska (Wolski et al. 2022). It is not similar in morphology to any northern hemisphere species.

PLASTEURHYNCHIUM

The scarce pleurocarp moss is found on shaded limestone rocks in sheltered woods.

Lesser striated feather moss (*Plasteurhynchium striatulum* syn. *Eurhynchium striatulum*) contains polyphenols and flavonoids that exhibit antioxidant activity (Erturk et al. 2015).

PLATYHYPNUM

Long-Beaked Water Feather Moss

The genus name derives from the Greek *platys*, "wide" or "flat," and *hypnum*, "moss," alluding to its prostrate, spreading habit.

Long-beaked water feather moss (*Rhynchostegium riparioides* syn. *Platyhypnidium riparioides*) enjoys living in and near running water. Various studies suggest this moss's use for bryo-monitoring heavy metals in streams and rivers (Monaci et al. 2021).

Various solvent extracts of this moss were tested for antimicrobial activity by Colak et al. (2011). Ethanol extracts were found to inhibit *Bacillus subtilis*, *B. cereus*, and *Salmonella* species. Methanol extracts inhibited these bacteria, as well as *Staphylococcus aureus*, *Pseudomonas aeruginosa*, and *Escherichia coli*. Work by Bukvicki, Veljic et al. (2012) found similar results, but included activity against *Micrococcus flavus* among the positive results.

PLEUROZIUM

Big Red Stem Mosses Red-Stemmed Feather Moss Schreber's Big Red Moss

The genus names is from the Greek *pleura*, "side," and *ozos*, branch, alluding to the pinnate branching.

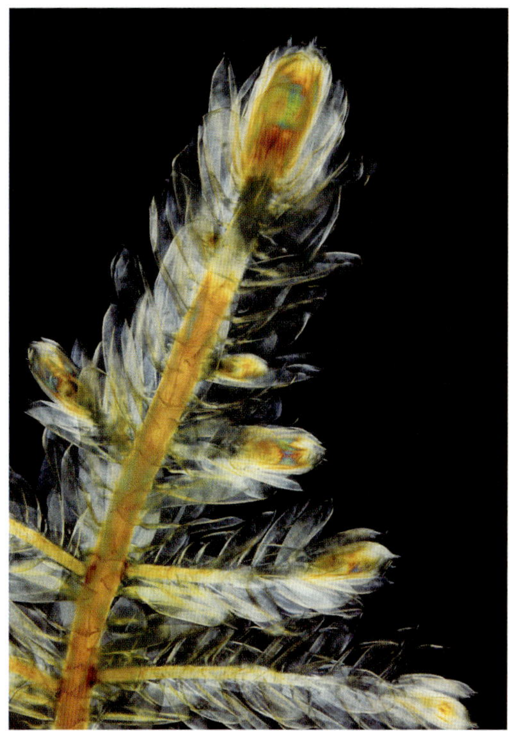

Pleurozium schreberi
(Big red stem moss)

Big red stem moss, red-stemmed feather moss, or Schreber's big red moss (*Pleurozium schreberi*) is common all over northern boreal forests.

This red-stemmed moss likely secretes species-specific chemo-attractants when limited by nitrogen access, which guide cyanobacteria to them, by which means they gain nitrogen. This signaling is regulated by the nitrogen demands of the moss and serves as a control of nitrogen input in boreal forests (Bay et al. 2013).

The moss exhibits antioxidant and antifungal activity (Chobot et al. 2008).

Big red stem moss inhibited at least one of the three cancer cell lines in work by Vollár et al. (2018). The research team selected 42 bryophytes and then did 168 water and organic extracts. They screened for activity against cervical epithelial adenocarcinoma (HeLa), ovarian (A2780), and invasive ductal breast (T47D) cancer cell lines. Ninety-nine of the extracts derived from 41 different species exerted more than 25% inhibition of at least one of the cancer cell lines at 10 µg/mL, and the n-hexane and cholorform extracts exhibited particularly significant inhibition. The water extracts showed no such activity. An earlier study by Klavina et al. (2015) found ethanol extracts exhibit significant inhibition of rat glioma (C6) cancer cell lines.

POGONATUM

Large-Leaf Moss
Pogonatum Mosses
Small-Mouth Moss
Small Spine Moss
Spike Mosses
Urn Haircap Moss

The genus name comes from the Greek *pogon*, "beard," alluding to the densly hairy calyptra. There are at least 156 species of *Pogonatum* worldwide. Spike moss is a common name.

Pogonatum cirratum is used for cardiovascular issues and neurasthenia in China (Harris 2008; Karim et al. 2014). The species name *cirratum* is derived from the Latin, meaning "curled" or "fringed hair." This moss, found in subtropical to tropical Asia, has been traditionally used in India as a laxative (Alam et al. 2015; Alam et al. 2012 "In Vitro Antifungal;" Chandra et al. 2017).

Water extracts of large-leaf moss, *Pogonatum cirratum*, exert cytotoxic effects and apoptosis against human T-cell acute lymphoblastic leukemia (CCL-119) cell lines, which suggests a potentially safer therapy for this disease, especially for children (Latif et al. 2019). The species is used in the Philippines for reducing fever, as a diuretic (to reduce edema), and for its laxative benefits, as well as for its hemostatic and anti-inflammatory activity (Azuelo 2011).

Pogonatum inflexum is sedative and hemostatic. It is traditionally used in wound healing, as well as for insomnia and heart palpitations (Harris 2008).

Small-mouth moss (*Pogonatum microstomum*) is used in Traditional Chinese Medicine for gallstones (Aruna and Krishnappa 2018). It contains

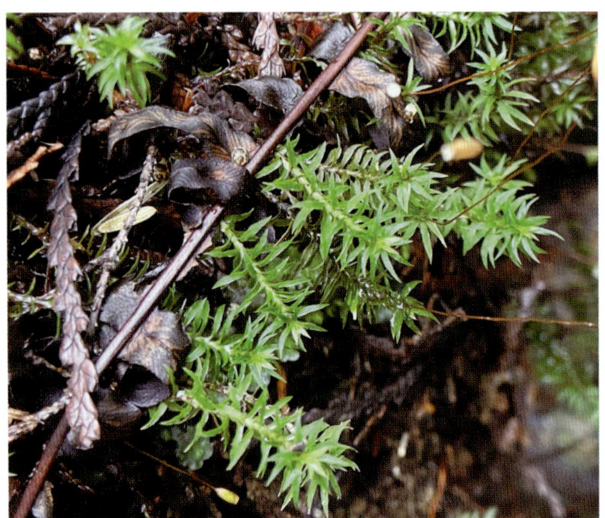

Pogonatum contortum
(Contorted Pogonatum Moss)
Photo by Graham Steinruck

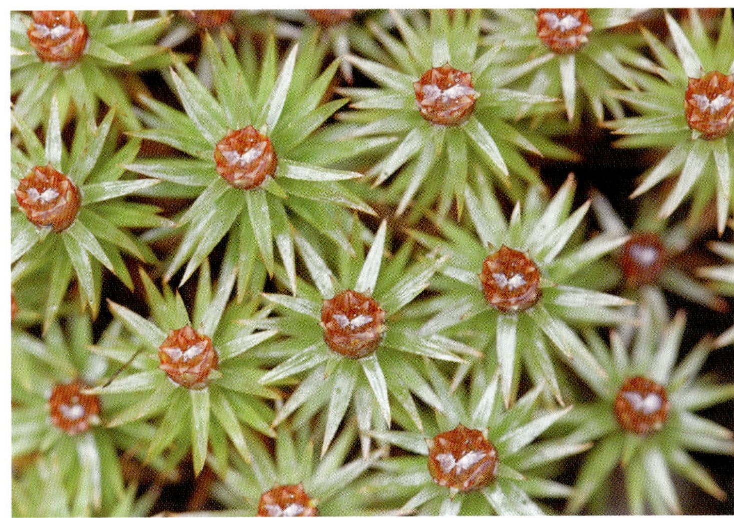

Pogonatum urnigerum (Urn Haircap Moss)

various flavonoids, glycosides, triterpenoids, phenols, and sterols. Moss extracts were found to be active against various microbes, including the bacteria *Agrobacterium tumefasciens*, *Streptomyces pneumonia*, *Escherichia coli*, *Klebsiella pneumoniae*, *Pseudomonas aeruginosa*, and the fungi *Candida albicans* and *Trichophyton rubrum*.

Small spine moss, *Pogonatum spinulosum*, contains pogonatones C and D. The former benzophenone derivative exhibits high cytotoxicity against pancreatic cancer (PANC-1) cell lines (Duan et al. 2023).

Extracts of urn haircap moss (*Pogonatum urnigerum* syn. *Polytrichum urnigerum*) show antifungal activity against *Trametes versicolor* and *Botrytis allii* (Wolters 1966). The species name derives from Latin *urna*, "urn," and *gerere*, "to bear," referring to the wide-mouthed capsule.

POHLIA

Nodding Thread Moss   Sponge Gourd Moss

The genus is named in honor of Johann Ehrenfried Pohl (1746–1800), a professor of botany at Leipzig University, where Johannes Hedwig (1730–1799) was professor of medicine until 1789. In that year Pohl moved to Dresden, and Hedwig was awarded his position, including directorship of the botanical garden there. The name is frequently mistakenly attributed to Johann Emanuel Pohl (1782–1834) an Austrian botanist working in South America. There are about 85 species identified to date.

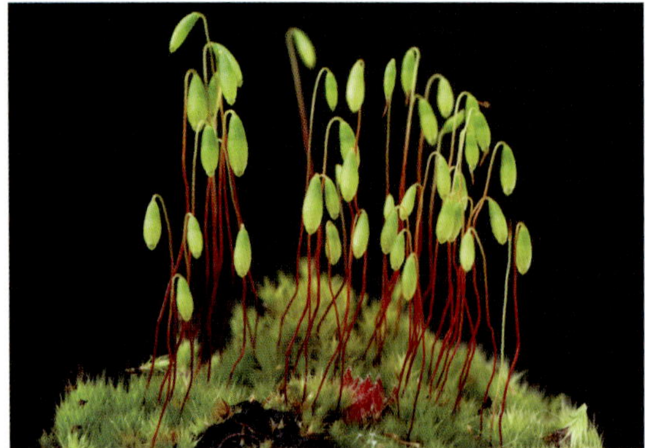
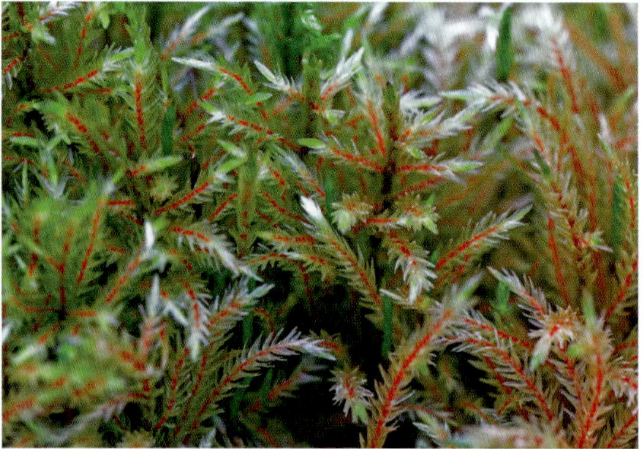

Pohlia nutans (Nodding Thread Moss)

The essential oil of nodding thread moss or sponge gourd moss (*Pohlia nutans*) contains nonanal (7.8%) and 2*E*-tetracecen-1-ol, as well as various aldehydes (33.4%) (Ücüncü et al. 2010). Chloroform and methanol extracts exhibit moderate activity against epithelial/cervical (HeLa) cancer cell lines (Vollár et al. 2018).

POLYTRICHASTRUM

Alpine Haircap Moss

The genus name is derived from a combination of *Polytrichum* (see below) and *astrum*, "star," alluding to the starlike form of this moss when viewed from above. About 20 species have been identified to date.

Alpine haircap moss (*Polytrichastrum alpinum*) has been traditionally used in parts of Europe for runny nose, coughs, and tearing eyes (Agelet and Valles 2003). In Traditional Chinese Medicine this moss is classified as a sedative and is used as a cough suppressant and hemostatic.

Similar to a few other bryophytes, *Polytrichastrum alpinum* contains ohioensins F and G. These compounds were obtained via methanol extract by Bhattarai et al. (2008, "In Vitro Antioxidant") and found to exhibit antioxidant activity.

The expression of cell adhesion molecules on vascular smooth muscle is responsible for leukocyte attachment and progression of atherosclerosis, a pattern of the disease arteriosclerosis that is characterized by the development of lesions on the walls of arteries. Ohioensin F inhibits activity against protein tyrosine phosphatase 1B and suppresses TNF α–induced adhesion by inactivation of the MAPK, Akt, and NF-kappaB pathways in vascular smooth muscle cells, suggesting a promising application for treatment of atherosclerosis (Byeon et al. 2012).

POLYTRICHUM

Haircap Mosses Silk Wood Moss

Geographic Range: North America and throughout temperate and boreal latitudes in the Northern Hemisphere; the Pacific Islands; New Zealand; Australia

Habitat: cool conifer forests in raised and transitional bogs; near decaying wood and tree bases

Practical Uses: baskets, bedding, brooms, brushes, crafts, curtains, landscaping, mats, rugs

Medicinal Applications: amenorrhea, antibacterial, antibiotic, anticancer, antifungal, antipyretic, diuretic, hair, hemostasis, kidney stones and gallstones, menopause, mouthwash, prostate issues, uterine prolapse, vulnerary

The genus name *Polytrichum* derives from the Greek *polys*, "many," and *thrix*, "hair," due to its hairy calyptra. There are 40 accepted species.

Common haircap moss (*Polytrichum commune*) is a readily overlooked yet valuable plant from the forest floor. The genus refers to its appearance of having many hairs, hence in the doctrine of signatures it is beneficial for the follicle challenged. Traditionally, decoctions and oil extractions of haircap moss were used to strengthen and beautify women's hair. This was probably due to the suggestion of the long hairs on the calyptra that cover the capsule. German physician and botanist Leonhart Fuchs (1501–1566) writes in his book *De Historia Stirpium Commentarii Insignes* ("Notable Commentaries of the History of Plants"),

> A decoction of this plant in water or lye strengthens the roots of the hair, and, therefore, in cases of alopecia, cover the bald head with hair. As a potion, it helps considerably with the extraction of thick and viscous material from the chest and lungs; it breaks up stones and is diuretic. It is helpful in epilepsy and ailments of the spleen (Drobnik and Stebel 2021).

The *Polytrichum* mosses contain rare benzo-naphthoxanthenones. Investigative work on bog haircap moss, *Polytrichum strictum* syn. *P. affine*, as well as the moss *Pogonatum jamesonii* has been published by Basile et al (1999). Seven flavonoids were isolated from these two moss species and four other mosses. The flavonoids were the flavone apigenin, apigenin-7-0-triglycoside, lucenin-2, luteolin-7-0-neohesperidoside, saponarine, vitex, and the biflavonoid bartramiaflavone. Some compounds showed significant inhibition of *Enterobacter cloacae*, *E. aerogenes*, and *Pseudomonas aeruginosa*, all gram-negative bacteria. Another compound, luteolin 4'-neohesperidoside (L4N), inhibits four antibiotic-resistant bacteria including MRSA, *Klebsiella pneumoniae*, the shiga toxin producing the *Escherichia coli* serogroup, and *Bacillus cereus* (El-Shiekh et al. 2023).

Also, significant synergistic activity against gram-negative bacteria was noted in cases of the use of L4N in conjunction with common antibiotics. With *Bacillus cereus*, for example, a combination of the standard drug vancomycin with L4N was highly effective, despite the pathogen being vancomycin-resistant. In vivo evaluation showed significant decrease in *Klebsiella pneumoniae* and shiga-toxigenic *Escherichia coli*s shedding and colonizing. Renal and pulmonary lesions in lab animals were remarkably enhanced, with significant decreases in bacteria-infected tissue. The study suggests L4N as a potential substitute for or perhaps an adjunct therapy (author observation) with traditional antibiotics.

Hairy cap moss or haircap moss (*Polytrichum commune*) is found in coniferous forests, sometimes in the same area as *Sphagnum* species. The moss

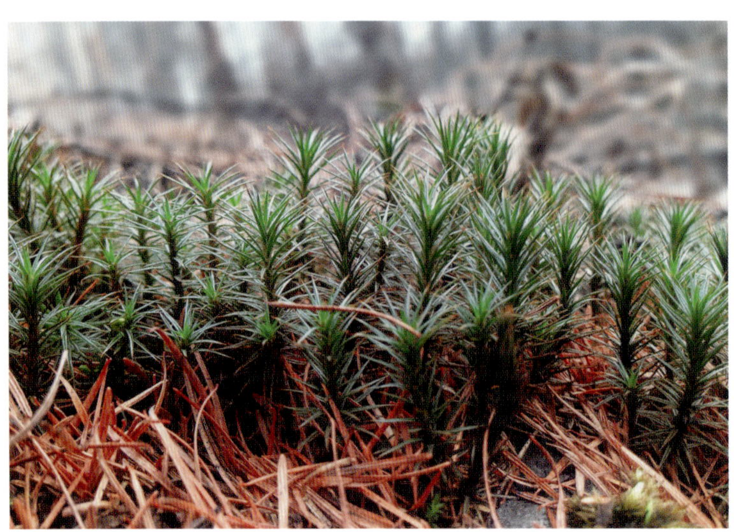

Polytrichum commune (Common Haircap Moss)

contains allantoin, sphagnol, silicon dioxide, communins A and B, benzonaphthoxanthenone, ohioensin A and H, 3-hydroxyphloretin oligomers, and methyl indoline-6-carboxylate (Fu et al. 2009).

Polytrichum commune essential oil's major constituents are biformene (13.6%), α-pinene (6.53%); and bornyl acetate (8.10%) (Yücel 2021).

Polytrichum commune is the best moss for craft projects. This could be a moss doormat, a traditional use in Scandinavia for wiping wet, muddy boots. It can also be used for making brooms, carpets, and sweeping brushes. I highly recommend Ulrica Nordström's book *Moss, from Forest to Garden* for more detailed instructions. She presents a plethora of ideas and great visual instructions to produce Saikei "planted landscapes" and a Kokedama "moss ball" for indoor enjoyment all year round.

The shoots and leaves of haircap moss are traditionally used by the Maori of New Zealand to decorate cloaks, alternating brown and black with *Polytrichadelphus magellanicus*, a Southern Hemisphere moss species (Beever and Gresson 1995). The Iroquois (the Haudenosaunee Confederacy, or "people of the long house") of eastern North America traditionally used this moss to treat wounds (Herrick 1995). Haircap moss is useful for quelling fever and to alleviate cuts and wounds by staunching the bleeding and encouraging clotting and regeneration of tissue. It also makes a useful mouth rinse in cases of gingivitis (Harris 2008).

In China, haircap moss is traditionally used to stop bleeding and night sweats associated with menopause. A tea made from this moss is used to treat uterine prolapse, which can affect bladder health and raise other concerns.

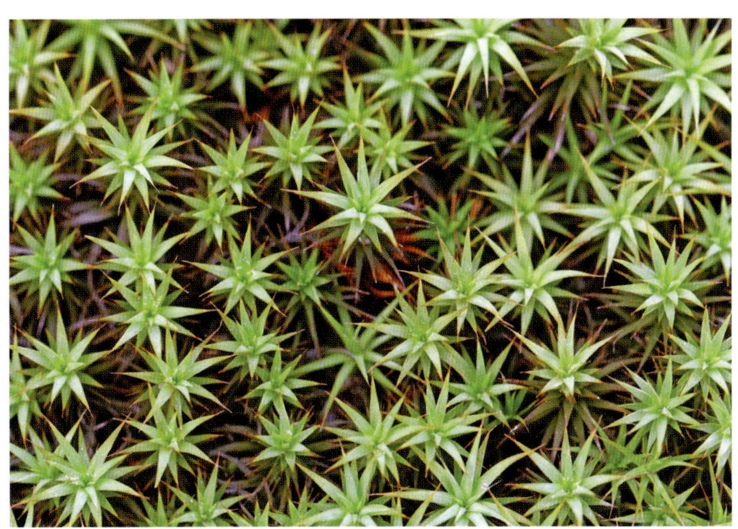

Polytrichum commune (Common Haircap Moss)

It is used in Traditional Chinese Medicine for fever, to staunch bleeding, for uterine prolapse, to address prostate concerns, and to treat lymphocytic leukemia. A tea made from the moss is also used to relieve and dissolve gallbladder and kidney stones (Chandra et al. 2017).

Eighteenth-century English priest and naturalist Gilbert White (1720–1793) wrote about "neat little bosoms which our foresters make from the stalk of the *Polytrichum commune*, or great golden hair, which they call silk wood, and find plenty in the bogs. When this moss is well-combed and dressed, and divested of its outer skin, it becomes a beautiful bright chestnut color; and being soft and pliant, is very proper for the dusting of beds, curtains, carpets, hangings, etc." (White 1837). In those former times, vegetable oil was mixed with the dry powdered moss, which has a hairy calyptra, for hair health (Glime 2013). Traditionally, *Polytrichum commune* was also used to make mats, rugs, and baskets. A partially finished *Polytrichum* basket dating from 86 AD was found during the excavation of an early Roman fort near Newstead, England.

The northern Scandinavian Sami use haircap moss for bedding. They select a large patch of plants, cut out an area, and separate them from the soil. This bed is rolled up and carried from place to place. In northern England it was once used to stuff mattresses and upholstery. Linnaeus recommended *Polytrichium* mattresses, as they didn't attract fleas and other pests.

Hairy cap moss was collected, dried, and combined with animal fat by the northern Cheyenne of Montana to relieve the pain of burns (Hart 1981). In New Zealand, the Maori weave the moss into their cloaks for insulation and

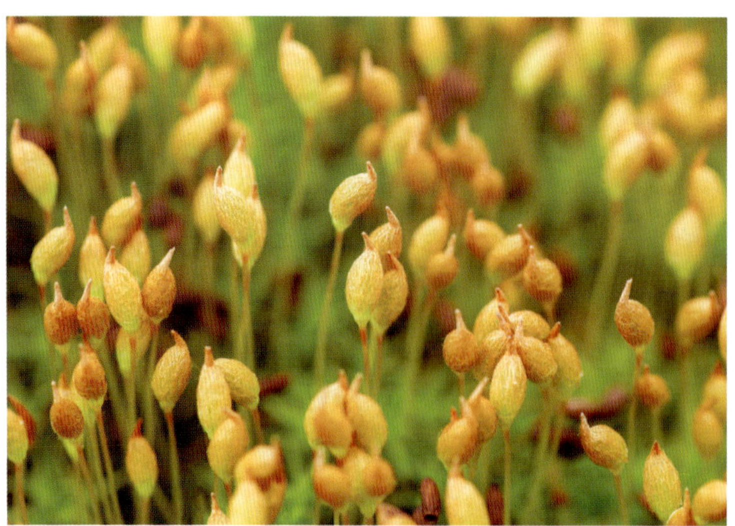

Polytrichum commune (Common Haircap Moss)

decoration. *Polytrichum commune* was used by the Nitinaht of Vancouver Island as a gynecological aid during pregnancy (Turner et al. 1983; Chandra et al. 2017). Women in labor would chew the moss stems to ease the pain of labor and speed up childbirth.

The spore-filled capsules of *Polytrichum* might be gathered and eaten as a survival food. Your author would probably prefer something else, or I would probably fast, which is a better survival strategy than nibbling on wilderness berries.

Allantoin, or 5-ureidohydantoin, a compound found in this moss, is also found in corn silk, comfrey, and other *Symphytum* species of flowering plants in the borage family. Allantoin is widely used in creams, salves, hand and hair lotions, and other skin-soothing cosmetics. The compound is a cell regenerator and inhibits collagenase, which causes collagen to break down. Recent work by Tzeng et al. (2022) examined allantoin's antioxidant, anti-inflammatory, and neuroprotective benefits. Allantoin was found to reduce abnormal hyperphosphorylation of tau, the microtubule-associated protein that forms insoluble filaments that accumulate as neurofibrillary tangles in Alzheimer's disease. This suggests this moss's potential for treating Alzheimer's and other neurodegenerative diseases.

Sphagnol is a common antiseptic found in nearly all mosses. In a 2022 study, moss extracts of *Polytrichum commune* that contain this compound inhibited *Bacillus cereus* and *Pseudomonas aeruginosa* (Rol et al.). When added to hand soap, which was then given to volunteers to wash their hands with, the results found significant reduction of microbials. This appears to be a much better solution than the antibacterial soaps currently on the market that contain triclosan, an endocrine disrupter that affects thyroid health. *Polytrichum commune* was widely used in sixteenth-century Europe. In Sweden it was called bear moss, as bears would use it to line their dens. Linnaeus wrote, "The bear collects this for his winter collection of berries." He also described how he cut two pieces of bear moss into a mattress and blanket with the mossy side against his body and claimed he slept better than in the softest of beds (Nordström 2019). Today it is used in Japanese bowl gardens and is sold in nursery squares to create checkerboard designs.

Extracts of the moss show activity against *Pseudomonas aeruginosa*, *Staphylococcus aureus*, *Bacillus cereus*, and *Escherichia coli* (Klavina et al. 2015; Belkin et al. 1952). Ethanol extracts contain 7,8-dihydroxy-5-methoxycoumarin-7-β sophoroside; p-coumaric acid; and minor amounts of benzoate derivatives and atraric acid, all of which shows antitumor and mitochondria-dependent cell apoptosis against cultured leukemia (L1210) cells, suggesting that Traditional Chinese Medicine's use of this moss for treating leukemia is based on empirical observation (Cheng et al. 2013).

Another compound found in this moss, ohioensin A, exhibits good binding to various pathways involved in treating osteoporosis (Liu et al. 2020). Ohioensin H did not show any cytotoxicity against five human cancer cells tested (Fu et al. 2009), however, communins A and B exhibit cytotoxicity against lung, hepatic, and gastrointestinal cancer cell lines, and demonstrate efficient activity against human breast cancer and human T-cell blood cancer cells.

An ethyl acetate extract was tested for cytotoxicity against a panel of leukemia cells in work by Yuan, Cheng et al. (2015), who found it triggers perturbations in intracellular homeostasis that regulate mitochondrial-dependent apoptosis. The extract is relatively rich in flavonoids (about 88.84%). This moss's anticancer and antimicrobial activities were also noted in a study by Klavina et al. (2015), wherein ethanol extracts exhibited moderate antiproliferative activity on six cancer cell lines.

A moss infusion of *Polytrichum commune* is traditionally used in China to dissolve kidney and gallbladder stones (Gulabani et al. 1974).

Newly found compounds in *Polytrichum commune* were investigated for their anti-neuroinflammatory activity against microglia cells, a type of glial cell located throughout the brain and spinal cord of the central nervous system (Guo et al. 2020). This protective effect may be due to the inhibition of compounds that promote the liberation of pro-inflammatory cytokines.

Recent work by Faleva et al. (2022) identified some dihydrochalcones in *Polytrichum commune* that possess high radical-scavenging activity. They possess low toxicity, leading researchers to suggest the possible applications as biologically active food additives and pharmaceuticals.

In the materia medica, this moss is mentioned as a treatment for prostate gland swelling and for amenorrhea (when the menses are absent). The latter is based on work by J. P. Bonnafoux, who in 1831 reported twelve cases of amenorrhea cured using an infusion of this moss in milk.

Extracts show antifungal activity against *Trametes versicolor*, *Botrytis allii*, *Fusarium bulbigenum*, and *Pyricularia oryzae* (Wolters et al. 1964). Neck rot is a postharvest disease in onions that occurs after storage. *Botrytis allii* is one of three members of the genus that cause problems for organic producers.

GREAT GOLDEN MOSS ESSENCE

This essence from *Polytrichum commune* anchors cosmic light into the second layer of DNA. It creates a powerful and magical linkage and connection with the Sacred Altars of the West and the places of true emotional well-being.

First Light Flower Essence of New Zealand produces No. 162, Great Golden Moss.

Another species, bank haircap moss (*Polytrichum formosum* syn. *Polytrichastrum formosum*) is common in cool conifer forests and in temperate rainforests of northern Europe and North America. Marques et al. (2021) extracted this moss with 70% ethanol and showed a dose-dependent inhibition of collagenase, which is associated with skin aging. A methanol extract showed mild inhibitory effect (44%) against tyrosinase, associated with inhibition of skin pigmentation. The responsible constituents are ohioensin A, and ohioensin C. *Nor*-ohioensin D was recently isolated by this same team, as was communin B. The results of their work indicate a potential application as a new, natural source of collagenase and tyrosinase inhibitors.

Polytrichum formosum exhibits strong antioxidant activity (Chobot et al. 2008). It also exhibits antibacterial activity against *Staphylococcus aureus*, *S. epidermidis*, *Bacillus cereus*, and *Escherichia coli* (Akatin et al. 2022).

In Turkey, extracts of the moss are used to repel the wheat weevil, *Sitophilus granaries*. The presence of compounds such as myristic, palmitic, and lauric

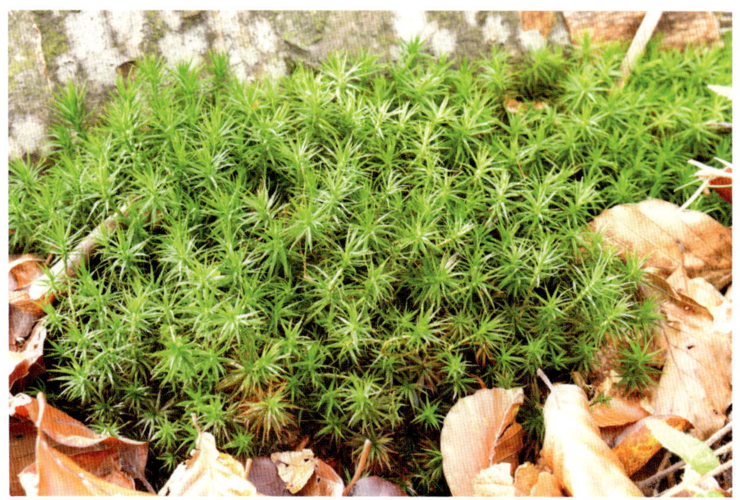

Polytrichum formosum (Bank Haircap Moss)

acids exhibit insecticidal activity against this common agricultural pest (Abay et al. 2013).

Work by Vollár et al. (2018) found various solvent extracts exhibit cytotoxicity against epithelial/cervical (HeLa) and ovarian (T47D) cancer cell lines.

Bank haircap moss possesses significant antioxidant activity (Smolinska-Kondla et al. 2022).

Bank haircap moss, *Polytrichum formosum*, along with nine other mosses out of twenty-three studied, exhibit good antimicrobial activity against *Paenibacillus* larvae isolates that cause American foulbrood diseases in honeybee larvae (Sevim et al. 2017). The other mosses showing benefit are *Polytrichum commune*, *Calliergonella cuspidata*, *C. lindbergi*, *Metzgeria conjugata*, *Isothecium alopecuroides*, *Syntrichia calcicola*, *S. montana* syn. *S. intermedia*, *Tortella densa*, and *Grimmia alpestris*.

Another species, *Polytrichum juniperinum*, commonly called juniper haircap moss, is found in coniferous forests, in raised and transitional bogs, and near decaying wood and tree bases. Its main attribute is as a powerful diuretic. According to Finley Ellingwood (1915), American doctor of eclectic medicine who was the author of the influential *American Materia Medica*, juniper haircap moss has been shown to remove twenty to forty pounds of water in a twenty-four-hour period in some people.

The northern Cheyenne used this moss species as a diuretic and to provide relief from prostate issues (Hart 1981). Taken as a strong infusion, it possesses very little smell or taste. It never produces nausea or any stomach issues. It is useful for removing uric acid and phosphate-based gravel from the system. It was traditionally taken as a tea for kidney and gallbladder stones and to treat common colds (Gulabani 1974). This should be noted by herbalists and naturopaths, as up to 80% of kidney stones are oxalic-acid based. Uric acid is also related to gout. This moss is effective in lessening urinary obstructions and suppression due to a chill or cold in the kidneys.

Ascites (fluid buildup as a result of cirrhosis), anasarca (generalized edema), and hydrops (fetal edema), especially of cardiac origin, are relieved with tea of *Polytrichum juniperinum* served at body temperature. Fever and inflammation are likewise treated with cool infusions of juniper haircap moss. Enlargement or inflammation of the prostate is helped by either an infusion or a tincture of this moss. This remedy is considered for old men suffering from bladder issues or an enlarged prostate or prostatitis. It may be safely used in dysuria (painful urination) associated with pregnancy and helps relieve urethra pain during urination.

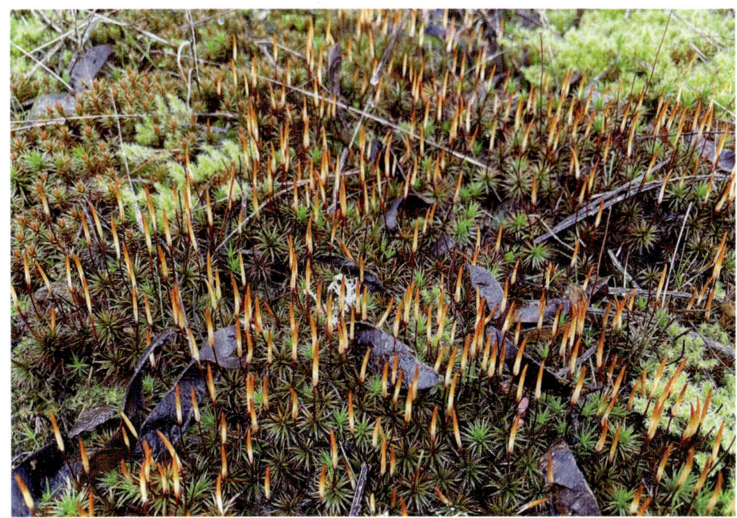

Polytrichum juniperinum (Juniper Haircap Moss)
Photo by Drew T. Henderson

Klavina et al. (2015) produced ethanol extracts and found the presence of 7,8-dihydroxy-5-methoxycoumarin-7-β sophoroside; atraric acid; 3-methoxy-4-hydroxybenzoic acid; and minor amounts of sphagnic, ferulic, and abscisic acids. Antiproliferative tests against six cancers were unimpressive, save for moderate activity against human lung (A549) cell lines.

Karpinski and Adamczak (2017) tested ethanol extracts of *Polytrichum juniperinum* against three gram-positive bacteria (*Enterococcus faecalis*, *Staphylococcus aureus*, and *Streptococcus pyogenes*) and two gram-negative bacteria (*Escherichia coli* and *Klebsiella pneumoniae*). They found the moss showed activity only against gram-positive bacteria.

In an earlier study, Savaroglu, Ilhan et al. (2011) found *Polytrichum juniperinum* active against five bacteria: *Bacillus subtilis*, *Enterococcus faecalis*, *Escherichia coli*, *Pseudomonas aeruginosa*, and *Staphylococcus aureus*.

Extracts of field-collected juniper haircap moss exhibit activity against *Bacillus cereua* and *Staphylococcus aureus*, and cytotoxicity against ovarian (CHO-K1) cancer cell lines (Ruiz-Molina et al. 2019).

This moss contains lunularic acid (also see the listing for the liverwort *Lunularia cruciata*, in chapter 2). It was used in the past for acute gonorrhea with severe burning pain upon urination. A case study recorded by Vermeulen and Johnston (2011) is given below:

> As in four days I shall be 81 years old [and] the most I can do is to make suggestions to others. Before I began the practice of medicine, *Polytrichum*

juniperinum was a domestic remedy for painful urination in old people, and I have made some sweeping cures with it [usually in the mother tincture], but generally considered it in inflammation of the bladder.

During my vacation in the country, I learned of a man of sixty-five who was living by himself and seriously ill. Being something of a "Samaritan," I visited him and found him suffering from prostatitis and bladder irritation. Sometimes [he] could introduce a catheter, other times he could not, and the doctor had given no relief. . . . I went to the field and gathered some of the moss [*Polytrichum*], told him to put the small quantity I gave him in one quart of water, steep it to one pint, and take one teaspoonful occasionally. . . . Three days later he said, "If I never feel worse than I do now I will never complain." Those who call me a "crank" for giving attenuated remedies ought to feel relieved now. To those who object to low preparations I will say it was all I could do, and I have ordered some attenuation made.

And a second case study by Vermeulen and Johnston:

I was called to see a lady of sixty-five years of age suffering from profuse bloody urination, apparently more blood than urine; with such excruciating pain she said she must die if not relieved soon. The pain was constant and so bad in her back that she was sure she had a serious kidney disease. Microscopic examination of the urine showed severe inflammation of the bladder, but no trouble with the kidneys. I gave her *Polytrichum juniperinum* mother tincture, four or five drops in one-half a glass of water, one teaspoonful once in two hours. In four days she was well and said every time she took a dose she felt better than she did two hours before. This is a sovereign remedy for painful urination of old people, when the disease is confined to the bladder.

The dried *Polytrichum juniperinum,* extracted with benzene yields 0.34% of an oil consisting mainly of a waxy ketone, 12-tricosanone.

Other *Polytrichum* species also exhibit cytotoxic activity. Ohio haircap moss, *Polytrichum ohioense*, contains ohioensins A–E, which in culture exhibit activity against murine leukemia (9PS) and certain human tumor cells, including breast cancer (MCF-7) (Zheng et al. 1993). The moss was also found to contain benzonaphthoxanthenones and bibenzyl derivatives that inhibit progression of melanoma (RPMI-7951) and glioblastoma multiforme (U-251) cancer cell lines

(Zheng et al. 1993). In an earlier study (Zheng et al. 1989), ohioensin A, derived from *Polytrichum ohioense*, exhibited activity against porcine kidney and human breast (MCF-7) cancer cell lines. Laboratory studies have shown extracts to possess weak antitumor effects against sarcoma 37 in mice (Belkin et al. 1952).

Mountain haircap moss (*Polytrichum pallidisetum*) contains three novel benzonaphthoxanthenones (ohioensins), 1-O-methylohioensin B; 1-O-methyldihydroohioensin B; and 1,14-di-O-methyldihydroohioensin B; and two novel cinnamoyl bibenzyls, pallidisetins A and B. Work by Zheng et al. (1994) tested the latter two compounds and found them to be cytotoxic against human melanoma (RPMI-7951), glioblastoma multiforme (U-251), and murine lymphocytic leukemia (P-388) cell lines. The compound 1-O-methylohioensin B is cytotoxic against human colon carcinoma (HT-29), human melanoma (RPMI), and human glioblastoma multiforme (U-251) cell lines. The compound 1,14-di-O-methyldihydroohioensin B inhibits lung (A549) and human melanoma (RPMI-7951) cancer cell lines.

The species commonly called bristly haircap moss, *Polytrichum piliferum*, has traditionally been used to stimulate hair growth and as a tea to encourage urination (Karpinski and Adamczak 2017). The researchers found activity against gram-positive bacteria.

Juniper Haircap Moss Tea

Decoct two ounces (60 grams) of dried moss in one liter of water down to half. Take four ounces at room temperature every eight hours or as needed. Stronger infusions are also effective.

Juniper Haircap Moss Tincture

One to two ml. of mother tincture three times daily. The mother tincture is made from the whole plant above ground of dry haircap moss.

JUNIPER HAIRCAP MOSS ESSENCE

Juniper Mist Moss Essence (from *Polytrichum juniperinum*) anchors cosmic light into the fifth layer of DNA. It creates a powerful, magical linkage and connection with the Sacred Altars of the West and the places of true emotional well-being. First Light Flower Essence of New Zealand produces No. 165, Juniper Mist Moss Essence.

RUBY FAIRY MOSS ESSENCE

This esssence (from *Polytrichum juniperinum*, red form) anchors cosmic light into the seventh layer of DNA. It creates a powerful, magical linkage and connection with the Sacred Altars of the West and the places of true emotional well-being.

First Light Flower Essence of New Zealand produces No. 167, Ruby Fairy Moss Essence.

BRISTLY HAIRCAP MOSS ESSENCE

This essence (from *Polytrichum piliferum*) helps one see goodness and beauty if one's thoughts have been negative. It gives another starting point and some rest.* This description is from the Mariana Essences company.

Homeopathy

The homeopathic remedy bank haircap moss from *Polytrichum formosum*, helps relieve eczema. A case study by homeopath Elisabeth Sehlinger, in Narayana Verlag's *Mosses and Ferns* (2021–22), helps one understand the benefits:

> A patient had severe eczema for twenty years along with recurrent vaginitis, colds, and abscesses of the sebaceous and lymph glands, as well as urinary incontinence with physical movement. She notes this person also had an electrical charge that messes up computers, drains batteries, and so forth. There is a fear of heights, crowds, and tunnels. She is a perfectionist but does not know her own needs or boundaries, is goal-oriented, very ambitious, and very sensitive about being ostracized.

The recommended dose is 30c to 200c.

The homeopathic remedy juniper haircap moss from *Polytrichum juniperinum*, is the go-to remedy for those who hold all their emotions inside. At times they feel they could explode but continue to suppress their tears. Crying is difficult, and oddly enough, frequent urination may provide an outlet for

*This essence is no longer commercially available. The Mariana Essences company, which is now Somos Life, is specializing in flower essences.

this emotional build-up. Painful urination often found in older people. Urinary obstruction, suppression, and prostatitis are all relieved by use of this moss.

The recommended dose is 5–10 drops of the mother tincture as needed in water (W. Boericke, 1927).

PSEUDOLESKEELLA

Nerved Leskea Moss

The genus derives from the Greek *pseudo*, meaning "false," and *leskea*, due to its resemblance to that genus. Four of the six species are found in North America.

Nerved leskea moss, *Pseudoleskeella nervosa* syn. *Leskeella nervosa*, shows antiproliferative activity against at least one of three hormone-sensitive cancer cell lines. Vollár et al. (2018) selected 42 bryophytes, including *Pseudoleskeella nervosa*, and did 168 water and organic extracts. The researchers then screened for activity against cervical/epithelial (HeLa), ovarian (A2780), and invasive ductal breast (T47D) cancer cell lines. Ninety-nine of the extracts derived from 41 species exerted more than 25% inhibition of at least one of the cancer cell lines at 10 µg/mL. Water extracts were found to moderately inhibit the breast cancer cell line, while only 19 samples of 15 taxa showed moderate antibacterial activity, with methicillin-resistant *Staphylococcus aureus* (MRSA) the most susceptible.

PSEUDANOMODON

Poodle Moss Slender Tail Moss Tree-Skirt Moss

The genus has only one species and is a member of the Neckeraceae family.

The cytotoxic agent ansamitocin P-3 has been isolated from slender tail moss, also known as tree-skirt moss, and poodle moss. *Pseudanomodon attenuatus* syn. *Anomodon attenuatus*. This compound is a polyketide antibiotic that shows potent cytotoxicity against human lung (A-549) and colon (HT-29) cancer cell lines (Suwanborirux 1990). It also shows cytotoxicity against murine lymphoma (P-388) cells after 48 hours. This compound was also found in *Thamnobryum subseriatum* syn. *Thamnobryum sandei*. Its cytotoxic action involves binding to tubulin at the maytansine-binding site to inhibit microtubule assembly, induce microtubule disassembly, and disrupt mitosis. Patents have been applied for its use in the treatment of gastric cancer and as an antitumor and antiviral drug.

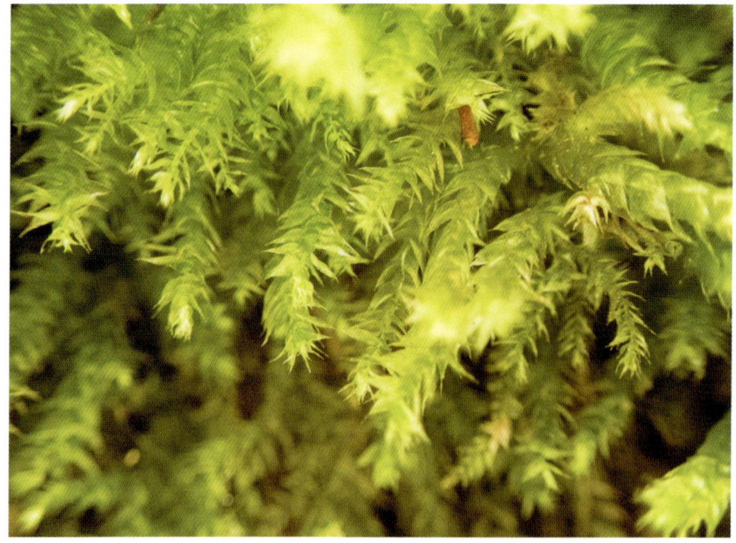

Pseudanomodon attenuatus (Tree-Skirt Moss)

PSEUDISOTHECIUM

Lesser Striated Feather Moss   Cat's Tail Moss

Lesser striated feather moss is epiphytic on tree trunks, branches, rock cliffs, and boulders at low to moderate elevations in Alaska, British Columbia, Alberta, Montana, Idaho, Oregon, and California in North America, as well as in Europe, Asia, and the Atlantic and Pacific Islands.

Pseudisothecium derives from the Greek *pseudo*, false, *isos*, "equal," and *theke*, "case," in reference to the symmetric capsule.

The Hesquiat of Vancouver Island use lesser striated feather moss, *Pseudisothecium stoloniferum* syn. *Isothecium stoloniferum*, for hand cleansing, probably after cleaning fish or game (Turner and Efrat 1982).

PSEUDOSCLEROPODIUM

Glasswort Hydnum Moss   Juicy Lucy   Neat Feather Moss

The genus name derives from the Greek *pseudo*, "false," added to the genus name *scleropodium*. There is only one species.

Neat feather moss was formerly used to stuff mattresses and pillows, most likely because many mosses are resistant to mold and act as insect repellants (Pant and Tewari 1989). Braids made from this moss and pieces from the *Neckera* and *Dicranum* species decorated ladies' hats in early Boston.

Neat feather moss (*Pseudoscleropodium purum* syn. *Scleropodium purum*), also called juicy Lucy and glasswort hydnum moss, was steam-distilled and analyzed by Tosun et al. (2015). The main compound in its essential oil is α-pinene (16.1%). The oil shows good activity against *Mycobacterium smegmatis*.

Work by Vollár et al. (2018) found solvent extracts exhibit cytotoxicity against epithelial/cervical (HeLa), ovarian (T47D), and breast (A2780) cancer cell lines.

Homeopathy

The homeopathic remedy neat feather moss from *Pseudoscleropodium purum* presents various themes in patients. When seeing a roadside, banishment and death marches may be envisioned. The patient drags themselves along, feeling responsible for companions, making superhuman efforts and having a strong will to survive. It is for people who have survived the worst and the children of such people, children who fight and don't give up. There is a love of life and physical and emotional stability years after a serious accident.*

PTILIUM

Knight's Plume Moss Ostrich-Plume Feather Moss

The name is derived from the Greek *ptilon*, "feather," alluding to its plumelike habit.

Ostrich-plume feather moss or knight's plume moss (*Ptilium crista-castrensis*) is found in sunny, mixed deciduous and coniferous forests having moderate humidity. The common names describe it well, as the fronds look identical to ostrich fern (*Matteuccia struthiopteris*) plumes.

Ethanol extracts contain 7,8-dihydroxy-5-methoxycoumarin-7-β sophoroside; and atraric, caffeic, sphagnic, abscisic, pimaric, and ferulic acids (Klavina et al. 2015). Abscisic acid is a hormone dating back to early living organisms, probably produced by early cyanobacteria. It is generally thought of as controlling plant growth, but nanomolar abscisic acid (ABA) controls the metabolic response to the availability of glucose in humans. It stimulates glucose uptake in skeletal muscles and adipose tissue that has an insulin-dependent process and increases energy use in brown and white adipose fat.

*Case study by Britta Dähnrich in Narayana Verlag's *Mosses and Ferns* (2021–22). Initial proving by Jan Scholten (2018, 172).

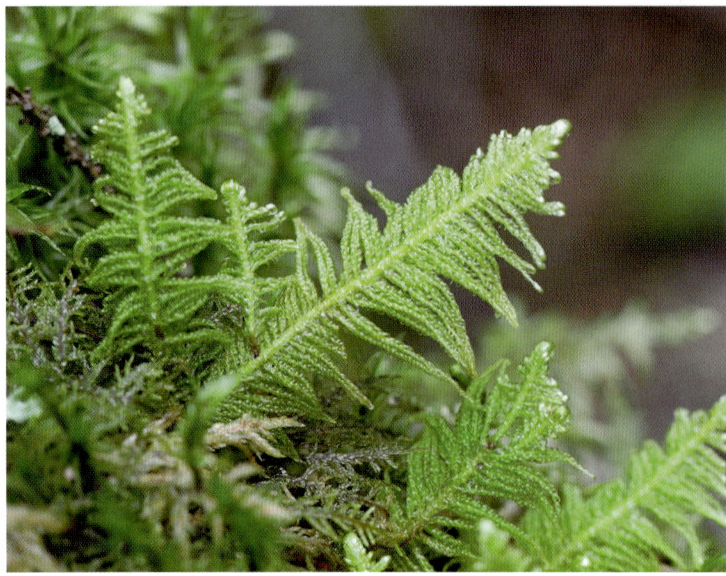

Ptilium crista-castrensis (Ostrich-Plume Feather Moss)

Work by Magnone et al. (2020) found micrograms per kilogram of weight of ABA improves glucose, blood glucose, lipids, and other factors in patients who are borderline for prediabetes and metabolic syndrome.

Klavina et al. (2015) found modest inhibition of rat glioma (C6) cancer cell lines.

PTYCHOMNION

Pipe-Cleaner Moss   Red Stem Moss

The Greek *ptychio* means "degree" or "diploma" while *mnion*, of course, means "moss." The common name derives from the dry appearance and prostrate, red stems of this moss. Maybe that's it. An academic degree or diploma is considered by some students as a "dry" form of education.

Pipe-cleaner moss, also called red stem moss (*Ptychomnion aciculare*) is one of the most widely known mosses, often found under beech trees in the Southern Hemisphere. It is ancient, as early fossils have been unearthed from Early Pleistocene sediments in western Tasmania.

RED STEM MOSS ESSENCE

This essence (from *Ptychomnion aciculare*) anchors cosmic light into the sixth layer of DNA. It creates a powerful, magical linkage and connection with the Sacred Altars of the West and the places of true emotional well-being.

It is available from First Light Flower Essence of New Zealand, as No. 166 Red Stem Moss.

PTYCHOSTOMUM

Tall Clustered Thread Moss

Tall clustered thread moss *Ptychostomum pallescens* syn. *Bryum pallescens*, was steam-distilled by Özdemir et al. (2010) and was found to yield an essential oil rich in nonanal (29.3%) and Z-phytol (8.9%), as well as various aldehydes (41.7%).

Ptychostomum creberrimum syn. *Bryum thomsonii* syn. *B. erythrinum* syn. *B. porphyroneuron* var. *giganteum* is used in the northwest Himalayas to heal wounds (Kumar et al. 2007). This moss is also used in Traditional Chinese Medicine and known as *juan ye zhen xian*.

PYLAISIA

Many-Flowered Leskea

The genus is named for French bryologist Auguste Jean Marie Bachelot la Pylaie (1786–1856). There are 15 recognized species.

Pylaisia falcata syn. *Stereodon falcatus* moss exhibits antioxidant activity (Téllez-Rocha et al. 2021). Falcata is derived from the Latin meaning "falcon-shaped" or "sickle-shaped;" a double-edged sword used in early times in Spain and Greece. The term was given for the moss's curved or hooked appearance.

The epiphytic moss many-flowered leskea (*Pylaisia polyantha*) grows on a wide range of trees, forming silky dense patches on bark. The exothecial cell walls are equally thickened, helping identification and separation from *Hypnum* species.

RACOMITRIUM

Fringe Mosses Rock Mosses

The name of the genus derives from the Greek *rhakos*, "rag" or "remnant," and *mitra*, "turban" or "little cap," alluding to the calyptra, which is split all around the base in some species, hence the common name fringe moss.

Racomitrium species can also be used to remediate diesel fuel spills.

Dense rock moss (*Racomitrium ericoides* syn. *Niphotrichum ericoides* syn. *Racomitrium ericoides*) and woolly fringe moss or hoary rock moss (*Racomitrium lanuginosum*) is a hardy, northern species. The moss was traditionally used by Indigenous people of Labrador, Canada, for lamp wicks (Bland 1971). Like many bryophytes, the species accumulate long-chain polyunsaturated fatty acids (l-PUFA) such as arachidonic acid (AA) and eicosapentaenoic acid (EPA). Work by Lu et al. (2023) examined the lipid composition of 39 species in Iceland and found the AA and EPA of six mosses, including *Racomitrium lanuginosum*, were abundantly distributed in the phospholipids and glycerolipids.

Work by Calder et al. (1986) found ethanol extracts moderately active against *Staphylococcus aureus*.

RACOPILUM

African Carpet Moss

The genus name derives from the Greek *rhakos*, meaning "rag" or "remnant," and *pilos*, "felt cap," alluding to the basally torn calyptra. About 44–63 species.

Racopilum africanum contains secondary metabolites that possess anti-inflammatory activity (Ayinke et al. 2015). Acetone extracts show strong inhibition of *Bacillus subtilis*, *Staphylococcus aureus*, and *Streptococcus pyogenes*, and ethanol extracts exhibit antifungal activity against *Microsporum gypseum* and *Aspergillus niger* (Oyesiku and Caleb 2015). *Microsporum gypseum* can cause inflammatory skin lesions such as tinea corporis, a fungal infection that is a type of ringworm in children and adults, companion animals, and even pandas.

RHACOCARPUS

Purple Rhacocarpus Moss

The genus name is derived from the Green *rhakos*, "rag" or "remnant," and *karpos*, "seed," referring to the raggedly split base of the calyptra.

Valarezo (2018) gathered, steam-distilled, and identified 94 constituents in 6 mosses found in Ecuador. The essential oil of *Rhacocarpus purpurascens* contains two main constituents, α cadinol (36.8%) and α-santalene (8.4%). Alpha-cadinol inhibits angiotensin-converting enzyme (ACE), involved in the formation of angiotensin II, which causes constriction of blood vessels and hypertension

(Tripathi et al. 2023). The compound, also found in common beans (*Phaseolus vulgaris*), exhibits more binding affinity for ACE than captopril, a drug used in the treatment of hypertension and some types of congestive heart failure.

RHIZOGONIUM

Thyme Leaf Moss

Rhizogonium distichum moss is endemic to New Zealand. The genus name *Rhizogonium* may derive from the idea that sporophytes appear to rise from the root, or rhizome, but in fact they are found on low stem branches at the base of the plant. The species' name derives from the plant's two-rowed insertion of leaves. Around 20 species have been identified worldwide.

The compounds dicranolomin (a biflavone) and five triluteolins (triflavones) have been identified. Two of the latter have been structurally identified and named rhizogoniumtriluteolin and distichumtriluteolin (Geiger and Seeger 2000). The other two are bartramiatriluteolin and strictatriluteollin, which exhibit inhibition of fungi and α-amylase, suggestive of antidiabetic activity (Yang, Lim et al. 2022).

RHIZOMNIUM

Common Hairy-Lantern Moss
Large Leaf Moss
Fan Moss
Thyme Mosses

The genus name derives from the Greek *rhiza*, "root," and *mnium*, "moss."

Fan moss or large leaf moss (*Rhizomnium glabrescens*) was traditionally used by Indigenous peoples of Canada for relief of blood blisters, boils, and breast abscesses (Harris 2008). Dotted thyme moss, also called thyme leaf moss and common hairy-lantern moss (*Rhizomnium punctatum*) is used for swelling by Native healers in the United States (Harris 2008).

THYME-LEAF MOSS ESSENCE

This essence (from *Rhizomnium punctatum*) evokes safe and potent embodiment. It increases our body consciousness so that we become aware of the living, breathing vitality of our physical self.

It is available from LightBringer Essences, a UK company.

RHODOBRYUM

Ariseamos Moss
Giant Bryum
Green Rose Moss
Rose Mosses
Rosy Thyme Tread Moss
Umbrella Moss

Geographic Range: nearly worldwide (except Antarctica) in temperate to tropical regions

Habitat: grasslands; sand dunes; rock ledges; around ant hills

Practical Uses: erosion control, beauty in shaded gardens, shelter for insects

Medicinal Applications: antiaging, antiangiogenic, anticancer, antidiabetic, antihypertensive, antimicrobial, antiobesity, antioxidant, antiproliferative, antipyretic, cardioprotective, diuretic, immune-modulating, neuroprotective, sedative

The genus name *Rhodobryum* derives from the Greek *rhodon*, "rose," and *byron*, "moss," alluding to the terminal leaf rosette. Virtually all species are found worldwide. Virtually all 19 accepted species are found worldwide, two in North America.

Rose moss or rose bryum (*Rhodobryum roseum*) is used in Traditional Chinese Medicine for angina and other cardiovascular conditions. It appears to protect the myocardium and cardiomyocytes. Ariseamoss is referenced from the Greek (Edwards 2012).

In parts of India, rose moss is used for sedation, neurasthenia, and cardiopathy (Asakawa 2007). Numerous studies on dogs and rabbits have been conducted in China on the prevention of atherosclerosis. Gao et al. (2004) investigated this moss for increasing blood flow and curing cardiovascular disease.

The related giant rose moss or umbrella moss (*Rhodobryum giganteum*) is antipyretic, diuretic, and anti-hypertensive, and is used for sedation, neurasthenia, psychosis, cardiopathy, and expansion of heart blood vessels (Alam et al. 2015). The Chinese know it as *hui xin cao,* meaning "return to heart herb," confirming its cardiovascular benefits, which are supported in early work by Wu (1977). It contains p-hydroxycinnamic acid and 7-8-dihydroxycoumarin, and a rat study found a 50% ethanol extract elicited a significant cardioprotective effect by lowering the levels of serum marker enzymes and lipid peroxidation. Somewhat later work by Wu (1982) found the extract, when given to white mice,

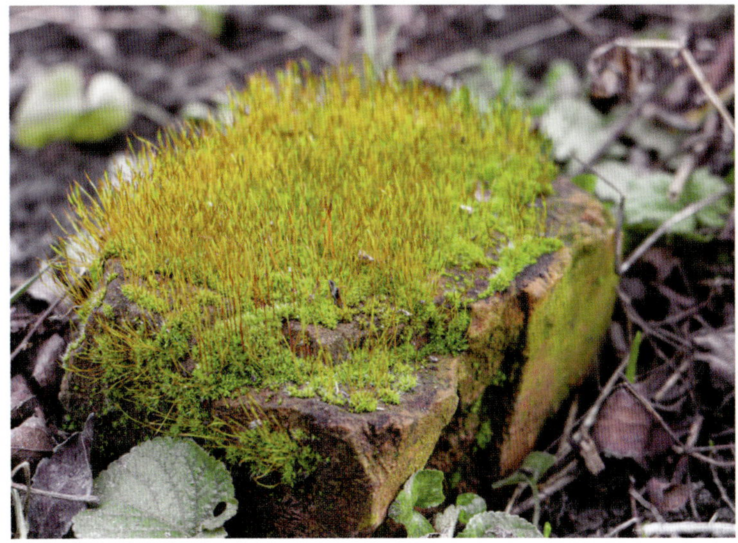

Rhodobryum roseum (Rose Moss)

reduced oxygen resistance by increasing the rate of blood flow in the aorta by over 30%.

Work by Sabharwal et al. (2023) found that *Rhodobryum roseum* syn. *Hypnum roseum* had activity against *Escherichia coli*, *Pseudomonas syringae*, and *Staphylococcus aureus*.

Two of the components of *Rhodobryum roseum*, piperine and methyl piperate, exert significant protective effects on cardiac myocytes (Hu et al. 2009). Piperine has been found to attenuate pathological cardiac fibrosis in a mice study (Ma et al. 2017). In fact, piperine, which is plentiful in black pepper (2–7.4%), is antiproliferative, antitumor, antiangiogenic, antioxidant, antidiabetic, anti-obesity, cardioprotective, antimicrobial, antiaging, and immune modulating (Ul Haq et al. 2021). As well, piperine is neuroprotective and inhibits acetylcholinesterase, indicating that it may be useful in the prevention or treatment of Alzheimer's disease (Khatami et al. 2020). Other compounds in *Rhodobryum roseum* are caffeic acid methyl ester; uracil glucoside; ursolic acid; 5α; 8α-epidioxy-methylcholesta-6; 22-dien-3β-ol and -methylcholesta-6,9(11); 22-trien-3β-ol; β sitosterol; and daucosterol (Wang, Liu et al. 2005). Ethanol and acetone extracts inhibit the bacteria *Athelia rolfsii*, the agent of "southern blight" disease in crops, and the fungus *Xanthomonas oryzae*, a serious pathogen on rice crops (Shivom et al. 2020).

A related species, *Rhodobryum ontariense*, is often mistaken for rose moss. If you count the leaves in the rosette you can tell the difference.

Rhodobryum roseum has 16 to 21 leaves in a single rosette, but *Rhodobryum ontariense* has 18 to 52. It too is a valuable cardiotonic moss. A study by Pejin, Bianco et al. (2012) found a total of eight fatty acids: 9,12,15-octadecatrien-6-ynoic acid (42.26%); α linolenic acid (20.32%); palmitic acid (14.31%); 9,12-octadecadienoic-6-*y*noic acid (13.31%); linoleic acid (5.25%); oleic acid (2.47%); and y-linoleic acid (0.92%). Two of these fatty acids have been found to possess cardioprotective activity: 9,12,15-octadecatrien-6-ynoic; and α linolenic acid. Though the researchers were unable to find the actual mechanism behind this moss's cardioprotective ability, their findings nevertheless support its traditional use for heart-related health concerns.

In a follow-up study, Pejin, Iodice et al. (2012) found additional benefits of *Rhodobryum ontariense* in the discovery of a new fructooligosaccharide sugar, 1-kestose, which acts as a prebiotic, helping improve healthy probiotics for gut health. Work by Tochio et al. (2018) confirmed this in that the researchers found 1-kestose promotes the growth of *Faecalibacterium prausnitzii*, which produces butyrate, a major metabolite of the gut microbiota that has many beneficial anti-inflammatory effects on metabolic health. And Endo et al. (2020) found in an in vitro human fecal batch culture model involving seven healthy adults, beneficial *Bifidobacterium longum* increased when fed 1-kestose.

A randomized, double-blind, placebo-controlled pilot study of 40 patients with mild to moderate ulcerative colitis involved giving 1-kestose or a placebo for eight weeks (Ikegami et al. 2023). The oral 1-kestose was well-tolerated and provided clinical improvement through modulation of the gut microbiome.

Sarcopenia is a deterioration of muscle mass (atrophy) that occurs in many seniors. Dysbiosis, which describes a disruption of the gut microbiome and a resulting imbalance, is associated with this functional disorder. To test the benefit of 1-kestose on elderly patients with sarcopenia, six seniors were given this unique sugar for 12 weeks. Not only did their level of *Bifidobacterium longum* significantly increase, but their skeletal muscle mass was greater, and their body fat percentage was lower (Tominaga et al. 2021). Watanabe et al. (2021) found that when 1-kestose was administered to obese-prone individuals, their fasting serum insulin level was significantly reduced compared to placebo. The researchers suggest 1-kestose supplementation has the potential to ameliorate insulin resistance in overweight people via modulation of gut microbiota.

Rhodobryum ontariense has been tested for heavy metal content (Pejin, Kien-Thai et al. 2012). Of particular note was the presence of organic manganese in the moss tea, which has traditionally been used to treat hypertension

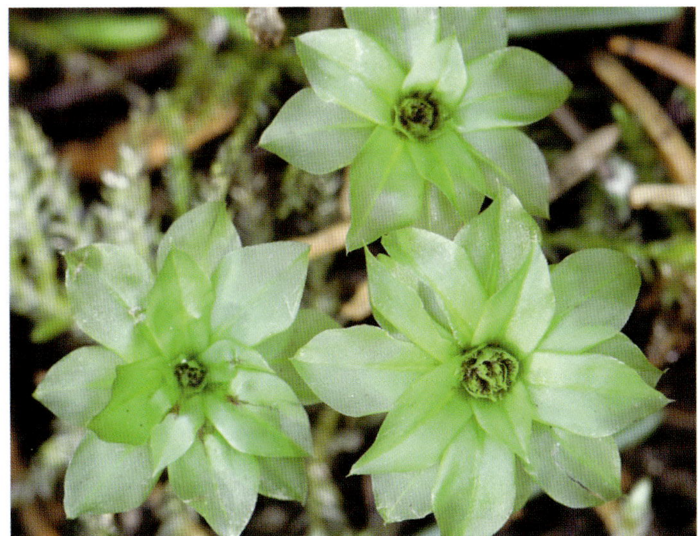

Rhodobryum roseum (Rose Moss)

and other heart disorders. This moss was gathered and hydro-distilled by Pejin et al. (2011). Thirteen compounds were identified, with the main ones being phytol (31.95%), a constituent of plant essential oils that often exhibits antimicrobial or cytotoxic activities; and 1-octen-3-ol (15.44%). Other minor constituents are cis-decahydronaphthalene, allo-hedycaryol, jasmone, and a carboxylic acid methyl ester. This amount of phytol is unusual for most mosses. Jasmone, of course, is found in jasmine essential oil and is both an attractant (for humans) and a repellant (for insects).

An endophytic fungus has been identified in *Rhodobryum giganteum*, umbrella moss. Work by Yang et al. (2020) found a number of constituents from a culture of *Botrysphaeria laricina*, a common pathogen of fruit trees that causes rot and decay. These include botrysphins G–I (isopimarane-type diterpenoids); 11,12-dihydroxylentiseusether (muurolane-type sesquiterpenoid); dechlorobotrysphone; 4,5-dihydroxy-3-methoxy-6-undecanoyloxy-2-cyclohexen-1-one; sphaeropsidin; lentideusether; and sphaeropsidone. Botrysphins G and H showed significant inhibitory activity of nitric oxide, a free radical.

Work by Hu et al. (2020) identified laricinin A; tricycloalternarenes X–Y; 3,4,7-trihydroxy-6-methylcoumarin; ethyl acetylorsellinate; diorcinol K; and tricycloalternarenes C–D. Tricycloalternarene Y and tricycloalternarenes C and D show significant quinone reductase activity in human hepatoma (Hepa 1c1c7) cancer cells. This was confirmed in a later 2017 study by Zhang et al., which identified botrysphones A–C, botrysphins A–F, as well as known sphaeropsidone, chlorosphaeropsidone, and sphaeropsidins A and B. Botrysphin D and sphaeropsidin A showed significant quinone reductase inducing activity against human hepatoma (Hepa 1c1c7) cancer cells.

RHYNCHOSTEGIUM

Feather Mosses

The genus name is derived from the Greek *rhynchos*, "beaked" or "nose," and stego, "cover" or "lid," referring to the rostrate opercula of the sporophyte.

Acetone extracts of *Rhynchostegium riparioides* (long-beaked water feather moss) were tested against 11 bacteria, including several pathogenic species, and found to be active against gram-negative bacteria (Basile, Vuotto et al. 1998).

Rhynchotegium serrulatum is found mainly in the Americas and able to grow under artificial light in areas devoid of natural sunlight. One example is the Niagara Cave in Harmony, Minnesota. It's a 60-meter-deep limestone cave with a 20-meter waterfall, complete with stalactites and stalagmites.

RHYTIDIADELPHUS

Electrified Cat's Tail Moss
Shaggy Mosses
Springy Turf Moss
Square Gooseneck Moss

Geographic Range: cool temperate and boreal zones in North America, Eurasia; Atlantic Islands; Pacific Islands; Australia

Habitat: lawns, golf courses

Practical Uses: art, bedding, clothing, insulation, wound healing

Medicinal Applications: anticancer, pain, vulnerary

Rhytidiadelphus derives from the genus *Rhytidium* and the Greek *adelfós*, "brother," alluding to the supposed close relationship between the two genera.

Rhytidiadelphus squarrosus is known as springy turf moss in the United Kingdom, while in the United States its name is square gooseneck moss. It is a grass-lover's worst nightmare, as it is the most common moss to invade the revered Kentucky Blue Grass. I say let it take over, as it will save you time and money, and will help protect the environment.

Rhytidiadelphus squarrosus was studied by Wolski et al. (2021), and extracts were found to exert a strong anticancer effect on mouse fibroblast line L929 at higher concentrations. Work by Vollár et al. (2018) found various solvent and water extracts exhibit cytotoxicity against epithelial/cervical (HeLa) and breast (A2780) cancer cell lines.

A similar species, little shaggy moss (*Rhytidiadelphus loreus*), was used by the Nuxalk (Bella Coola) for wounds, abscesses, and boils (Turner 1973). To survive extreme cold and retain cell fluidity, it accumulates various fatty acids. Little shaggy moss is the main species covering the grounds of the Bloedel Reserve's famous moss garden in Washington State.

Like many bryophytes, *Rhytidiadelphus* species accumulate long-chain polyunsaturated fatty acids (l-PUFA) such as arachidonic acid (AA) and eicosapentaenoic acid (EPA). Work by Lu et al. (2023) examined the lipid composition of 39 species in Iceland and found the AA and EPA of six mosses, including *Rhytidiadelphus loreus*, were abundantly distributed in the phospholipids and glycerolipids. Ethanol extracts are rich in 7,8-dihydroxy-5-methoxycoumarin-7-β sophoroside; atraric acid; and 4-hydroxybenzoic acid. Work by Klavina et al. (2015) tested the extracts against six cancer cell lines and found weak activity.

SPRING TURF MOSS ESSENCE

This essence, from *Rhytidiadelphus squarrosus*, is for those who fear the dark spaces within themselves. As with the childhood fears of darkness, many people fear the uncharted areas within their own beings. It is available through Yorkshire Flower Essences.

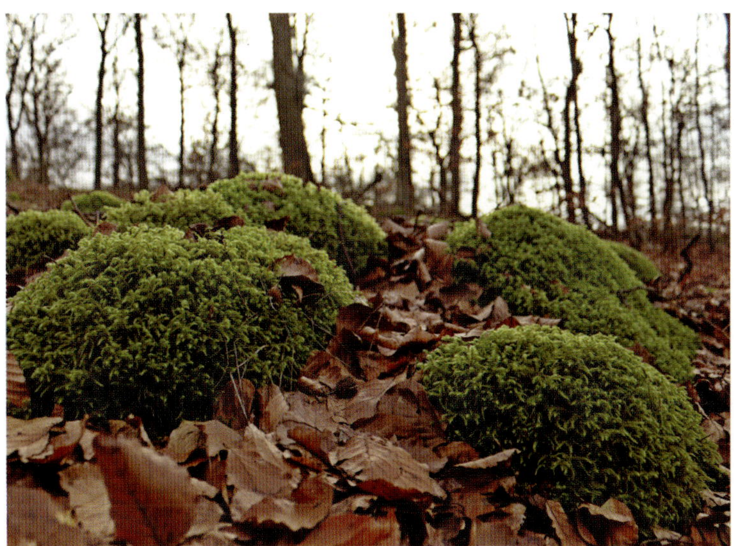

Rhytidiadelphus loreus (Little Shaggy Moss)

RHYTIDIUM

Crumpled-Leaf Moss Wrinkle-Leaved Feather Moss

Crumpled-leaf moss or wrinkle-leaved feather moss (*Rhytidium rugosum*) is common in my part of the world, northern Alberta, Canada. It is the only terrestrial moss in the region that has rugose leaves, hence the species name.

Work by Vollár et al. (2018) found various solvent extracts, including *Rhytidium rugosum*, exhibit moderate cytotoxicity against epithelial/cervical (HeLa), ovarian (T47D), and breast (A2780) cancer cell lines.

ROSULABRYUM

Capillary Thread Moss

Capillary thread moss has a cosmopolitan range, growing on dry grassland and rocks in dry areas. The common name derives from the leaves of the main rosette twisting in a spiral around the stem. There are 75–80 species worldwide.

Capillary thread moss (*Rosulabryum capillare* syn. *Bryum capillare*) was used externally by the Seminole of Florida for fever, fungal infections, and body pain (Sturtevant 1954; Harris 2008; Chandra et al. 2017). Other common names are descriptive of this bryophytes's appearance and habitat: rooftop moss, twisting thread moss, spiral web tooth, and screw bryum. This moss exhibits antibacterial and biofilm inhibition against *Staphylococcus epidermidis*

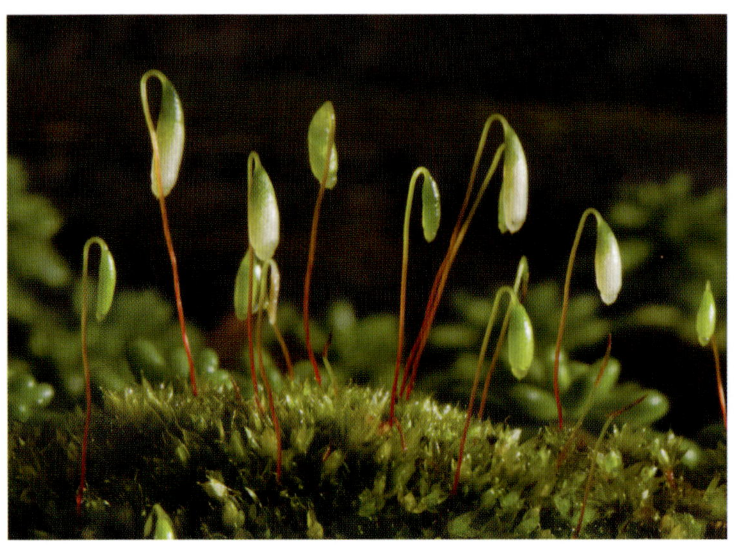

Rosulabryum capillare (Capillary Thread Moss)

and cytotoxicity against breast (SKBR 3) and cervical/epithelial (HeLa) cancer cell lines. Cytotoxicity against human mammary epithelial (MCF-12A) cells was mild (Onbasli and Yuvali 2021).

Various solvent extracts of *Rosulabryum capillare* inhibit *Bacillus cereus*, *Salmonella* sp., *Staphylococcus aureus*, and *Pseudomonas aeruginosa* (Elibol et al. 2011). The same study found *Plagiobryoides cellularis* syn. *Bryum cellulare* ethanol extracts active against *Escherichia coli*, *Pseudomonas aeruginosa*, *Klebsiella pneumoniae*, and *Staphylococcus aureus*. Distilled water extracts inhibited growth of *Escherichia coli* and *Salmonella typhi*.

Work by Deora and Guhil (2016) identified antifungal activity against *Curvularia lunata*, which causes seed germination problems in corn, rice, millet, and sugar cane. In humans, it is the main cause of phaeohyphomycosis, an opportunistic fungal pathogen that can severely affect immune-compromised individuals, those on steroid drugs (including transplant recipients), as well as AIDS and cancer patients. It is also implicated in asthma, rhinitis, sinusitis, and various bronchial infections. Ethanol extracts were found to inhibit various fungi, including *Aspergillus niger*, *Fusarium moniliforme*, and *Rhizoctonia bataticola*, at nearly two-thirds the rate of antifungal medication nystatin.

Recent work by Onbasli and Yuvali (2021) investigated *Rosulabryum capillare* and found poor activity against *Staphylococcus epidermidis* biofilm, but significant cytotoxicity against human breast (SK-BR3, 60%) and human epithelial/cervical (HeLa, 76%) cancer cell lines. However, the extract rated poorly against the breast cancer cell line MCF-12A (18%).

Syed's thread moss, flabby thread moss, or armpit (or hair) moss (*Rosulabryum moravicum* syn. *Bryum moravicum* syn. *B. laevifilum*) is found on living hardwoods as well as on rotting logs. Water extracts exhibit moderate antioxidant activity; one milligram showed the equivalent of 84 µg of ascorbic acid (Pejin et al. 2013). Work by Vollár et al. (2018) found solvent and water extracts of 42 bryophyte species, including *Rosulabryum moravicum*, exhibit cytotoxicity against epithelial/cervical (HeLa), ovarian (T47D), and breast (A2780) cancer cell lines. Water extracts did not inhibit the breast cancer cell line.

Marsh bryum, elbow-shaped thread moss, or triangular bryum (*Rosulabryum perlimbatum* syn. *Bryum pseudothyridium*) is a northern moss rich in fatty acids that maintain cell fluidity. Like many bryophytes, this moss accumulates long-chain polyunsaturated fatty acids (l-PUFA) such as arachidonic acid (AA) and eicosapentaenoic acid (EPA). Work by Lu et al. (2023) examined the lipid composition of 39 species in Iceland and found the AA and EPA of six mosses, including *Rosulabryum perlimbatum*, were abundantly distributed in beneficial phospholipids and glycerolipids. This moss also accumulates high concentrations of equally beneficial PUFA-containing triacylglycerols.

SANIONIA

Circle Leaf Moss   Sickle-Leaved Hook Moss

The genus was named by German bryologist Leopold Loeske (1865–1935) to honor Carl Gustav Sanio (1832–1891), a Prussian botanist and professor of botany at the University of Königsburg, best known for his work on wood anatomy, particularly the nature of compression wood. Five species are recognized.

Sickle-leaved hook moss or circle leaf moss, common names of the antarctic moss *Sanionia uncinata*, contains antioxidant and photoprotective activity against UV radiation. A residual water fraction from an extract absorbs the UV-visable spectrum, suggesting that *S. uncinata* presents a good potential for skin photoprotection against UV-radiation (Fernandes et al. 2019). The SPF was low (2.5), but the SPF values of benzophenone-3 and octyl-methoxycinnamate increased three and four times respectively in association with the water fraction. This moss also exhibits antioxidant activity equivalent to standard butylated hydroxytoluene (Bhattarai et al. 2008, "Antioxidant Activity"). Extracts are active against *Staphylococcus aureus*, inhibit acetylcholinesterase and are cytotoxic to breast and prostate cancer cell lines (Teodoro et al. 2024).

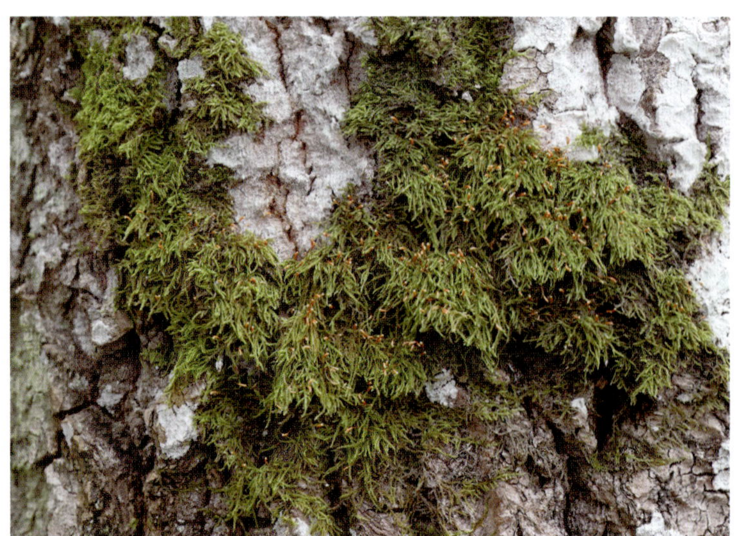

Sanionia uncinata (Sickle-Leaved Hook Moss)

The antarctic moss *Sanionia georgicouncinata* contains sanionins A and B. Work by Ivanova et al. (2007) found these compounds exhibit activity against gram-positive bacteria, mycobacteria, multidrug-resistant *Staphylococci*, and vancomycin-resistant *Enterococci*. Low cytotoxicity and anti-inflammatory activity were also noted.

SCHISTIDIUM

Grimmia Mosses   Steel Ring Moss

The genus name is derived from the Greek *schisto*, "divided," and the diminutive *idion*, alluding to the splitting of the calyptra at the base. *Schistidium* and *Grimmia* are members of Grimmiaceae family. The former are often found on rocks near water and the latter are more common in drier locations.

The antarctic moss *Schistidium antarctici* contains the endophytic fungus *Mortierella alpina*. Work by Melo et al. (2014) isolated high levels of polyunsaturated fatty acids (PUFAs), including gamma-linolenic acid and arachidonic acid, representing nearly half the total fatty acid content. The extracts demonstrated significant antioxidant activity and strong antibacterial activity against *Escherichia coli*, *Pseudomonas aeruginosa*, and *Enterococcus faecalis*.

Karpinski and Adamczak (2017) found thick point grimmia (*Schistidium crassipilum*) showed significant inhibition of *Streptococcus pyogenes*, *Staphylococcus aureus*, *Escherichia coli*, *Enterococcus faecalis*, and *Klebsiella pneumoniae*.

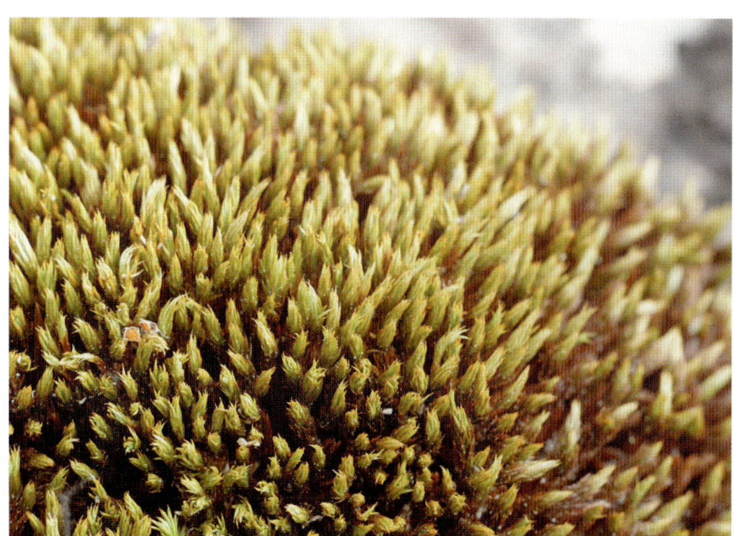

Schistidium maritimum (Seaside Grimmia)

Work by Vollár et al. (2018) found various solvent extracts, including those from *Schistidium crassipilum*, exhibit moderate cytotoxicity against epithelial/cervical (HeLa), ovarian (T47D), and breast (A2780) cancer cell lines.

Seaside grimmia (*Schistidium maritimum*), formerly known as steel ring moss in Sweden, is found along the coastlines of northern Europe, North America, and Asia. In fact, it is the only moss capable of living on rocks on the seashore, thriving despite saltwater spray and brackish water that other mosses cannot tolerate (Nordström 2019). There may be up to 120 species in the genus.

SCHISTOSTEGA

Gold Mosses Luminescent Moss

The genus name derives from Greek *schistos*, meaning "divided," and *stego*, "cover" or "concealed," alluding to the mistaken observation that the operculum splits.

Luminescence has been attributed to the cave-dwelling moss known as dragon's gold, goblin's gold, or luminescent moss (*Schistostega pennata*). This moss is able to grow in low light situations by using spherical cells in the protonema that act as a lens, collecting and concentrating whatever light is available. This gives the moss a greenish-gold radiance. It is found in caves in Asia, Europe, and North America.

Kimmerer (2003) writes a wonderful chapter on her adventures with goblin's gold in a cave.

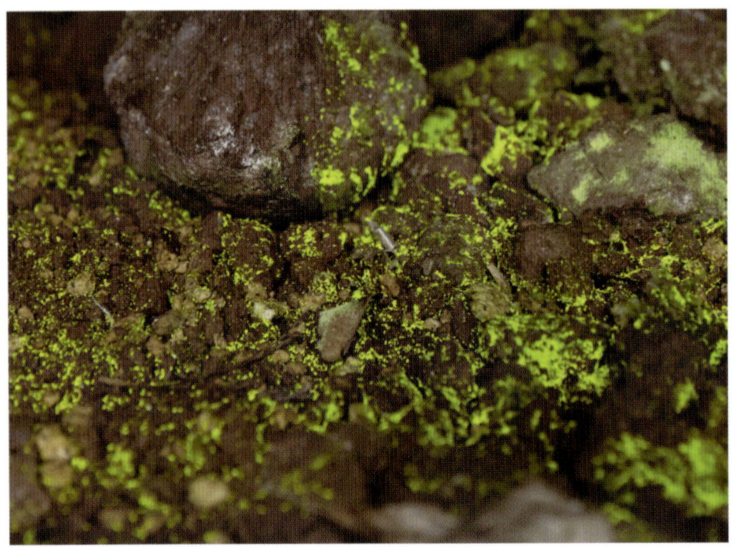

Schistostega pennata (Goblin's Gold)

According to a Japanese legend, this moss once saved a man's life. This myth has since become part of a Japanese opera. In Hokkaido, a monument to this moss is placed outside a tiny cave where the moss is abundant.

Austrian botanist Anton Kerner von Marilaun (1831–1898) wrote of goblin's gold,

> On the level floor of the cave, innumerable golden-green points of light sparkle and gleam, so that it might be imagined that small emeralds had been scattered . . . When it is brought into the bright daylight . . . one can easily understand how the legends have arisen of fantastic gnomes and cave-inhabiting goblins who allow the covetous sons of earth to gaze on the gold and precious stones, but prepare a bitter disappointment for the seeker of the enchanted treasure; that, when he empties out the treasure which he hastily raked together in the cave, he sees roll out of the sacks, not glittering jewels, but only common earth (von Marilaun 1863).

SCOPELOPHILA

Tongue-Leaf Copper Moss

The genus name may derive from the Greek *skopelos*, meaning "crag, " or the Latin *scopus*, meaning "target," and the Greek *philia*, meaning "fondness," alluding to its fondness for rocky habitats. Note that the name of the city of Philadelphia contains the same root, hence its famous moniker "City of Brotherly Love."

SEMATOPHYLLUM

Signal Mosses

The genus name derives from the Greek *sematos*, diminutive of *sema* meaning "mark" or "character," and *phyllon*, "leaf" (Dixon 1954). This is due to the distinct alar cells of the leaf structure observed in over 200 species worldwide.

Sematophyllum adnatum was used as a medicinal tea in the Yucatán, "suggesting an in-depth traditional knowledge of some of this moss's phytochemical properties and ecological features," according to Hernández-Rodriguez (2020).

Prostrate signal moss (*Sematophyllum demissum*) is found in certain confined areas of Asia, Europe, and South America, and is widely found in eastern North America. Work by Kirisanth et al. (2020) looked at six different air-dried

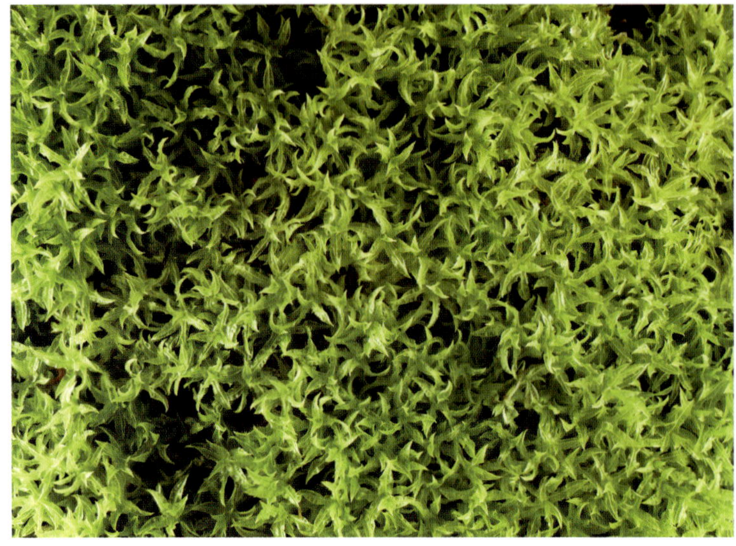

Sematophyllum homomallum (Bronze Signal Moss)

bryophytes, including *Sematophyllum demissum*, which were cold-extracted with three different organic solvents. They were screened against three bacteria and one fungus. Six out of eighteen were active against gram-positive bacteria, and two extracts were active against the fungal strain. Ethyl acetate extracts showed α-amylase inhibition in half of the mosses ranging from 8% to 30%.

SPHAGNUM

Ball White Moss
Bogmosses
Drowned Kittens
Peat Mosses

Geographic Range: worldwide

Habitat: acidic soil, bogs, marshes, peatland, sandy creek banks, wetlands

Practical Uses: bandages, clothing, environmental remediation, fermentation, conservation agent (art and archeology)

Medicinal Applications: anemia, antibacterial, anticancer, antifungal, anti-hepatic, anti-inflammatory, antipyretic, antiseptic, antiviral, aphrodisiac, cardioprotective, eyes, fertility, hemorrhoids, hemostasis, hypertension, immunomodulatory, neuroprotective, reproductive diseases, skin, vulnerary

Warning: Sporotrichosis can result from moss's exposure to a wound, causing fungal pulmonary and lymphatic infections.

The genus name derives from the Greek *sphagnos*, referring to a now indeterminate plant and applied by German botanist Johann Jacob Dillen Dillenius (1684–1747). There are about 300–380 species of sphagnum worldwide.

Sphagnum mosses contain terpenoids, flavonoids, essential oils, carotenoids, fumic and fulvic acids, sphagnol, and iodine. Various species contain unique minor constituents.

Sphagnum moss is sold in herb shops in China, where decoctions are used to cure acute hemorrhage and eye diseases.

Choi et al. (2014) found that because water extracts of peat moss exert anti-inflammatory and antioxidant effects, the result is a reduction of inflammation and prevention of cellular damage.

Work by Painter (2003) found sphagnum wound dressings three to four times more absorbent than cotton dressings. Such dressings react chemically against various proteins, thereby immobilizing whole bacterial cells as well as enzymes, exotoxins, and lysins secreted by various pathogens. This effect is due to the pectin complex in the cell wall of this moss, which is structured in a similar manner to the immune-enhancing pectin from tracheophytes.

Sphagnol extracted from peat moss is used for hemorrhoids and various skin problems such as psoriasis, eczema, and acne. A peat extract has been used successfully to treat ear infections in children as well.

Tolpa Peat Preparation (TPP) was invented and patented in 1994 by Polish botanist Stanislaw Tolpa (1901–1996). TPP was probably inspired by the use of peat in medicated baths and as poultices in Austrian health spas in the 1800s. This evolved into a branch of balneotherapy, or therapeutic bathing, in Europe by the 1950s (Drobnik and Stebel 2020). Nowadays the healing properties of hot peat baths are well known in health spas throughout Europe. From muscle injuries to infertility, peat baths are taken at high temperatures that would be close to scalding if the bath were simply water. In peat, heat is transferred molecule to molecule, not by convection the way it is in water. Thus, a temperature of 45–48° C can be tolerated, which would be unbearable to a person bathing in water. After thirty minutes in a peat bath, a patient's body temperature rises one degree, dramatically increasing circulation of blood to injured areas and reducing pain.

The antiseptic properties of peat tars date back to as early as 1902 with the use of distilled tars at an Irish peat-fueled generator. Peat moss was used extensively in military hospitals during World War I for fighting infections, and before that it was similarly used in the Russo-Japanese War (1904–1905).

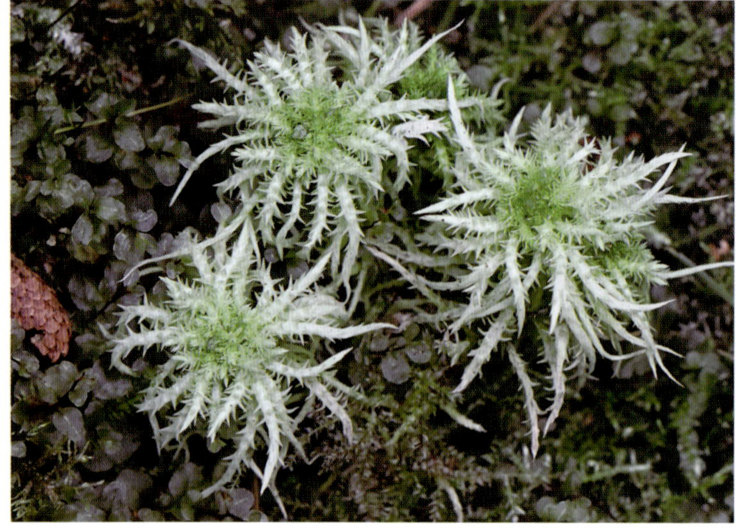

Sphagnum squarrosum (Spiky Bogmoss)

It is estimated that the British army used about a million pounds of dressings a month during World War I. The wounds healed better, with fewer infections than sterile surgical bandages, as sphagnum is cooler, softer, and less irritating.

Frahm (2004) tested alcohol extracts of 20 bryophytes, one of which was *Sphagnum* sp., for antifungal activity. He reported curing a fungal infection of the skin with a bryophyte extract. This success was reported on television, in magazines, and in a published book, with many people using the extract for their own fungal infections. Reputedly, one could cure athlete's foot by walking barefoot through a peat bog.

Polysaccharides, a pectin-like polymer isolated from sphagnum moss, comprise over 4% of sphagnan in dry weight. Work by Zaitseva (2009) found the extracted polysaccharides to be strongly acidic (pH 2.8) and soluble in water and various solvents. Antibacterial activity was noted for *Escherichia coli* and *Pseudomonas aeruginosa* (gram-negative strains), but not for *Staphylococcus aureus* (a gram-positive strain). The extracts were tested on 17 fungi isolated from ethnographic museum objects and archaeological objects excavated in the Canadian Arctic. Twelve species were susceptible. The application of sphagnan as a preservative agent in art and archeological conservation waxes was also tested. After three weeks' exposure of wax to *Aspergillus* spp., 44% of the wax was consumed, but when 0.1% of *Sphagnum* extract was mixed with wax, the weight loss was only 4% in the same time frame.

Work reported more recently in Ireland by Lewington (1990) has shown six *Sphagnum* species possess activity against both gram-positive and gram-negative bacteria. The antibacterial activity may be due to associated endophytes such as *Penicillium* species or associated cyanobacteria such as *Nostoc* spp. Maybe.

Sphagnum possesses the potential to immobilize bacterial cells, enzymes, exotoxins, and lysins secreted by pathogens. Once immobilized, they are inactivated by a Maillard reaction, a nonenzymatic reaction between sugars and proteins that occurs upon heating, an effect that produces, for example, the browning of some foods like meat and bread. Animal products preserved in peat bogs are due to the Maillard reaction inhibiting microbes by sequestering amino acids, peptides, and ammonia, so that the end products (melanoidins) inhibit growth. This process is due to cross-linking the polypeptide chains and sequestering essential multivalent metal cations. The preservative ability correlates with α-keto-carboxylate groups in sphagnan (glycuronoglycan), which is more than 60% of the holocellulose in the hyaline cell walls (Painter 2003). For example, the Maillard reaction is responsible for suppressing the virulence gene expression operon in *Listeria monocytogenes* (Sheikh-Zeinoddin et al. 2000). As a result, sphagnum peat has been investigated as a source of stimulants for microbial fermentation processes.

A medicinal product made from peat is Torfot, a Soviet preparation developed at the Filitov Institute of Eye Diseases and Tissue Therapy of the National Academy of Medical Sciences of Ukraine. Torfot's active constituents are probably phenols and amines. Its main application is in the treatment of ophthalmic conditions such as progressive myopia, myopic chorio-retinitis, opacification of vitreous humor, opacification of the cornea resulting from keratitis, and early retinal degeneration. For these purposes it is administered both topically and subcutaneously. More recently this product is being used to treat anemia, hepatitis, and various skin, nerve, and reproductive diseases. Tolpa Peat Preparation (TPP) uses are referenced in work by Piotrowska et al. (2000).

A drinkable peat bog preparation from Germany called Trinkmoor can be purchased online. It contains humic acid and trace minerals.

Of long-term importance may be derivatives of steroids and triterpenoids, with β-sitosterol and β-sitostanol accounting for half the steroids recovered from peat. The other half has been partially examined, with small amounts of estrone, estradiol, and estriol present. These may act as phytoestrogens.

In the 1920s, Rudolph Steiner suggested that substances made from peat could offer protection and healing to humanity. In the 1940s, Dr. Rudolph Hauschka, an Austrian chemist and inventor and the founder of the skin-care company that bears his name—and who was, like Steiner, an anthroposophist—began to manufacture peat products to help people suffering under chaotic environmental changes. This includes stress associated with electromagnetic radiation.

Solum uliginosum is an oil produced by collecting peat liquid, storing it in a dark incubating chamber for seven days, and then exposing it rhythmically to the rising and setting sun. It is then stored for two to three months to help dissipate the sulphurous odor. The remaining fiber can be carded and spun with silk or wool. Johannes Moss has a small factory located in Rydoebruk, Sweden, where he has harvested peat scraps and formed a fiber, which is woven into garments by a farming community for developmentally disabled aduts in Copake, New York.

Sphagnum peat contains fulvic acid that has been found useful in the prevention and treatment of allergies (Yamada et al. 2007). Peat also contains several humic acids that are active against the polio virus (Witthauer et al. 1976). Humic acid also shows antiviral activity against herpes simplex types 1 and 2 by interfering with the adsorption (that is, adhesion) of viruses to host cells (Klöcking et al. 1976).

Sphagnum moss inhibits the growth of *Sarcina lutea* syn. *Micrococcus luteus*, a gram-positive bacteria found in soil, the human gut, and elsewhere. It is rarely harmful except in immune-compromised persons and may prove useful in other applications. Norwegian researchers examined the bacteria in Trondheim Fjord and found it possesses a rare and highly sought-after pigment that can absorb long-wavelength UV radiation (in the range of 350–475) to provide the ultimate in skin protection. A patent has been applied for by Promar AS, a Norwegian fishing supply company, to manufacture and use the light-filtering substance extracted from this bacterium. It contains a particular carotenoid, sarcinaxanthin, which absorbs sunlight at exactly the right wavelength. The solar radiation is absorbed by the sun cream before reaching the skin. Known as UVAblue, it has been in commercial production since 2013.

Research in Lithuania by Jarukas et al. (2021) examined the composition of humic and fulvic acids and humin in black, brown, and light peat and sapropel. Sapropel is a thick sediment that is rich in fatty acids and waxes. The term is derived from the Greek *sapros*, meaning "putrefaction," and *pelos*, meaning "mud" or "clay." The highest amounts of fulvic acid (1%) and humic acid and humin (15.3%) were found in pure brown peat. The dominant organic compound was bis(tert-butyldimethylsilyl) carbonate, which ranged from 6.9% to 25.68% in peat extracts. The highest mass fraction of malonic acid amide was in the sapropel extract (12.44–26.84%). Significant amounts of acerohydroamic, lactic, and glycolic acids were also found.

When peat is extracted with potassium hydroxide, the result is 25.87% humic acid and 0.7% fulvic acid. Leonardite, an intermediate stage between peat and lignite, is less oxidized than soft coal and contains from 30% to 80% humic acid. This compound is named after geologist A. G. Leonard (1865–1932), who did early research on the substance. Leonardite is rich in humic acid, and improves the ability of crops to absorb nutrients, giving higher yields, faster growth, and healthier plants. Humintech, a company based in Grevenbroich, Germany, researches and produces various products sold to over 70 countries around the world.

Humic substances possess antioxidant activity. Work by Csicsor and Tombacz (2022) based on various extraction methods screened humic, fulvic, and himatomelanic acids for this activity and found that "the extraction method affects not only the physico-chemical properties, but also the free radical scavenging activity of the fractions."

Niewes et al. (2022) compared traditional alkaline extraction of humic substances found in peat with an ultrasound-assisted alkaline extraction method to gauge the efficient extraction of fulvic and humic acids. They found using peat as a raw carbon material for humic substances extraction using ultrasound technology provided higher efficiency.

Humic substances exhibit antioxidant activity similar to vitamins C and E (Klein et al. 2021). Moreover, peat moss humic acids are not only antioxidant but also cytoprotective in 3T3-L1 cell cultures associated with adipocyte formation, which plays a critical role in energy balance according to Zykova et al. (2022). The researchers conclude that "remarkable antioxidant and cell protective activity of humic acids makes them a promising natural source of new pharmaceutical substances that feature a wide range of biological effects."

Humic acid derived from bog peat increases the production of IL-4 and IL-10 and reduces production of IL-2 and IFN*y* by peripheral mononuclear cells taken from healthy donors, suggesting a beneficial influence on the development of the Th1/Th2 immune response (Trofimova et al. 2022). Earlier work by Trofimova et al. (2020) found that humic acid extracted from high-moor peat improves the humoral immune response in mice.

Natural humic substances possess activity against the HIV-1 virus when compared to water-soluble matter isolated from shilajit (Zhernov et al. 2021).

Fulvic acid contributes to cognitive health by preventing the accumulation of tau protein associated with Alzheimer's disease (Cornejo et al. 2011).

WATER MOSS ESSENCE

This essence from *Sphagnum palustre* helps when you are avoiding intimacy, appearing open and able to give, but only on a material and superficial level. The symptoms may manifest as intolerance toward others or appearing superior or aloof. Extreme cases may manifest as phobias, inertia, or reclusive behavior concealing weaknesses rather than confronting, revealing, and healing them.

Water Moss essence lets you learn to exist for yourself, moving away from survival as a way of being; it's all about communication. Throat, ears, thyroid, mouth, teeth, gums, and neck problems can all be eased. Realignment with this essence means reaching for the stars, uniting in spiritual goals, and experiencing a true feeling of belonging and an absolute sense of connection.* This description is from Olive Flower Essences.

Fulvic acid weakens resistin-induced adhesion of colorectal (HCT-116) cancer cells to endothelial cells (Huang et al. 2015).

This acid attenuates atopic dermatitis caused by type 2 helper T-cell inflammation. Work by Wu et al. (2023) found that the mechanism behind this organic substance derived from humus reduces symptoms and serum levels of CCL17 and CCL22, thereby providing anti-inflammatory, antibacterial, and immunomodulatory effects.

To investigate the anti-allergic effect of Canadian sphagnum peat and to test for inflammatory and allergenic responses, fulvic acid was extracted and purified from a sample and characterized by using an element analysis meter, Fourier transform infrared spectroscopy, electron spin resonance spectroscopy, and nuclear magnetic resonance spectroscopy (Yamada et al. 2007). The results showed that sphagnum peat may be useful for the treatment or prevention of allergic diseases.

Both humic and fulvic acids inhibit the human melanoma (A375) cell line, in part through cell-programmed death (Salehi et al. 2022).

*This product is no longer available commercially.

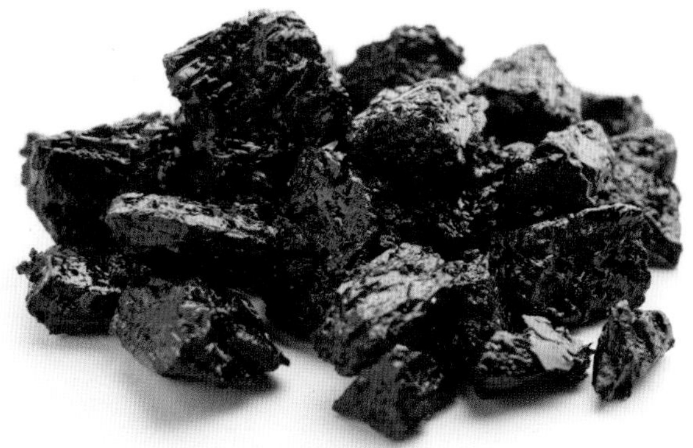

Shilajit, an organic mineral product of mostly biological origin

Shilajit, a powerful antioxidant, is a brown-black exudation from layers of rocks in mountain ranges around the world, especially in the Himalayas, and, like peat moss, is rich in fulvic and humic acids. It has been used in Ayurvedic medicine for thousands of years as well as in traditional Iranian medicine for the prevention of osteoporosis and improving bone health. Some people believe shilajit is not from an organic source, but of course it is. Coal, petroleum, oil, and natural gas are all organic by definition. Studies done on shilajit provide a good comparison with peat moss, which is also rich in fulvic and humic acids, hence shilagit is a good indicator of the properties of sphagnum moss.

A randomized, double-blind, placebo-controlled trial of postmenopausal women with osteopenia examined the benefits of this traditional Ayurvedic medicine. Sixty women aged 45–65 years with osteopenia were given one of three treatments for 48 weeks: a placebo, 250 mg of shilajit, and 500 mg of shilajit. Bone mineral density (BMD) of the lumbar spine and femoral neck were measured before, during, and at the completion of the investigation. In the placebo group, the BMD progressively decreased. The shilajit groups showed significant increased levels (Pingali and Nutalapati 2022).

Shilajit also shows potent antiviral activity against herpes simplex 1 and 2, human cytomegalovirus, and human respiratory syncytial virus. Both the extract and humic acid displayed a similar activity, including partial virus inactivation and interference with virus attachment (Cagno et al. 2015).

A randomized, double-blind, placebo-controlled trial by Pandit et al. (2016)

looked at testosterone levels in healthy male volunteers aged 45 to 55 years. A dose of 250 mg of shilajit taken twice daily for three months showed significant increased total testosterone, free testosterone, and dehydroepiandrosterone compared to placebo. Gonadotropic hormones levels were also well-maintained.

Shilajit possesses parasympathetic effects as well. A study on rat corpus cavernosum suggests this may be part of the mechanisms associated with its traditional role as an aphrodisiac (Kaur et al. 2013). Both men and women possess corpus cavernosum tissue, the former penile, and the latter clitoral. By relaxing the tissue, more blood flow can create better erections and clitoral engorgement.

Eight weeks of shilajit supplementation increased type 1 collagen synthesis, an important structural protein of skin, eyes, bones, ligaments, tendons, and muscles. Thirty-five athletic males were divided in a randomized control trial, and after eight weeks of supplementation there was a significant increase in levels of serum pro-c1*a*1, a biomarker of type 1 collagen synthesis (Neltner et al. 2022).

An animal trial found shilajit supplements potentiate the effects of chemotherapy drugs but mitigate the metastasis-induced liver and kidney damage in osteosarcoma (Jambi and Alshubaily 2022).

An alternative source of humic acid can be extracted from a "green source"—cow dung powder. This is a simple, cost-effective, eco-friendly source of humic acid (Barot and Bagla 2009). Yield is about 10%. Don't laugh too loud! Japanese scientists have found a way to extract vanillin from the same source, and it may be coming to an ice cream parlor near you.

Sphagnum cristatum is an alpine moss common in New Zealand at higher elevations. Work by Calder et al. (1986) found ethanol extracts moderately active against *Escherichia coli*. *Sphagnum falcatulum* is another species found in the Southern Hemisphere, in Australia and South America. The same group of researchers found ethanol extracts have significant activity against *Escherichia coli* and moderate activity against *Staphylococcus aureus*.

Ethanol extracts of flat-topped bogmoss (*Sphagnum fallax)* were tested against six cancer cell lines and showed antiproliferative activity against C6 (rat glioma) and mouse melanoma cancer cell lines (Klavina et al. 2015).

Wolters et al. (1964) found that solvent extracts of fringed bogmoss, *Sphagnum fimbriatum*, and pale bogmoss, *Sphagnum nemoreum*, show antifungal activity against *Coniophora cerebella*, *Trametes versicolor*, *Fusarium oxysporum* f.sp. *lycopersici*, *Fusarium bulbigenum*, and *Magnaporthe grisea* syn. *Pyricularia*

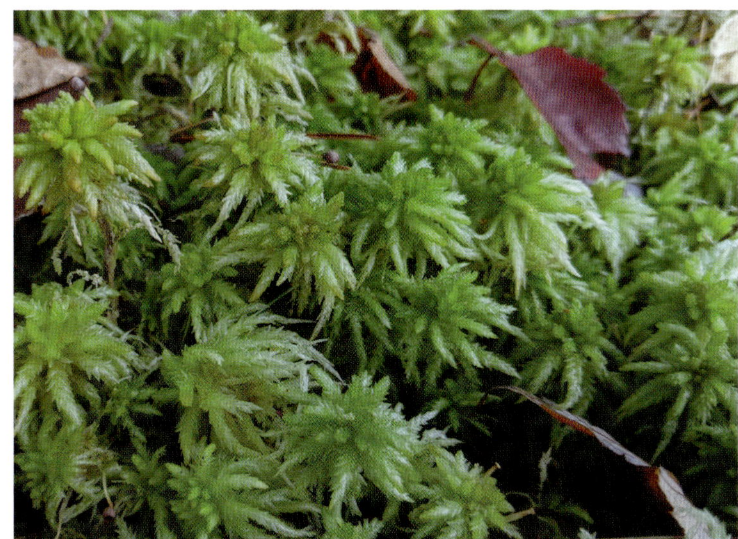

Sphagnum fimbriatum (Fringed Bogmoss)
Photo by Drew T. Henderson

oryzae. Joshi, Singh et al. (2022) found these mosses inhibit both fungi and bacteria and possess antioxidant potential as well. In a later study by Joshi et al. (2023), water-methanol compounds were found to have antiviral activity.

Fringed bogmoss, *Sphagnum fimbriatum*, has been traditionally used for hypertension, cardiac conditions, and as an antipyretic (Muhammad et al. 2018).

White-toothed peat moss (*Sphagnum girgensohnii*) is used for surgical dressings in China (Harris 2008; Pant 1998; Ando and Matsuo 1984; Ding 1982). The species name honors Gustav Karl Girgensohn (1786–1872), an Estonian bryologist and court counselor in Tartu.

Sphagnum junghuhnianum ethanol extracts were tested on five gram-positive and six gram-negative bacteria and eight fungi. Activity against virtually all the organisms was confirmed (Singh et al. 2007).

An ethanol extract of *Sphagnum magellanicum*, commonly called magellanic bogmoss or large-leafed red peat moss, was dried, weighed, and dissolved in distilled water. It was then tested against various gram-negative bacteria, including *Azotobacter vinelandii*, *Erwinia carotovora* subsp. *carotovora* (now *Pectobacterium carotovorum*), *Enterobacter aerogenes*, *Escherichia coli*, *Pseudomonas aeruginosa*, *Salmonella typhi*, and *Vibrio cholerae*; and against gram-positive *Staphylococcus aureus* subsp. *aureus* and *Streptococcus* group B (Montenegro et al. 2009). The extract also shows antibacterial activity against the bacterium *Pectobacterium carotovorum*, whose species name means "carrot-eater," which causes beet vascular necrosis and blackleg in postharvest potatoes.

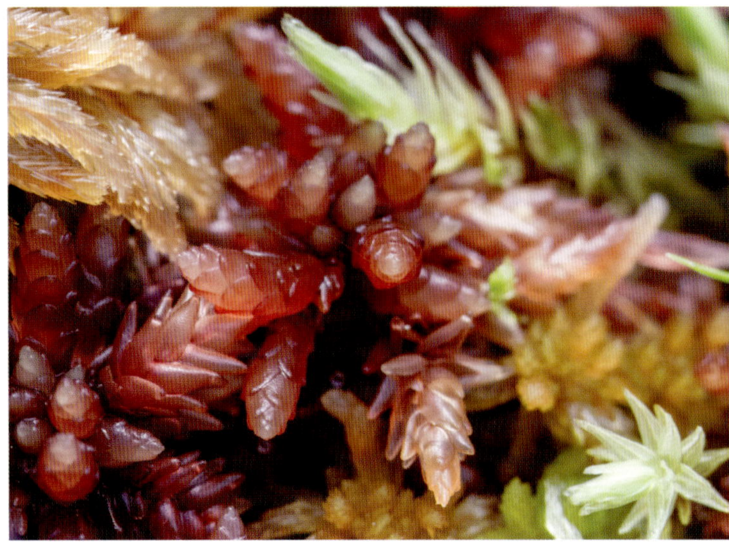

Sphagnum magellanicum (Magellanic Bogmoss)

Sphagnum magellanicum is mentioned by Harris (2008) and other bryologists as the main moss used by Indigenous peoples of Canada for sanitary pads, diapers, and home insulation.

Montenegro et al. (2009) studied *Sphagnum magellanicum* and identified vanillic, chlorogenic, syringic, caffeic, gallic, 3-4 hydroxybenzoic, p-coumaric, and salicylic acids. They also identified this moss's antioxidant activity. The investigation showed the growth of the cultures of the bacteria *Erwinia carotovora* subsp. *carotovora* and *Vibrio cholerae* were inhibited by ethanol extracts of this species, as were the cultures of *Escherichia coli*, *Salmonella typhi*, *Staphylococcus aureus* subsp. *aureus*, and *Streptococcus* type beta.

Bacteria associated with *Sphagnum magellanicum* and *S. fallax* were screened for antagonistic activity against a variety of human pathogenic fungi (Opelt et al. 2007). The team identified 493 bacterial isolates, with the majority in the genera *Serratia* (15%), *Burkholderia* (13.5%), *Staphylococcus* (13.5%), and *Pseudomonas* (10%). This suggests not only compounds with biological control of plant pathogens, but also possible benefit against opportunistic human pathogens.

Klavina et al. (2015) tested ethanol extracts of a dozen mosses, including four *Sphagnum* species, and found very significant antiproliferative activity against rat glioma (C7) and significant activity against human epidermoid (A431) cancer cell lines.

Blunt-leaved bogmoss (*Sphagnum palustre*) is used in China for surgical dressings and to treat eye diseases. Some other names for this common moss are rose peat moss, rusty peat moss, ball white moss, and drowned kittens. Not sure the origin of the last name.

Sphagnum portoricense and *Sphagnum strictum* mosses show antibacterial activity against *Staphylococcus aureus* and *Pseudomonas aeruginosa* (Madsen and Pates 1952).

Sphagnum quinquefarium inhibits *Botrytis cinerea* fungus found in wine grapes, as well as *Alternaria solani*, a fungal blight found in tomatoes and potatoes (Mekuria et al. 2005).

Both *Sphagnum rubellum* and *Sphagnum tenellum*, found in the middle and along the edges of bogs, respectively, were tested against six cancer cell lines and were found to exhibit antiproliferative activity against A549 (lung) and MCF-7 (breast) cancer cells in former, and C6 (rat glioma), A549 (lung) and $CaCO_2$ (colorectal) cells by latter (Klavina et al. 2015).

Lustrous bogmoss, brownish bogmoss, and plume-leaved bog moss are some of the common names of *Sphagnum subnitens*. Calder et al. (1986) found ethanol extracts of this species moderately active against *Escherichia coli*.

Rigid bogmoss or small squarrose peat moss (*Sphagnum teres*) is used in China for hemorrhoids and eye diseases (Ding 1982; Glime 2007).

Bryologist John A. Eastman points out an unusual feature of peat bogs, "Sphagnum bogs also produce methane gas: often a hollow rod inserted into a bog will nurture a flame. Small clouds of released methane sometimes spontaneously ignite, producing those mysterious, hovering 'bog-lights' or 'will of the wisps' seen over a bog at night" (Eastman and Hansen 1995).

Caution: Fungal-caused sporotrichosis is a hazard to nursery workers and sphagnum harvesters. Sphagnum species can be dangerous to use as a bandage, as pulmonary sporotrichosis (a fungal lung infection) can result. Be careful! The fungus believed to be responsible is *Sporotrix schenckii*. If the fungus enters a cut, it can create a slightly nodular sore in one to ten weeks. The fungus then travels through the lymphatic system, leaving a red streak and a series of nodules on the skin of the arms. In some cases it finds a way to the joints and bones. It can be treated with potassium iodide and antifungal medications, including *Usnea* (a genus of fruticose lichens) creams.

SPHAGNUM MOSS ESSENCE

This essence from *Sphagnum* spp. is for releasing the need for an unbalanced or harsh judgment of one's healing journey. It creates a space of unconditional acceptance in the heart so that core issues can emerge and heal. It is a call to life, helping one understand the evolving journey of life and inner growth. It is for those whose past is emerging with a fresh understanding and a release of deep core issues. It brings new levels of freedom and a greater expression of oneself.

It is available through Alaska Essences.

SPLACHNUM

Dung Mosses Petticoat Moss Yellow Mushroom Moss

Dung moss or petticoat moss is known for its entomophily, or insect pollination, commonly found on dung or dead, decomposing animals. The genus name derives from the Greek *splachnos* meaning "guts" or "entrails." The top of the dry plant's asexual spores is often red and wrinkled. The plant produces a fecal odor to attract coprophagic insects. There are 11 species identified at present.

Small capsule dung moss (*Splachnum ampullaceum*) is common in the boreal forest of North America and elsewhere. It produces a yellow or pink-colored hypophysis that releases volatile compounds to attract flies. An abundance of plastids have been found in the fly attractant which differentiate during moss maturation and form over 50 volatile oils including aromatic acetophenone and p-cresol (McCuaig et al. 2015).

Red parasol and yellow mushroom moss (*Splachnum rubrum* and *S. luteum*) are two of the most spectacular mosses of the north. They grow on

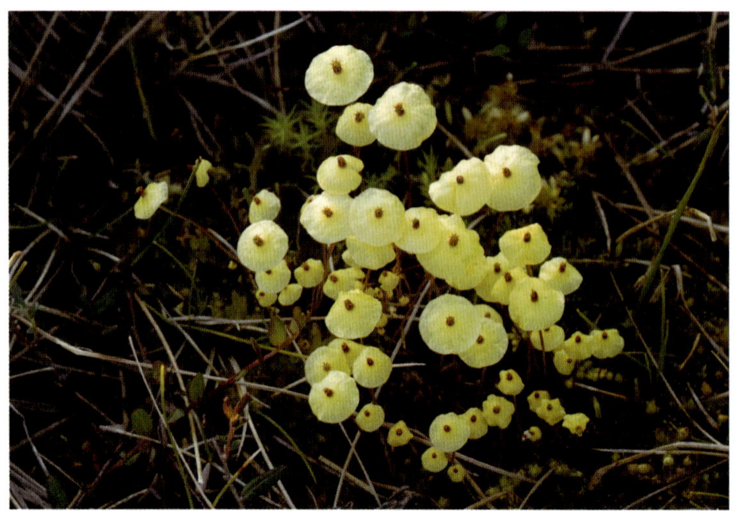

Splachnum luteum (Yellow Moosedung Moss)

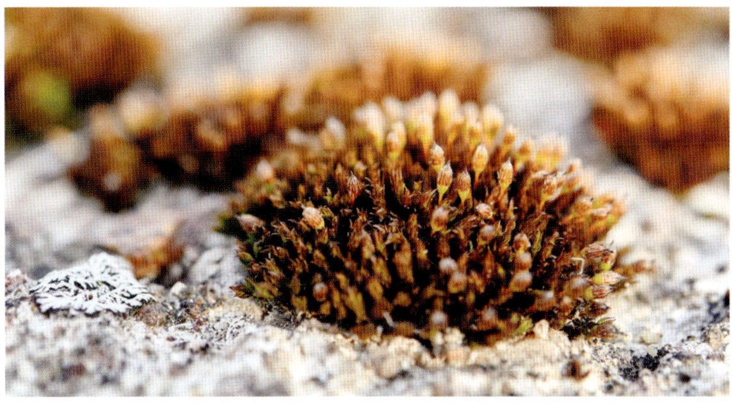

Splachum rubrum (Yellow Mushroom Moss)

moose dung in fens and bogs of the boreal forest and resemble fairy rings. Flies and mosquitoes use the caps as landing pads, attracted by the scent of ammonia and butyric acid, and help disperse spores to the next dung pile. Pretty clever! Red parasol or brilliant red dung moss is noted for its brilliant magenta-red sporangia.

Despite their source of nutrients, both contain interesting volatile oils including octanol, 3-octanone, 3-octanol, trans-2-octenal, 1-octen-3-ol, 1-octanol, and 2-octen-1-ol.

Splachnum rubrum has much higher levels of octanol, with the male gametophyte containing large concentrations of valeric and isovaleric acids.

SPIRIDENS

Noble Moss

Spiridens reinwardtii is a climbing, epiphetic forest moss that can reach up to three meters in length in southeast Asia, Australia, Philippines and other Pacific islands. The famous botanist William J. Hooker used the word "noble" in his description. The genus contains ten species.

STEREODON

Curly Hypnum Moss

Stereodon species grow in moist, shaded forests. Curly hypnum moss is native to northern California and in one isolated part of the San Francisco Bay Area.

Curly hypnum moss (*Stereodon subimponens* syn. *Hypnum subimponens*) contains two terpene synthases that exhibit antimicrobial activity on *Escherichia coli*, *Staphylococcus aureus*, and the plant pathogen *Pseudomonas syringae* which is virulent to tomatoes. The species name of the latter is derived from *Syringa vulgaris* (lilac tree) from which it was first isolated (Hu et al. 2021). This species is an atmospheric biological ice nucleator and found inside hailstones. It may be useful in the production of artificial snow.

SYNTRICHIA

Screwmosses Star Moss Twisted Moss

The genus name derives from the Greek *syn*, "plus," "together," or "joined," and *trichos*, "hair," alluding to the attachment of the hairlike peristome teeth on the bases to the inner membrane. There are 87 species worldwide, 10 in Canada.

In a 2017 study, both *Syntrichia calcicola* and *Syntrichia montana* syn. *S. intermedia* and 7 other mosses out of 23 exhibited good antimicrobial activity against *Paenibacillus* larvae isolates that cause American foulbrood diseases in honeybee larvae (Sevim et al.). The other mosses showing benefit were *Polytrichum formosum* and *P. commune*, *Calliergonella cuspidata* and *C. lindbergi*, *Metzgeria conjugata*, *Isothecium alopecuroides*, *Tortella densa*, and *Grimmia alpestris*.

Syntrichia caninervis syn. *Tortula caninervis* is the most dominant species, thriving on the soil crust of the Mojave Desert; on the arid soil of the Great Basin; and on the Columbia Plateau of Eastern Washington and northern Oregon, where intense solar heat and freezing nights provide challenging conditions for the survival of plants and where quartz rock sand blocks light transmission intensity down to 1.2%, helping the related *Tortula inermis* survive. In work by Ekwealor and Fisher (2020), *Syntrichia caninervis* was more likely to be found on the surface of desert soils, suggesting extreme desiccation tolerance. Plants that coat themselves in sand, which is known as psammophory, have a survival adaptation.

The essential oil of *Syntrichia intermedia* contains 9.9% E-2-tetradecen-l-ol, and 8.3% nonanal, as well as 18% aldehydes (Özdemir et al. 2010).

Twisted moss or star moss (*Syntrichia ruralis* syn. *Tortula ruralis*) gets its name for its unique twisted shape when dried out. Other common names suggesting the appearance of this bryophyte are sandhill screwmoss and great hairy screwmoss.

Syntrichia ruralis grows abundantly throughout western forests. It is being investigated by bryologist Melvin Oliver, adjunct professor of plant sciences at

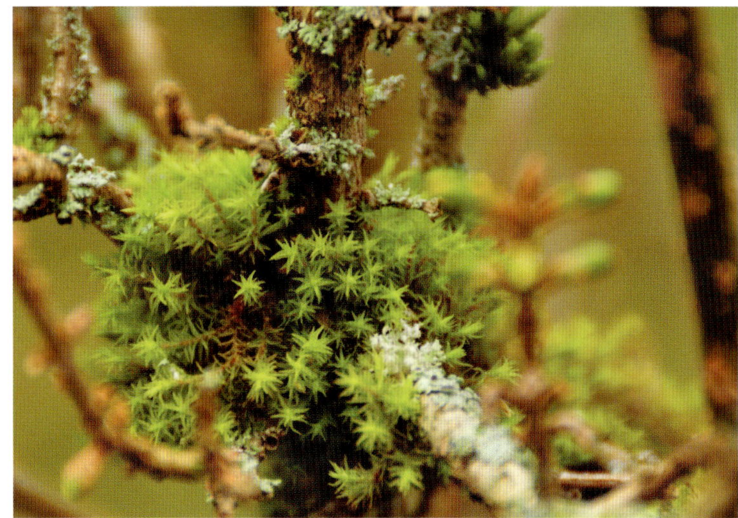

Syntrichia ruralis (Twisted Moss)

the University of Missouri, for its relatively untapped gene pool that may lead to more drought-resistant crops. As soon as a few drops of water are poured on *Syntrichia ruralis*, what seems like a brown Brillo pad becomes lush green with individual starlike branches (hence the common name star moss). Viewed through an electron microscope, the dry moss shows massive cell damage that is repaired within minutes. Oliver envisions lawns, rangelands, and pastures that could do the same. "We're talking about using genetic engineering to create a grass that can approach the capability of the star moss to completely dry up, turn brown, and recover quickly when it rains," he says.

Oliver reasons that clues to the drought-repair gene begin with those proteins that increase during the recovery period. He has found 74 proteins that increase significantly within two hours of rewetting. Oliver is pleased that what was once an academic interest of his while teaching and completing his Ph.D. at the University of Calgary may now change forever the meaning of crop drought tolerance.

Work by Özerkan et al. (2022) evaluated ethyl alcohol extracts of *Syntrichia ruralis* and four other mosses on 5-fluorouracil–resistant colorectal cancer lines (HCT116 and HT29). All bryophytes tested were found to possess cytotoxicity.

Work by Vollár et al. (2018) found various solvent and water extracts of *Syntrichia ruralis* exhibit moderate cytotoxicity against epithelial/cervical (HeLa), ovarian (T47D), and breast (A2780) cancer cell lines.

Karpinski and Adamczak (2017) tested ethanol extracts of *Syntrichia ruralis* against *Enterococcus faecalis*, *Klebsiella pneumonia*, *Staphylococcus aureus*, and *Escherichia coli.* They found the moss showed activity against only the gram-positive bacteria, *E. faecalis* and *S. aureus.*

Elibol et al. (2011) found ethanol and methanol extracts of *Syntrichia ruralis* to be active against *Escherichia coli* and *Salmonella* species.

Wolski et al. (2021) found an extract of *Syntrichia ruralis* stimulates human foreskin fibroblast line HFF-1 proliferation and skin wound healing.

This moss is used in Antarctica to monitor the ozone layer (Faburé et al. 2010).

SYNTRICHIA RURALIS MOSS ESSENCE

This essence from *Syntrichia ruralis* is useful when the soul is lost and disconnected, and receptivity is to be enhanced, and reconnection found. This is essential for the inner growth of the soul and our attunement to all life; it allows you to see life as you never have before.* This description is from Canadian Forest Essences.

TAKAKIA

Impossible Moss   Puzzling Moss

The genus name honors the Japanese bryologist Noriwo Takaki (1915–2006).

Takakia lepidozioides was originally classified in Marchantiophyta (liverwort) family. The *Takakia* genus has been reclassified, however, based on the resemblance of the male sporophyte of the related *Takakia ceratophylla* to that of some mosses. Moreover, the secondary metabolites of *Takakia lepidozioides* are eudesmane-type sesquiterpene lactones and hydrocarbons that are markers for liverworts. The Japanese name *nanjamonja-goke*, "impossible moss," alludes to its confusing identification. Knowing taxonomists as I do, it may take a few more decades to sort this out and of course help Ph.D students write a paper or two.

This moss is often found near rocks, waterfalls, and tundras in the Himalayas, Taiwan, Borneo, Japan, Alaska, and British Columbia.

Takakia lepidozioides produces a small amount of hop-22(29)-ene and coumarin, which release this moss' characteristic woody, piney, rustic, and earthy odor, characteristic in highly, hopped beer.

---

*This product is no longer commercially available.

This moss contains volatile compounds such as dihydrocoumarin; 1,4-hydroquinone; dihydrobenzofuran; α-asarone; and α tocopherol. This suggests it is more likely a liverwort than a moss (Asakawa et al. 2015). Time will tell.

TAXIPHYLLUM

Scale Leaf Moss

The genus name may derive from the Latin *taxus*, referring to the genus of coniferous trees known as yews; and *phyllon*, "leaf." Some authors believe it derives from the Greek *taxis*, "arrangement" or "rank," but in that case *Ditaxiphyllum* would be a more logical name, as the leaves are more or less two-ranked. Scale leaf moss (*Taxiphyllum taxirameum* syn. *Isoterygium geophilum* syn. *I. taxirameum*) is common in the southeastern United States and is the most common species in South America of the 59 found worldwide.

In India it is used for hemostasis and external wounds. It is anti-phlogistic, meaning it possesses anti-inflammatory properties (Alam et al. 2015). In Traditional Chinese Medicine it is used as a hemostat and to reduce inflammation (Du 1997).

TETRAPLODON

Skull Moss Slender Cruet

The genus name is derived from the Greek *tetraplo*, "fourfold," and *odon*, "tooth," alluding to the arrangement of the peristome teeth (Dixon 1954).

Slender cruet or skull moss (*Tetraplodon mnioides*) is used in Traditional Chinese Medicine to treat stroke, epilepsy, and to provide a sedative benefit (Ding 1982).

THAMNOBRYUM

Foxtail Feather Moss

The genus name derives from the Greek *thamnos*, meaning "bush" or "shrub," alluding to the untidy, bushy growth form; and *bryon*, "moss."

Foxtail feather moss (*Thamnobryum alopecurum*) was used traditionally to pack eggs before the invention of egg cartons (Nicholson 1914).

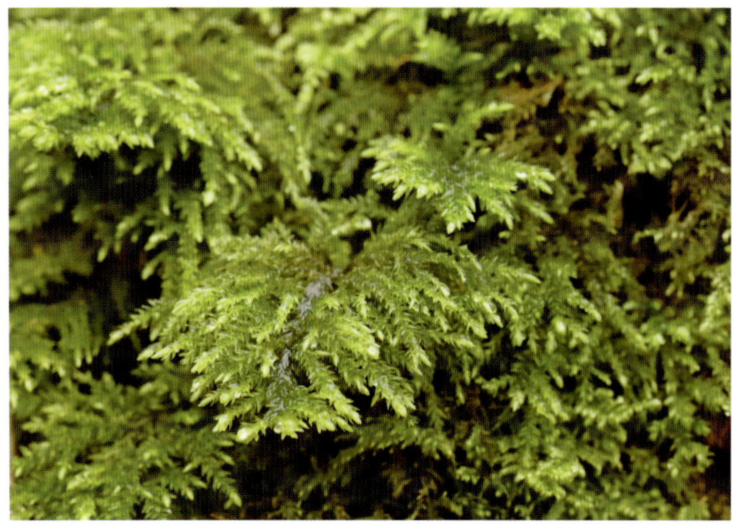

Thamnobryum alopecurum (Foxtail Feather Moss)

This moss is cytotoxic to several cancer cell lines. Work by Vollár et al. (2018) found various solvent extracts of *Thamnobryum alopecurum* exhibit moderate cytotoxicity against epithelial/cervical (HeLa), ovarian (T47D), and breast (A2780) cancer cell lines. Water extracts showed no inhibition.

The endemic Japanese moss *Thamnobryum subseriatum* contains maytansinoids 1, 3, and 4; and 15-methoxyansamitocin P-3. These compounds are potent cytotoxins (Sakai et al. 1988). Another compound, trewiasine, is cytotoxic against ascitic tumors, lymphoma (U937), murine cervical (U14), and Lewis lung carcinoma (Yue et al. 1992).

THUIDIOPSIS

Furry Thuidium

Furry thuidium moss is widespread in both forests and grasslands of Australia, New Zealand, and various Pacific islands.

Thuidiopsis furfurosa, formerly classified as *Thuidium furfurosum*, shows significant inhibition of *Staphylococcus aureus* according to Calder et al. (1986).

THUIDIUM

Delicate Fern Moss
Delicate Tamarisk Moss
Eastern Weft Moss
Log Moss
Philibert's Tamarisk Moss
Sheet Moss

Geographic Range: North America, Central America, South America, West Indies, Europe, Asia

Habitat: damp grasslands, heaths, moist acidic soil; a few species prefer calciferous soil

Practical Uses: mattress and pillow stuffing; moss garden

Medicinal Applications: antianxiety, antibacterial, anticancer, antidiabetic, anti-inflammatory

The genus name *Thuidium* is derived from a combination of the Latin diminutive *idium* and the genus *Thuja*, alluding to the feathery, branched fronds. In turn, *Thuja* is probably a corruption of what fourth-century Greek philosopher Theophrastus, in his *Enqiury into Plants*, called *thya*, referring to thyine wood, which in turn is derived from the Greek verb *thyo*, "I perfume," suggesting the use of cedarwood for incense. Over 230 species are found worldwide.

As Robin Wall Kimmerer says in her book *Gathering Moss* (2003), "Rural folks are more like *Thuidium delicatulum*—we need a lot of room and shady moisture to flourish, choosing to live along quiet brooks rather than busy streets. Our pace of life is slow, and we are much less tolerant of stress. In a city, that lifestyle would be a liability."

Various *Thuidium* mosses are used in China for their antibacterial and anti-inflammatory activity.

Extracts of eastern weft moss, *Thuidium cymbifolium*, were tested for inhibition against a variety of bacteria (Bodade et al. 2008). Ethanol extracts inhibited *Escherichia coli*, *Klebsiella pneumoniae*, *Proteus vulgaris*, *Pseudomonas aeruginosa*, and *Staphylococcus aureus*. Distilled water inhibited *Escherichia coli* to a larger zone than an ethanol extract. Various fungi were also susceptible to acetone, ethanol, chloroform, and distilled water extractions.

Delicate fern moss, *Thuidium delicatulum*, also called log moss, sheet moss, and delicate tamarisk moss is found in the Americas from Alaska to Brazil as well as Asia and Europe. The twice-branching pinnate plant with tiny leaves looks delicate but is very hardy. It makes an excellent choice for a moss garden.

Marques et al. (2022) investigated the beneficial anti-inflammatory effects of 32 species of bryophytes and found *Thuidium delicatulum* significantly inhibited nitric oxide production in LPS-stimulated RAW 264.7 murine macrophages. Other research by Altuner and Cetin (2009) found antibacterial activity against *Yersinia enterocolitica*, *Staphylococcus aureus*, and *Candida albicans*.

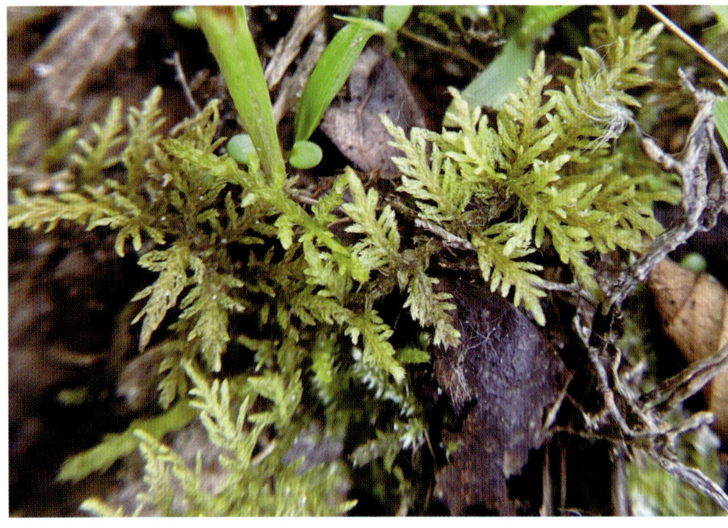

Thuidium delicatulum (Delicate Fern Moss)
Photo by Graham Steinruck

A growing concern is the explosion of insulin resistance, or type-2 diabetes, in which insulin continues to be secreted by beta cells in the pancreas, but blood sugar is not efficiently transferred to red blood cells. Lowering leptin levels is beneficial, as elevated numbers are related to the accumulation of body fat and weight gain. A 70% ethanol extract of *Thuidium kanadae* was given to mice fed a high fat diet (Shin et al. 2016). The researchers found the moss reduced blood serum lipid levels as well as insulin and leptin levels. Radical scavenging ability and the lowest antioxidant activity was found in the 70% ethanol extracts, while deionized water extracts exhibited higher antioxidant potential.

Valarezo (2018) gathered, steam-distilled, and identified 94 constituents in 6 mosses found in Ecuador, including *Thuidium peruvianum*, whose essential oil contains 21.7% phytol and 10.1% valerenol. The latter compound is also found in the medicinal herb valerian. In an earlier 2009 study it was discovered that valerenol enhances the response to GABA (A) receptors, exerting antianxiety behavior in a mice study (Benke et al. 2009).

Philibert's tamarisk moss (*Thuidium assimile* syn. *T. philibertii*) was examined by Vollár et al. (2018). The researchers found various solvent and water extracts exhibit moderate cytotoxicity against epithelial/cervical (HeLa), ovarian (T47D), and breast (A2780) cancer cell lines.

Pelekium schistocalyx syn. *Thuidium schistocalyx* syn. *Cyrto-hypnum schistocalyx* is decocted and cooled and used as a tea by the Chácobo of Bolivia to relieve headache (Boom 1996).

Tamarisk moss (*Thuidium tamariscinum*) is named for the leaf shape, which resembles the leaves of the tamarisk tree. In the Azores this moss was traditionally used to stuff pillows and mattresses, sometimes combined with the mosses *Pseudoscleropodium purum* and *Hypnum cupressiforme*. Work by Chobot et al. (2008) found this moss's extracts exhibit nitric oxide free-scavenging activity, while Mohandas and Kumaraswamy (2018) found its terpenoids exhibit antioxidant activity similar to ascorbic acid. Greeshma and Murugan (2018) showed that terpenoid extracts inhibited *Staphylococcus aureus* and *Escherichia coli* and showed remarkable antifungal activity as well.

LESSER TAMARISK MOSS ESSENCE

This essence from *Thuidium recognitum* is for the love of life. It is for nourishing the old places that have become crippled, bringing rebirth, growth, and joy. It brings a zest for living, discovery, and expansion, and the desire to seek and search for new paths. It fosters a trust in oneself to experiment and be open to the unknown.*

TORTELLA

Crispmosses Frizzled Screwmoss

Geographic Range: Western US, Western Canada, South America, West Indies, Europe, Africa, Asia

Habitats: moist, cool, upland slopes dominated by large coniferous trees and streams and lake banks in higher elevated boreal forests; sandy soil in rocky uplands, rockslides, and at the base of sandstone outcrops, cliff crevices, ledges, in drainage basins of lakes and rivers

Practical Uses: refuge for beneficial insects

Medicinal Applications: antibiotic, anticancer, antifungal, digestive, vulnerary

The name of the genus is derived from the Latin *tortus*, "twisted," and the diminutive *ella*, alluding to the characteristic twisting of the long peristome teeth.

*This product is no longer commercially available.

Dense crispmoss (*Tortella densa*) and nine other mosses out of twenty-three tested, exhibited good antimicrobial activity against *Paenibacillus* larvae isolates that cause American foulbrood diseases in honeybee larvae in a study by Sevim et al. (2017). The other mosses showing benefit are *Polytrichum formosum*, *Polytrichum commune*, *Calliergonella cuspidata*, *C. lindbergi*, *Metzgeria conjugata*, *Isothecium alopecuroides*, *Syntrichia calcicola*, *S. intermedia*, and *Grimmia alpestris*.

Side-fruited crispmoss (*Tortella squarrosa*) is decocted as a tea for stomachache in Mexico. The warmed moss is also placed on wounds (Hernández-Rodriguez 2020).

A tea prepared from side-fruited crispmoss (*Tortella* syn. *Pleurochaete squarrosa*) is traditionally used to relieve stomachache and applied as a compress to heal wounds (Hernández-Rodriguez and López-Santiago 2021).

An acetone extract was tested against 11 bacteria strains and found to be active against a few gram-negative strains (Basile, Sorbo et al. 1998). Work by Elibol et al. (2011) was more specific; this team found solvent extracts inhibited growth of *Bacillus cereus*, *Escherichia coli*, and *Saccharomyces cerevisiae*.

Frizzled crispmoss or frizzled screwmoss (*Tortella tortuosa*) is found on calcareous rocks in moist, cool, upland slopes dominated by large coniferous trees as well as on streams and lake banks in higher elevated boreal forests.

Tortella tortuosa extracts show activity against *Candida albicans* (Elibol et al. 2011). The moss contains palmitic, 4-hydroxy benzoic, salicylic, gallic, caffeic, and gensitic acids (Yaghuglu et al. 2017). Work by Özerkan et al. (2022)

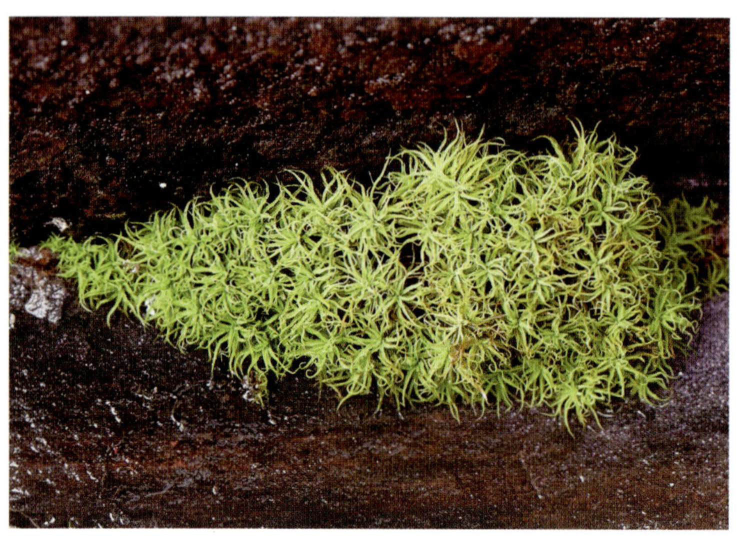

Tortella tortuosa (Frizzled Crispmoss)

evaluated ethyl extracts of this and four other mosses on 5-fluorouracil-resistant colorectal cancer lines. All bryophytes tested were found cytotoxic.

The bacterium *Bacillus atrophaeus* was isolated from *Tortella tortuosa* in a study by Aleti et al. (2016). It produces fengycins, iturins, and surfactins, all of which possess antifungal activity and can thereby protect tomato, lettuce, and sugar beets from *Rhizoctonia solani* infection. The researchers identified the variant surfactin C, which differs from surfactin A produced by *Bacillus subtilis*. The subtle difference gives varying signal strengths on biofilm formation and root colonization.

Savaroglu, Ilhan et al. (2011) found this moss active against three fungal species and five bacteria, including *Escherichia fergusonii*, a strain related to its more infamous cousin *Escherichia coli* and was named for William W. Ferguson, an American microbiologist. Some strains can infect open wounds and cause bacteraemia or urinary tract infections. They are highly resistant to the antibiotic ampicillin, and in some cases gentamicin and chloramphenicol.

Homeopathy

The homeopathic remedy frizzled crispmoss, from *Tortella tortuosa*, is for those quickly overwhelmed by stress. The person feels totally shrunken after being humiliated, degraded, and destroyed. The trauma makes them smaller and more compact. They may lack self-esteem. Jan Scholten (2018) notes the more shortsighted they are, the better this moss remedy will suit them.

The recommended dose is 30c.*

TORTULA

Screwmosses

The genus name is derived from the Latin *tortus*, meaning "twisted," which describes the spiral twisting of the peristome (Dixon 1954). An amusing, rather condescending name in this genus is pointless screwmoss (*Tortula inermis*).

The essential oil of summer screwmoss (*Tortula muralis*) contains nonanal (18.3%) and tetradecanol (4.3%) (Ücüncü et al. 2010). Along with three other mosses—*Homalothecium lutescens*, *Hypnum cupressiforme*, and *Pohlia nutan*—it was tested for antimicrobial activity against various bacteria and

*Case study is provided by Christina Ari in Narayana Verlag's *Mosses and Ferns* (2021–22).

fungi, including *Candida albicans* and *Saccharomyces cerevisiae*, with results showing antimicrobial activity only against the fungi.

Wolski et al. (2021) found that the moss extract stimulates human foreskin fibroblast line HFF-1 proliferation and consequent wound healing.

TRICHOSTELEUM

Hairy Moss

The genus name derives from the Greek *trichos*, "hair" or "hairlike," and *stele*, "pillar" or "column," alluding to the long, slender seta in about 200 species.

Trichosteleum papillosum is used by the Chácobo of Bolivia to relieve rheumatism (Boom 1996).

Trichosteleum species methanol extracts have been found to inhibit *Listeria monocytogenes*, *Escherichia coli*, *Bacillus cereus*, and *Pseudomonas aeruginosa* bacteria, as well as zucchini yellow mosaic virus in a study by Abdel-Shafi et al. (2017). When combined with tetracycline, the moss extract is antagonistic against the bacterium *Pseudomonas aeruginosa*. *Imbribryum* species are also synergistic.

WEISSIA

Green-Tufted Stubble Moss Pigtail Moss

The genus name is in honor of German botanist, lichenologist, and mycologist Friedrich Wilhelm Weiss (1744–1826). About 97 species to date.

Green-tufted, stubble moss or pigtail moss (*Weissia controversa* syn. *W. viridula*) is widespread. In parts of India a tea is prepared from this moss to treat intermittent fever (Asakawa 2007). It is also used for sinus inflammation, rhinitis, and as an antipyretic (Ding 1982), as well as a treatment for coughs and colds (Pant 1998).

WEYMOUTHIA

Mouse Ear Cress

The genus is named in honor of William Anderson Weymouth (1842–1928), an English-born botanical collector who lived in Tasmania. Upon arriving in Launceston, a town in the north of Tasmania, he worked on newspapers and later became an insurance agent.

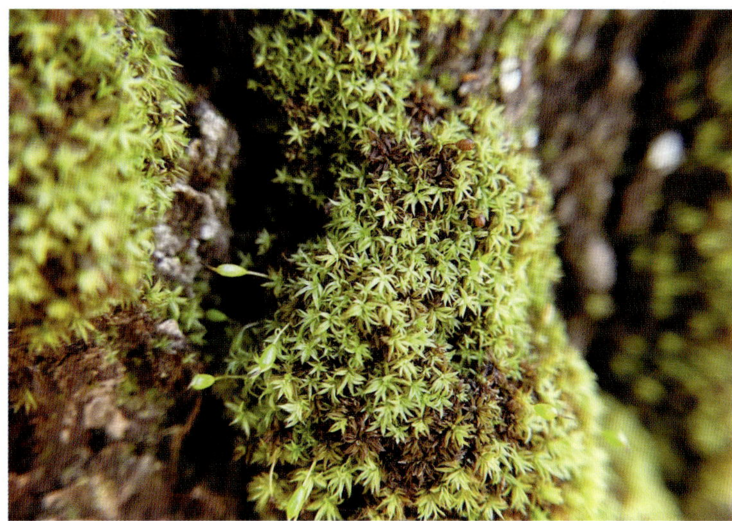

Zygodon sp. (Yoke Mosses)
Photo by Graham Steinruck

Mouse ear cress (*Weymouthia cochlearifolia*) is a Southern Hemisphere moss that is very common in Australia and South America. The species name is derived from its spoon-shaped leaves that resemble scurvy grass. Work by Calder et al. (1986) found ethanol extracts moderately active against *Escherichia coli.*

ZYGODON

Nowell's Limestone Moss   Yoke Mosses

Slender yoke-moss or Nowell's limestone moss (*Zygodon gracilis*) is one of the rarer mosses on the planet. It was first discovered and named after British bryologist John Nowell (1802–1867), who discovered it in 1860. It grows in isolated regions of Europe on dry limestone cliffs, and in one location on Haida Gwaii, British Columbia, as well as other locations in North and South America, Mexico, Europe, the West Indies, Asia, Africa, the Pacific Islands, and Australia. Just one square meter in size, it is listed as endangered in Haida Gwaii. John Nowell was believed to be the last person to see the moss fruiting, but research in England in 2003 examined 500 clumps and found 70% of these mosses were female, and they uncovered just one fruiting body. So it may not be too late!

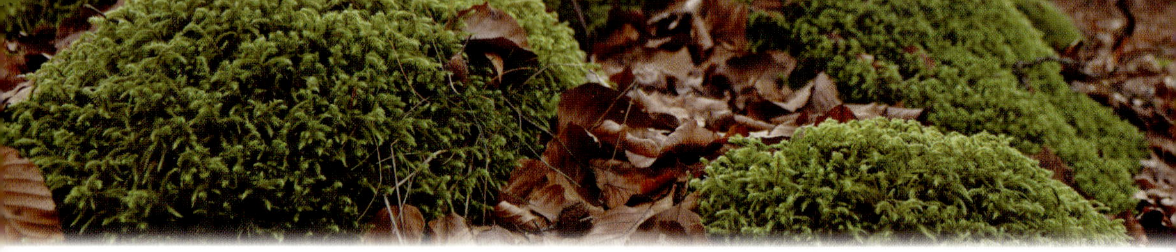

2 Liverworts

Marchantiophyta

With the advent of the autumn rains, the whole country quickly turned green,
And a profusion of liverworts such as I had never seen before,
Appeared on the green ground.

Douglas Houghton Campbell (1859–1953),
plant morphologist

GOOD LUCK, LOVE, AND MEDICINE

Liverworts are widespread globally but ignored by most laypersons walking through the woods. They should not be confused with the herbaceous perennial flowering plant genus *Hepatica*, sometimes misleadingly referred to as a liverwort but is actually an herbaceous perennial in the buttercup family. Almost all liverworts possess beautiful blue, yellow, colored, and colorless essential oil bodies with hundreds of terpenoids, acetogenins, and other aromatic compounds, including flavonoids with more than 40 new carbon skeletons.

Liverworts have a cellular oil body that produces an abundance of aromatic compounds, with many of the sesquiterpene and diterpenoid enantiomers (a pair of chemical compounds whose molecular structures have a mirror-image relationship to each other) of those found in "higher" plants. The aromatic compounds bibenzyl and bisbenzyl are rich in liverworts. Bibenzyls are steroidal ethane derivatives that resemble the structure of bioactive dihydro-stilbenoids or iso-quinolone alkaloids. They form mainly as secondary metabolites as a byproduct of the flavonoid biosynthetic pathway. They have numerous biological activities and possess antimicrobial, antifungal, antiviral, cytotoxic, insecticidal, and muscle-relaxing benefits.

Liverworts contain oil cells that exhibit remarkable essential oil capacity. In fact, some liverworts produce female sex pheromones that are also present in brown algae. Brown algae female gametes release sex pheromones, such as fruit-scented ectocarpene—that can be detected by humans when emitted into the ocean—to attract male gametes for reproduction and fertilization. Ectocarpene is also found in *Capsicum* fruit, and possesses antimicrobial, antifungal, and antitumor properties.

Common liverwort, umbrella liverwort, or lung liverwort (*Marchantia polymorpha*) is often found as a garden weed and as a pest in tree nurseries, where it can kill young seedlings.

The liverwort is both a good luck charm and a love medicine to a number of First Nations peoples. It can be chewed, sprinkled on objects, or drunk as a tea, the latter ensuring the consumer will think only of the secret admirer that fixed the tea!

An older English herbal author, Nicolas Culpeper (1653), commented on *Marchantia* based on its liver-shaped leaves that illustrate the doctrine of signatures: "It is a singular good herb for all the diseases of the liver, both to cool and cleanse it, and helps the inflammations in any part, and the yellow jaundice likewise." Most liverwort leaves are three-lobed, like the human liver, and hence they have long been associated with liver health. Liverworts have also been used for boils and abscesses, also due to the doctrine of signatures—the young archegoniophore resembles a boil when it first emerges from the thallus. Liverworts have also been widely used to treat pustules, wounds, fever, diuresis (increased urine flow), and hypertension.

Snake liverwort, *Conocephalum conicum*, is so named for the hexagonal markings on its leaf that resemble a snakeskin. It has a very pleasant odor when crushed. In the Pacific Northwest, the Haida people call it *xud t'aangal*, or hair seal's tongue, while the Kwakiutl name is tongue on the ground. First Nations people such as the Ditidaht of Vancouver Island use it as an eye medicine.

According to Canadian ethnobotanist Nancy Turner et al. (1983), various groups used snake liverwort to stop the flow of urine. One of her informants mentioned that it was eaten by people with recurrent dreams of sex with the dead. If the treatment did not stop this nighttime occurrence, it was believed that the dreamer would soon be joining their ancestors.

This liverwort is antifungal and has been used traditionally to treat gallstones.

Bryophytes such as *Conocephalum conicum* bioaccumulate lead.

This species is one of the largest thalloid liverworts, often found after a wildfire or at old campfire sites. It is considered by some a nuisance weed in greenhouses and tree nurseries. The fresh paste can be applied topically to treat skin inflammation. Other liverworts also accumulate cadmium, copper, and zinc and may also be suitable candidates for bryoremediation. *Scapania* species can survive an acidic pH of 3.9 and hyperaccumulate zinc, lead, and cadmium.

In India, where it is known as *patharshali* (Kumar et al. 2000), fresh *Plagiochasma appendiculatum* is applied as a thick poultice to treat a variety of skin conditions. This liverwort, as well as *Conocephalum conicum* and the mosses *Bryum argenteum* and *Mnium marginatum* were studied by Singh et al. (2000) for their ability to treat burn infections.

The thallus of orobus-seed liverwort, *Targionia hypophylla*, is widespread globally. Its scabby appearance led to its use in India for various dermatological issues, including scabies and itchy skin.

Leafy liverwort (*Frullania ericoides*) is widely found. In India, a thick paste is used to treat head lice.

There are nearly 140 *Riccia* species found worldwide. In India, children with ringworm are given a mixture of jaggery, an unrefined cane sugar, and ground thallus as a remedy (Shirsat 2008). Again, this is due to the doctrine of signatures, as it grows in a ring, resembling a ringworm infection.

The widespread glaucous crystalwort, *Riccia glauca*, has traditional use as an antipyretic, laxative, diuretic, anti-inflammatory, and to treat hypertension.

MEDICINAL CONSTITUENTS

Liverworts generally contain mainly monoterpines, sesquiterpines, and diterpenoids, as well as lipophilic aromatic compounds, oligosaccharides, polysaccharides, sugar alcohols, amino acids, fatty acids, aliphatic compounds, and prenylquinones. Individual liverwort species contain a variety of interesting compounds.

The more than 220 aromatic compounds and 700 terpenoids and other compounds found in liverworts exhibit cytotoxic, immune-modulating, and auto-immune efficacy (Sharma et al. 2022).

A mixture of common and snake liverworts in vegetable oils is prepared for insect bites, boils, burns, cuts, eczema, and wounds.

Various liverworts exhibit cytotoxic, antifungal, antiviral, and antimicrobial activity. They possess superoxide anion radical release inhibitory activity, muscle-relaxing activity, and cardiotonic and vasopressin antagonist activity.

Liverworts have seventeen biological characteristics (Alam et al. 2015):

1. Distinctive odor.
2. Tanginess and sourness.
3. Allergenic contact dermatitis inhibitory action.
4. Cytotoxic, anti-HIV, and DNA polymerase β (Pol B)–inhibitory; Pol B is linked to cancer and its inhibition is a potential target. Prunisin, found in leaves of *Prunus* species, including almonds, peaches, and apricots, is also a Pol B inhibitor.
5. Antifungal and antimicrobial.
6. Antifeedant activity against insects, mortality, and nematocidal activity.
7. Superoxide anion radical release inhibitory activity. The production of oxygen free radicals, especially superoxide anion (O_2) creates dysfunction in hypertension.
8. Inhibits 5-lipoxygenase. This blocks the activity of the 5-LO enzyme, crucial for the production of inflammatory leukotrienes in asthma, pain, and cancers.
9. Inhibits calmodulin The Dengue virus NS2A, for example, binds directly with calmodulin, which plays a key role in viral replication.
10. Inhibits hyaluronidase. This enzyme that breaks down hyaluronic acid, an important part of the extracellular matrix. Inhibition helps prevent the spread of toxins, bacteria, viruses, and venom throughout body tissue.
11. Inhibits cyclooxygenase, which would otherwise cause inflammation.
12. Inhibits piscicidal contamination to fish populations; piscicides are chemical substances poisonous to fish, used to control invasive species.
13. Neurotrophic activity.
14. Muscle-relaxing activity.
15. Cathepsins B and L inhibitory activity; cathepsins are enzymes that degrade proteins in animals and plants. Cathepsin B is a cysteine protease involved in Alzheimer's disease and cancer, while. Cathepsin L exhibits much stronger endoproteolytic activity and is involved in cancer cell metastasis, cardiovascular and kidney disease, and arthritis.
16. Cardiotonic and vasopressin antagonistic activity. Vasopressin is released by the pituitary gland, and antagonist may reduce the progression of polycystic kidney disease.
17. Anti-obesity activity.

More than 125 bis-bibenzyls have been found in liverworts to date, and these protective molecules possess antimicrobial, antifungal, cytotoxic, and muscle-relaxant benefits, as well antioxidant, tubulin polymerization inhibition and antitrypanosomal activity. Tubulin polymerization inhibitors disrupt microtuble formation leading to cancer cell cycle arrest and death. Trypanosomiasis, or sleeping sickness, is caused by the protozoa *Trypanosoma* brucei. Chagas disease is caused by the parasitic protozoa *Trypanosoma cruzi*. (Asakawa, Nagashima et al. 2022). Macrocyclic bis(bibenzyl)-type phenols exhibit significant potent activity against methicillin-resistant *Staphylococcus aureus* (MRSA) strains.

A number of liverworts possess cytotoxicity against lymphocytic leukemia cell lines. Diethyl ether extracts of *Bazzania pompeana*, *Kurzia makinoana*, *Lophocolea heterophylla*, *Makinoa crispata*, *Marsupella emarginata*, *Apopellia endiviifolia*, *Plagiochila fruticosa*, *Plagiochila ovalifolia*, *Porella caespitans*, *Porella japonica, P. perrottetiana, P. vernicosa*, and *Cladoradula perrotteti* all exhibit activity against this cancer cell line (Asakawa 1995a).

Liverworts emit volatile terpenoids or aromatic compounds when crushed. These are responsible for their intense scents, which can be sweet-woody resembling turpentine, fungus, carrot, and seaweed; these compounds also give liverworts their strong, hot, pungent taste.

The oil bodies in liverwort are easily extracted with various solvents and carrier oils. The volatile oils help the plant avoid being eaten by insects, slugs, snails, and other small fauna creatures.

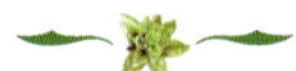

ACROBOLBUS

Kidney-Leaved Liverwort

Acrobolbus renifolius syn. *Tylimanthus renifolius* contains some interesting secondary metabolites. These include (-)-α-herbertenol; (-)-herbertene-1,12-diol; (-)-gamma-herbertenol; 9-acetoxy-10-hydroxyaromadendrane; 5,15-rosadiene-3,11-dione; and 2Z-phytene-1,15,20-triol. Several flavones and flavanones were also identified in work by Feld et al. (2003).

Ether extracts of *Acrobolbus renifolius* produces humulane-type sesquiterpene alcohol and its esters of 2,4-hexadienedioic acid; 3,4-dihydroxy-2,5-diphenyl-gamma lactone; (+)-3,11-eudesmadiene; and (-)-4(15),11-eudesmadiene (Toyota et al. 2004).

ACROLEJEUNEA

Acro is derived from the Greek meaning "highest" or "top" or "peak." *Acropolis* means "high city." *Lejeunea* is named in honor of Belgian physician and botanist Alexandre Louis Simon Lejeune (1779–1858).

The Chinese liverwort *Acrolejeunea sandvicensis* syn. *Trocholejeunea sandvicensis,* contains nine pinguisane sesquiterpenoids. Work by Zhu et al. (2022, "Pinguisane Sesquiterpenoids") found one of them displays moderate anti-inflammatory activity both in vitro (RAW 264.7 murine macrophage) and in vivo in a $CuSO_4$–induced transgenic zebrafish model.

ADELANTHUS

Lindenberg's Featherwort

The genus name *Adel* originates from the Hebrew, meaning "noble," and *Anthos,* meaning "flower" or "bloom." In Greek mythology, Anthus was the son of Autonous and Hipodamia. In the course of caring for his father's horses out of hunger they devoured him, and Zeus and Apollo, out of pity for Anthos's grieving family, transformed all of them into birds. His servant, who failed to protect him, was turned into a white heron—the *Anthus* genus.

Lindenberg's featherwort (*Adelanthus lindenbergianus*) is found in North America but is today considered rare in Scotland and parts of Ireland. This liverwort contains eleven *ent*-clerodanes, anastreptin, and orcadensin (clerodane diterpenes), three eudesmane sesquiterpenes, and two acetophenone derivatives (Bläs et al. 2004).

ANASTREPTA

Orkney Notchwort

Orkney notchwort (*Anastrepta orcadensis*) contains the bitter compound anastreptin (see also *Adelanthus*). This liverwort is common throughout Canada and the United States, especially on the inner Aleutian Islands above 300 meters. The common name derives from its first identification in 1808 near Hoy, one of the Orkney Islands in Scotland.

The major essential oil compounds are anastreptene and β-barbatene.

ANEURA

Fossickwort Ghostwort Small Greasewort

The genus name derives from the Greek *a*, "not," and *neuron*, "nerve," alluding to the absence of a midrib in the thallus. There are 54 species.

Fossickwort or ghostwort (*Aneura mirabilis*) is a parasitic liverwort that takes advantage of a mycorrhizal connection between a mushroom and its host tree. It is the only known parasitic seedless land plant with a nonphotosynthesis existence. The common name *fossick* means "sift," "scour," "rummage," or "forage"—typically for gold and other gemstones. And *wort* is the Anglo-Saxon term for "plant." *Fossick* was a term used in New Zealand and Australia in the 1850s, perhaps derived from British *fussock*, meaning "to fidget" or "bustle about." To fossick means to pick over abandoned gold or gemstone mines. *Mirabilis* derives from the Latin, meaning, "amazing," "wondrous," or "remarkable."

This liverwort is completely dependent on fungi, which it parasitizes by tapping into the mycelium linking tree species. Beerling (2019) notes it has learned which mycorrhizal fungi are amenable and can be encouraged or tricked into supplying carbon delivered by a host tree. It prefers pine and birch trees and avoids all other species. The tripartite arrangement of liverwort, fungi, and tree is found among numerous myco-heterotrophs, such as the perennial flowering plant ghost pipe (*Monotropa uniflora*), which is a white plant devoid of any chlorophyll and therefore unable to feed itself.*

Small greasewort (*Aneura pinguis*) is a fairly common liverwort. It contains a number of volatile compounds, including sesquiterpene hydrocarbons, oxygenated sesquiterpenoids, and linear aliphatic hydrocarbons. The main compound is pinguisone, followed by deoxopinguisone, and then isopinguisone and methyl norpinguisonate (Wawrzyniak et al. 2018). Pinguisone exhibits insecticidal activity against the cotton leafworm, *Spodoptera littoralis*, a species of moth that feeds on 87 plant species of economic importance (Wada and Munakata 1971; Benesova et al. 1969).

*Those interested may find out more about this interesting plant in my chapter on ghost pipe in *Herbal Allies: My Journey with Plant Medicine* (Rogers 2017).

APOPELLIA

Endive Pellia

Endive pellia, *Apopellia endiviifolia*, moves its chloroplasts around depending on temperature and sunlight. Phototropin, a blue light-activated serine/threonine protein kinase, is responsible for the response and movement via a simple signaling pathway (Yong et al. 2021). Actin filaments are associated with dark-induced chloroplast relocation in light and cold environments. The phototropin gene has been inserted into the JC polyomavirus as a valuable tool in detecting the virus in granule cell neuronopathy, encephalopathy, meningitis of immune compromised individuals. Many multiple sclerosis patients treated with immune modulation drugs develop progressive multifocal leukoencephalopathy (Dang et al., 2015).

ARCHILEJEUNEA

Archilejeunea ludoviciana subsp. *porelloides* liverworts were decocted by the Indigenous Chácobo people of Bolivia to relieve chest pain (Boom 1996). The related species *Spruceanthus olivaceus* syn. *Archilejeunea olivacea* contains the volatile compounds olivacene, a sesquiterpene hydrocarbon; ß-monocyclonerolidol; and (-)-spathulenol (Toyota et al. 1997).

ASTERELLA

Starwort Palmer's Asterella

Species of *Asterella* and other bryophytes are major constituents of shilajit. *Asterella* species contain indole or skatole-like compounds (20%), giving this liverwort a fishy or scat-like odor in many of its 53 species.

Starwort (*Asterella wallichiani* syn. *Asterella angusta*) contains dihydroptychantol; marchantins H, M, and P; riccardins B and D; perrottetin E; asterelins A–B; 11-O-demethylmarchantin; and adibenzofuran. Marchantins, riccardins, and perrottetin E are discussed under various liverworts in this chapter. Perrottetin E, for example, exhibits inhibitory activity against thrombin, a serine protease that contributes to hemostasis and can amplify inflammation (Nagashima et al. 1996). Asterelins A–B shows moderate activity against *Candida albicans*, a very common clinical fungus (Qu et al. 2007).

Starwort contains dihydroptychantol A (DHA), which shows

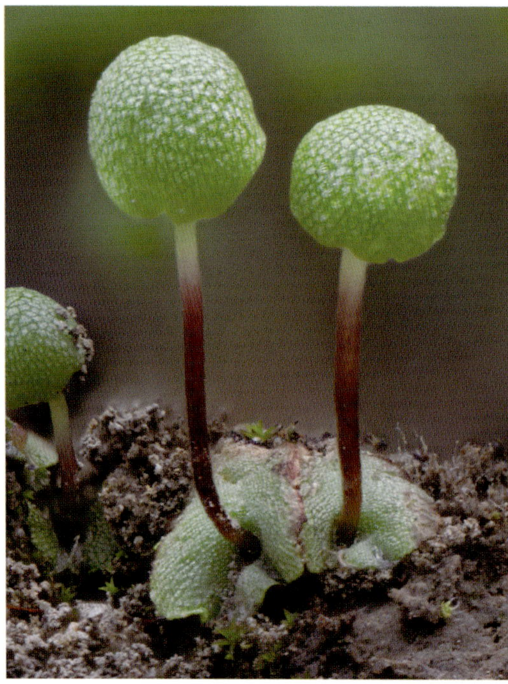

Asterella palmeri
(Palmer's Asterella)
Photo by
Alan Rockefeller

dose-dependent cytotoxicity enhancement of the chemotherapy drugs doxorubicin, vincristine, and paclitaxel. This includes doxorubicin-resistant leukemia (K562/A02), vincristine-resistant oral (KB/VCR), and paclitaxel-resistant lung (H460/tax) cancer cell lines (Li et al. 2009). DHA also possesses antifungal properties and induces autophagy, followed by apoptosis, in human osteosarcoma (U2OS) cell lines. It should be noted that quercetin also inhibits the migration and invasions of oral cancer (KB/VCR) cells. It induces apoptosis by suppressing expression of Bax and inducing the expression of caspase-3 and Bcl-2 (Yuan, Wang et al. 2015). The introduction of liposome quercetin to the market suggests a possible positive adjunct therapy.

Marchantin M has been isolated from this liverwort. Work by Zhang, Xing et al. (2015) found it reduces xenograft tumor growth in nude mice and induces endoplasmic reticulum stress in prostate (PC-3) cancer cells. Methanol extracts of *Asterella wallichiana* inhibit the *Escherichia coli*, *Bacillus subtilis*, and *Staphylococcus aureus* (Sawant and Karadge 2010).

Essential oil derived from *Asterella africana* is rich in monoterpenes, including α-pinene and myrtenyl acetate. Myrtenyl acetate is the main component in essential oil derived from the leaves of the common myrtle shrub, *Myrtus communis*. This oil inhibits the biofilm of *Staphylococcus aureus* and may be useful for multidrug-resistant *S. aureus* (MRSA), *Escherichia coli*, *Pseudomonas aeruginosa*, and *Listeria monocytogenes*. Work by Caputo et al. (2022) found myrtenyl acetate exhibits potential cytotoxicity against neuroblastoma (SH-SY5Y) cell lines as well as anti-acetylcholinesterase activity.

Alpha-zeorin isolated from *Asterella blumeana* exhibits cytotoxicity against leukemia (P-388) cell lines (Neves et al. 1998).

Asterella venosa ether extract contains geranyl acetate, β-myrcene, α-pinene, and myrtenyl acetate.

BALANTIOPSIS

Dangling Face Liverwort

The genus name derives from the Latin *balant*, meaning "sprouting" or "budding," and Greek *opsis*, "likeness" or "appearance."

Balantiopsis rosea and other species of this genus contain phenyl trans-β-methythioacrylate, β-phenethyl trans-β-methythioacrylate, 2-methoxyphenyl trans-β-methythioacrylate, as well as benzoate and cinnamate compounds (Nagashima, Kuba et al. 2006).

Another species, *Balantiopsis cancellata*, contains four 2-phenylethanol ethers and a phenylethanediol benzoate. Antifeedant activity toward *Spodoptera littoralis*, the African cotton leafworm, also known as Mediterranean brocade or Egyptian cotton leafworm, one of the most destructive insects in subtropical and tropical agriculture, as well as inhibition of the common fungi *Cladosporium herbarum*, is mainly due to the presence of trans-β-methythioacrylate 4 (Labbé et al. 2005). *Cladosporium herbarum* is a black-colored mold mainly found outdoors but can find its way inside homes in humid climates. It is not considered toxic to humans. The black mold that is toxic in homes belongs to the *Stachybotrys* species.

BARBILOPHOZIA

Greater Pawwort

The genus name is obscure but may derive from the Greek *barbelo*, the first emanation of God in Gnostic cosmogony; or from *barb*, meaning "pointed," and *Lophozia*, referring to the liverwort genus (see listing in this chapter).

Greater pawwort (*Barbilophozia lycopodioides* syn. *Jungermannia lycopodioides*) is found in most parts of Canada and elsewhere.

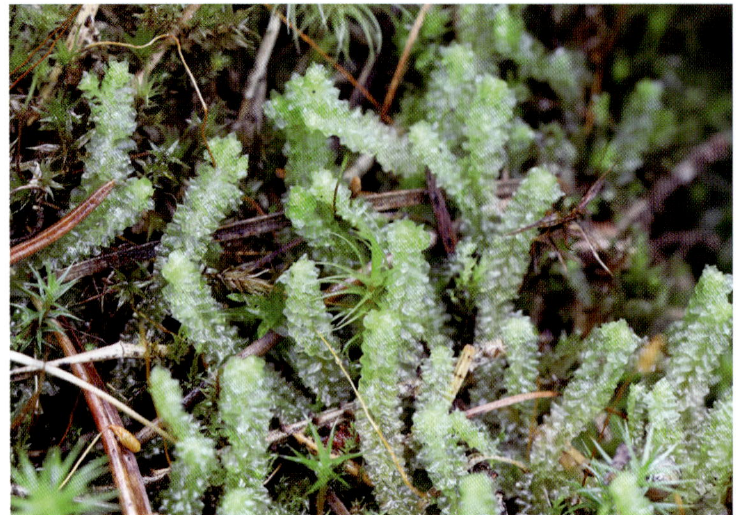

Barbilophozia lycopodioides (Greater Pawwort)

It contains the bitter compound barbilycopodin. The species name is likely related to its similar resemblance to *Lycopodium* clubmosses.

BAZZANIA

Three-Lobed Bazzania   Whipworts

Geographic Range: temperate forests of the northern hemisphere
Habitat: cool; moist; shady climates with high humidity
Practical Uses: cosmetics, insecticides
Medicinal Applications: antibiotic, anticancer, antifungal

The genus is named in honor of Matteo Bazzani (1674–1749), an Italian botanist and professor at the University of Bologna. Worldwide, there are nearly 280 species that climb on rocks and tree branches.

The genus *Bazzania* can be divided into two distinct chemotypes: albicanyl (drimenyl)-caffeate-cuparane; and calamenane. The former species include *Bazzania decrescens*, *B. fauriana*, *B. japonica*, and *B. yoshinagana*. The latter calamenane-rich species are *Bazzania nitida*, *B. tricrenata*, and *B. trilobata*.

Some *Bazzania* species, including *B. japonica* contain cyclomyltaylyl-3-caffeate, which hinders the release of superoxide anion radicals from rabbit and guinea pig peritoneal macrophages (Asakawa, Toyota et al. 1991). This suggests benefits in allaying oxidative stess and cellular damage.

Bazzania albifolia has been researched for bioactive compounds by Liu,

Guo et al. (2012). One sesquiterpenoid, chiloscyphenol A, exhibits cytotoxicity against human breast cancer (MCF-7) cell lines. Antifungal activity of this sesquiterpenoid against *Candida albicans* is due to both mitochondrial dysfunction and plasma membrane destruction. This suggests a human clinical potential (Zheng et al. 2018). Other compounds found in *Bazzania albifolia* are albifolione, delta-cuparenol, fusicoauritone, and chiloscyphenol B. The most common compound found in its essential oil is bazzanene.

Cuparenes, a compound isolated from *Bazzania decrescens*, shows inhibition of lipopolysaccharide (LPS)-induced production of nitrate (Harinantenaina, Kurata et al. 2005).

The major component of essential oil from *Bazzania francana* is ziera-12(13),10(14)-dien-5-ol. Work by Métoyer et al. (2018) identified three different chemotypes. The liverwort's chemotypes are based on diterpenes cuprane, *y*-maaliane, and monocyclofarnesane.

Bazzania harpago contains caffeic acid, (-)-gymnomitr-3(15)-en-4β-ol, and cneorubin X. The latter compound is the first recorded from nonvascular plants; it inhibits *Haliphthoros sabahensis* and *H. milfordensis* fungi (Ng et al. 2021).

Bazzania japonica has a sweet, balsamic, tree-moss like odor. This liverwort was steam-distilled by Lu et al. (2003) and found to contain the nor-sesquiterpenes 4-epi-11-nor-aristola-1(10),11-diene; 4-epi-11-nor-aristola-1,9,11-triene; 3-epi-11-nor-aristola-9,11-diene; and one oxygenated sesquiterpene, (-)-aristol-1(10)-en-12-ol. The compound (+)-himachala-2,4-diene is also present. Fuscumols A and B (eremophilane-type sesquiterpenoids) were identified in work by Fukada et al. (2023). They both exhibit moderate repellant activity against the adult population of the rice weevil, *Sitophilus zeamais*.

Fuscumol may also help attract and trap invasive *Tetropium* beetles, including the brown spruce longhorn beetle (*T. fuscum*), a European species found in Point Pleasant Park, Nova Scotia, since 1980, and since 2015, found in Scotland as well. This insect has a voracious appetite for red spruce. I spent many wonderful days in my early childhood in a park in Halifax, Nova Scotia, long before its destruction by this devastating invader. Fuscumol, which resembles male-produced pheromones (Sweeney et al. 2010), may also be useful in trapping the black spruce beetle (*Tetropium castaneum*), a European species gaining a foothold in North America.

The Southern Hemisphere liverwort *Bazzania longicaulis* was collected, distilled, and studied for volatile compounds (Koid et al. 2022). It contains 1-hexanol, 2-ethyl (26%); pentanoic acid (16.7%); 2,2,4-trimethyl-3-carboxyisopropyl;

isobutyl ester; dodecane (14.1%); limonene (12.9%); and some minor components. The related species *Bazzania loricata* was examined by the same team and was found to contain pentanoic acid (27.5%); 2,2,4-trimethyl-3-carboxy-isopropyl; isobutyl ester; nonanal (8.3%); decanal (9.4%); limonene (3.3%); linalool (2.7%); and other minor compounds.

Bazzania madagassa contains five cyclomyltaylanoids; 1R,5R-diacetoxycyclomyltaylan-10-one; and (+)-globulol, and ent-4β,10α-dihydroxyaromadendrane (Harinantenaina, Takahara et al. 2006).

A liverwort from Malagasy, *Bazzania nitida*, has been studied by Harinantenaina and Asakawa (2007). One compound, myltayl-4(12)-ene-2-caffeate, shows potent inhibition of nitric oxide in LPS-induced RAW 264.7 cells associated with murine leukemia (P-388).

Naviculyl caffeate, isolated from *Bazzania novae-zelandiae*, exhibits cytotoxicity against murine leukemia (P-388) cancer cell lines (Burgess et al. 2000).

Bazzania pompeana has an oakmoss-like scent prized in perfumery. It contains the sesquiterpene alcohols: bazzanenol, bazzanenyl caffeate, and isobazzanenol. The major component of the essential oil is bazzanene (Hayashi and Matsuo 1970).

Bazzania spiralis contains *ent*-8β-hydroxy-eudesma-3,11-diene; and *ent*-β-silene.

Extracts of greater whipwort, also called three-lobed bazzania (*Bazzania trilobata*) possess antifungal activity against *Botrytis cinerea*, *Cladosporium cucumerinum*, *Phytophthora infestans*, *Pyricularia oryzae*, and *Septoria tritici*.

Work by Scher et al. (2004) examined *Bazzania trilobata* and isolated and identified the antifungal sesquiterpenes bazzanins B and S; 5- and 7-hydroxycalamenene; as well as (-)-drimenol; drimenal; viridiflorol; and gymnomitrol. The researchers also identified three bisbibenzyls: 6',8'-dichloroisoplagiochin C; isoplagiochin D; and 6'-chloroisoplagiochin D.

Bazzanene is the major volatile component in this liverwort. A 70% ethanol extract possesses anti-collagenase activity, suggesting possible benefit as a natural ingredient in cosmetics. Other compounds include gynomitr-8(12)-en-4-one; and 7.8-dihydroxycoumarin-7-O-β-D-glucuronide. *Bazzania trilobata* inhibits *Botrytis cinerea*, *Alternaria solani*, as well as *Phytophthora infestans*, all fungi that affect tomatoes.

The isolated compound (-)-drimenol, a phytochemical, is antibacterial, with activity against *Staphylococcus aureus*, *Bacillus cereus*, *Escherichia coli*, *Pseudomonas aeruginosa*, and *Acinetobacter baumannii*. The latter bacterium is

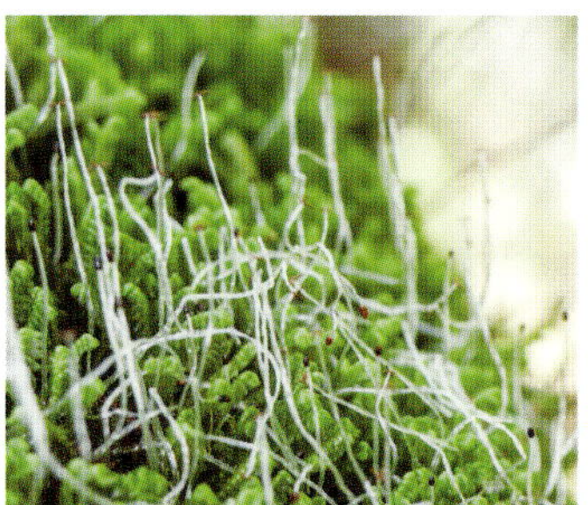

Bazzania trilobata (Three-Lobed Bazzania)

a major hospital-acquired bloodstream infection and the cause of 34 to 43% of deaths in ICUs (Mekuria et al. 2005). Drimenol decreases the proliferation and growth of melanoma (A2058 and A375) cancer cell lines (Russo et al. 2019). Drimenol was synthesized by Araque et al. (2023) into 13 compounds. One of them was evaluated for in vitro activity against prostate (PC-3), colon (HT-29), breast (MCF-7), and immortalized nontumor (MCF-10) cell lines. This phytochemical was found to be 100 times more selective than the standard drug fluorouracil against breast cancer cell lines, and 20 times more selective on prostate cell lines. It induces apoptosis by caspases 3/7 activity and inhibition of topoisomerase I. According to a study by Burgos et al. (2020), drimenol reduces monocyte adhesion to stimulated human endothelial cells, suggesting its use in the potential development of a drug for inflammatory vascular disease.

The phytochemical viridiflorol, isolated in *Bazzania trilobata*, was tested against a line of cancer cells by Akiel et al. (2022). It proved cytotoxic to breast (MCF-7), lung (A549), and brain (Daoy) cancer cells. The latter two were more sensitive to viridiflorol compared to the cancer drugs temozolomide and doxorubicin.

The lignan derivatives trilobatins D–K and jamesopyrone are present in *Bazzania trilobata* (Scher et al. 2003, "Lignan"). Trilobatin induces apoptosis in gefitinib-resistant lung cancer cells, possibly through inhibition of NFkB activity (Li, Xu et al. 2022). Gefitinib, a generic cancer drug sold under the brand name Iressa, is generally indicated after a first failed chemotherapy treatment for nonsmall-cell lung cancer. Other research papers suggest trilobatin's benefit in promoting angiogenesis after stroke as well as for alleviating nonalcoholic

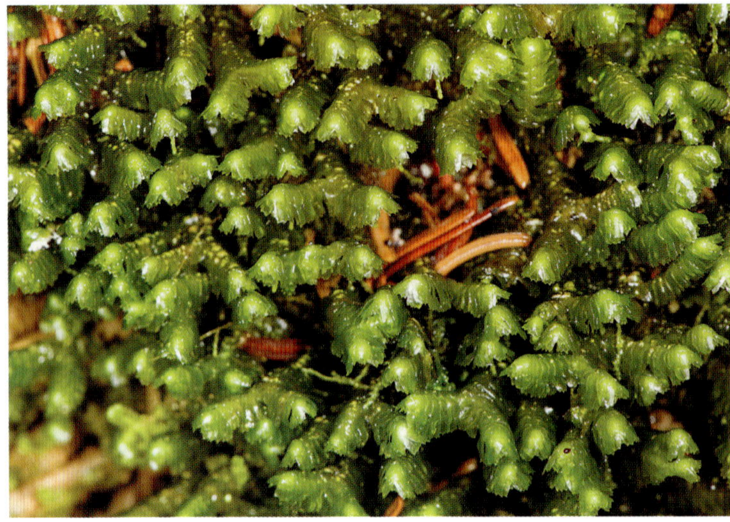

Bazzania sp. (Whipworts)

fatty liver disease, ameliorating insulin resistance, inhibiting HIV entry, preventing cisplatin-induced kidney damage, and alleviating cognitive deficits and pathology in an Alzheimer's disease mouse model.

Gymnomitriol, found in *Bazzania trilobata* and the liverwort *Gymnomitrion obtusum*, inhibits the agricultural fungi *Phytophthora infestans*, *Pyricularia oryzae*, and *Zymoseptoria tritici* (Scher et al. 2004).

Lesser Whipwort (*Bazzania tricrenata*) contains bazzanene, barbatane, calamenane, cuparane, drimane, tenuiorin, chamigrane-type sesquiterpenes, and three chlorinated bis-bibenzyls (Asakawa et al. 2008).

Bazzania tridens contains tridensenal, a sesquiterpene aldehyde, (-)-tridensone, (+)-aristol-9-en-12beta-al, (+)-aristol-9-en-12beta-oic acid, (=) cyclocolorenone, (-)-6S,7S-alpha bisabolol (Wu et al. 1992).

Bazzania vitatta contains vittatin, a compound with a bibenzyl backbone (Métoyer et al. 2018). It also contains aromadendrane, cuparane, pinguisane, alpha-pinguisene, 4,4-dimmethyl-3-(3-methylbut-3-enylidene)-2-fusicocca-2,5-diene, monocyclofarnesane, methylenebicycloheptane, viridifloral, neophytadiene, ethyl p-ethoxybenzoate.

BLASIA

Common Kettlewort

The genus and only species is named in honor of Blasius Biagi (1670–1735), an Italian botanist and clergyman from Vallombrosa, Italy.

Common kettlewort, *Blasia pusilla*, contains shikimic acid, riccardins C and F, and pusilatins A–D (Yoshida et al. 1996). Pusilatins B and C possess DNA β-polymerase inhibition and moderate cytotoxicity against human mouth epithelial cancer cells and weak HIV-RT inhibition.

High HDL levels relate to lower atherosclerotic conditions. Riccardin C functions as a liver X receptor (LXR) α agonist and (LXR) β antagonist. In a mouse study it was found to increase plasma HDL levels without elevating triglycerides. It also enhances cholesterol efflux from THP-1 cells (Tamehiro et al. 2005). One gram of riccardin C can be obtained by extraction from 1.25 kilograms of dried liverwort. Riccardin C, when combined with antifungal drug fluconazole, modifies resistant strains of *Candida albicans*. Riccardin F possesses in vitro antifungal activity against fluconazole-sensitive and resistant strains of *Candida albicans* (Xie et al. 2010).

Work by Millar et al. (2007) found *Blasia pusilla* retards fungal sporulation.

Tenuiorin is found in several species of lichens but also found in *Blasia pusilla*. The compound is weakly antioxidant but shows weak to moderate reduction and proliferation of human pancreas (PANC-1) and colon (WIDR) cancer cell lines (Ingólfsdóttir et al. 2002).

A *Nostoc* cynobacteria species, strain KVJ20, was isolated from this liverwort by Halsor et al. (2019). The cyanobacterium exhibits both antibacterial and anticancer inhibition.

BLEPHAROSTOMA

Hairy Threadwort

The genus name may derive from the Greek *bleph*, meaning "eyelid," and *stoma*, "mouth" or "opening," as in a stomach. This liverwort is very small, often found mixed in with other bryophytes on rocks or bark.

Blepharitis is an inflammation of the eyelids related to a vitamin D deficiency, or when combined with a dry mouth may be related to Sjogren's syndrome, an autoimmune condition. Hairy threadwort (*Blepharostoma trichophyllum*) contains blepharostol and five ent-labdane diterpenoids. The species name derives from the Greek *thrix*, meaning "hair," and *phyllon* "leaf," hence hairy leaf, or hairy threadwort.

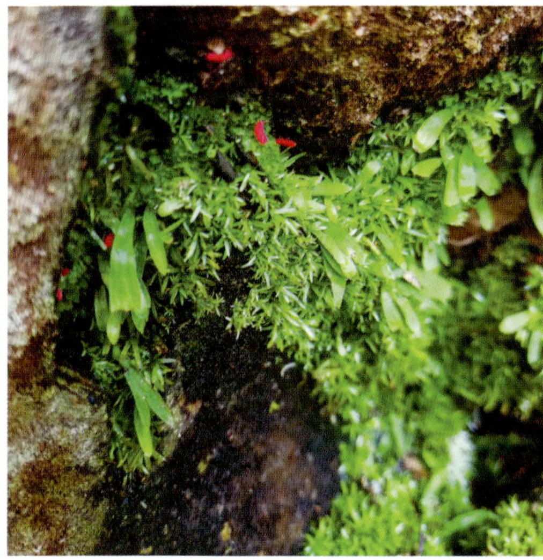

Blepharostoma trichophyllum (Hairy Threadwort)

CALYPOGEIA

Notched Pouchwort

The genus name may derive from the Greek *kalymma* meaning "veil" and *pog'eia*, a "peg-like ingrowth."

The growth and production of *Calypogeia granulata* compounds in suspension culture was investigated by Takeda and Katoh (1981). The level of compounds in culture form was similar to what is found in wildcrafted liverworts. The major volatile produced was 1,4-dimethylazulene, which is also found in

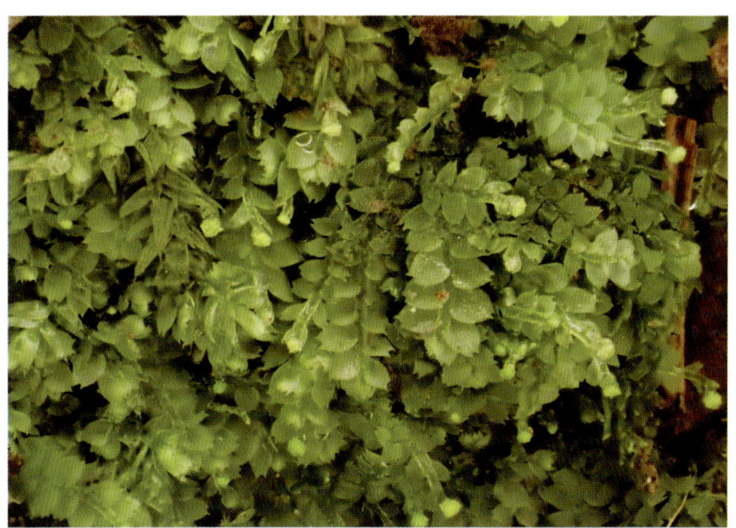

Calypogeia arguta (Notched Pouchwort)

the liverwort *Plagiochila aerea* syn. *P. bursata*; also isolated were bicyclogermacrene and tetrahydro-1,4-dimethylazulene. The total yield of essential oil was 2 to 3.3% from the dry liverwort.

Notably, bicyclogermacrene is a common compound in a wide variety of essential oils. Work by Grecco et al., (2015) found it may be responsible for cytotoxicity against murine melanoma (B16F10-Nex2), human glioblastoma (U-87), human cervical (HeLa), human cervical tumor (Siha), human colon (HCT), and human breast (MCF-7) cancer cell lines.

The lipophilic (fat-loving) compounds in *Calypogeia muelleriana* are maali-1,3-diene; two sesquiterpene alcohols with an aromadendrane skeleton; as well as 3-hydroxyledene and 4,5-dehydroviridiflorol (Warmers et al. 1998).

CEPHALOZIELLA

Threadworts

As strange as it sounds, the genus name may derive from the Greek *hephalo* or the Latin *cephalo*, meaning "head," and the Slavic *ziel*, for cabbage. This is highly unlikely, but cabbage head liverwort has a certain ring to it. About 80-90 species are found in the genus.

Ethanol extracts of *Cephaloziella kiaeri*, now reclassified as *Cylindrocolea kiaeri*, reveal the presence of cephaloziellins A–P and two known analogs (Li, Zhu et al. 2013).

CHANDONANTHUS

The genus has only four species found in North America, Europe, central Africa, eastern Asia, and Australasia. The *hirtellus* species is imperiled in British Columbia.

According to Ng et al. (2016a), chandonanones A, B, D, E, and F have also been isolated from *Chandonanthus hirtellus* syn. *Plicanthus hirtellus*. Methanol extracts isolated chandonanol, along with known chandonanthone, isochandonanthone, anastreptene, and (6R,7S)-sesquiphellandrene. Chandonanol exhibits potent antibacterial activity against *Staphylococcus aureus* and *Escherichia coli*. Anadensin, also isolated from this liverwort (Kraut and Mues 2014), exhibits weak activity against leukemia (HL-60) cancer cell lines. Dicranolomin, a biflavone, was also identified in this study.

CHEILOLEJEUNEA

Shield Liverwort

The liverwort *Cheilolejeunea trapezia* syn. *C. heilolejeunea imbricata* has a strong, milklike odor due to a mixture of (R)-dodec-2-en-1, 5-olide, and (R)-tetradec-2-en-1,5-olide (Toyota et al. 1997).

CHIASTOCAULON

Crossed-Stemmed Liverwort

Chiastocaulon caledonicum, endemic to New Caledonia, contains chiastocaulins A and B, dimers based on two myltaylane units, four barbatane, and three myltaylane-type sesquiterpenes (Métoyer et al. 2020).

CHILOSCYPHUS

Pale Liverwort
St. Winifred's Moss Liverwort
Square-Leaved Crestwort
Tourmentine Mâle

Square-leaved crestwort, pale liverwort, or St. Winifred's moss liverwort (*Chiloscyphus polyanthos*) is found throughout Canada and elsewhere, where it is sometimes referred to as tourmentine mâle.

This liverwort contains the pungent *ent*-dipolphyllolide, *ent*-diplophyllolide, *ent*-diplophyllin, *en*t-3-oxodiplophyllin, and 7β-hydroxy-*ent*-diplohylllolide; as well as cyperane- and eudesmane-type sesquiterpenes. The cyperane-type could inhibit cell proliferation and extracellular matrix accumulation in high glucose cultured mesangial cells, suggesting possible benefit in antidiabetic nephropathy (Zhang et al. 2018).

Chiloscyphus pallidus, which has been renamed *Cryptolophocolea pallida*, has an intense scent similar to stink bugs, but at the same time is camphorous, strongly mushroomlike. The major components are *cis* and *trans*-2 hexenals, but the stink bug smell is due to (E)-dec-2-enal, (Z)-dec-2-enal, and (E)- and (Z)-pent-2-enals.

Chiloscyphus polyanthos has been tested with various solvent extracts and found to be cytotoxic, but not genotoxic, suggesting a possible medicinal application (Kara et al. 2020).

Chiloscyphus polyanthos var. *rivularis* syn. *Chiloscyphus rivularis* contains the compound 13-hydroxychiloscyphone, which exhibits cytotoxicity against lung (A549) carcinoma cell lines (Wu et al. 1997). It was also tested against a few yeast strains and found to be a selective DNA-damaging agent that is neither a topoisomerase I nor II inhibitor.

A sesquiterpenoid derived from *Chiloscyphus polyanthus* var. *rivularis* exhibits cytotoxicity against lung (A549) cancer cell lines (Zhang et al. 2016). This species also exhibits antileukemic activity (Asakawa et al. 2013, "Cytotoxic and Antiviral"). *Chiloscyphus polyanthos* syn. *Jungermannia polyanthos* is widespread across Canada and is also found in Pennsylvania, Wyoming, and Vermont. It is probably more widespread in North America. It is also found in Europe, North Africa, Siberia, the Himalayas, and in Japan. A sesquiterpenoid from *Chiloscyphus polyanthos* var. *rivularis* was tested by Zhang et al. (2016) and found to be cytotoxic against lung carcinoma (A549) cell lines.

CLASMATOCOLEA

The pan-tropical liverwort *Clasmatocolea vermicularis* has been found on the tiny, sub-Antarctic Prince Edward Island in the Indian Ocean and is claimed by South Africa. I find this interesting as the Canadian province of Prince Edward Island is my birthplace. Both were named to honor Prince Edward, Duke of Kent, the fourth son of King George III. He later became the father of Queen Victoria. The liverwort is also found in tropical Ecuador.

Work by Lorimer, Burgess et al. (1997) identified the sesquiterpene lactone diplophyllolide A, which exhibits cytotoxicity against the murine lymphoma (P-388) cell line. This compound is found as well in *Mastigophora diclados* and exhibits cytotoxicity against leukemia (HL-60) and epidermoid carcinoma (KB) cell lines.

COLURA

Cowlworts

The *Colura* genus contains about 80–90 species, mainly distributed in tropical regions. Like bladderwort (*Utricularia* spp.), many have formed fused leaf margins that trap ciliates, suggesting a carnivorous lifestyle as a source of nitrogen. For example, *Colura ornithocephala* syn. *C. zoophaga* captures ciliates in water sac traps, similar to the bladder traps of bladderwort (*Utricularia* spp.). It is unknown if this liverwort is carnivorous or if the presence of ciliates is accidental. The epiphytic liverwort is only several millimeters in size and grows on *Cliffortia nitidula* tree branches and trunks in highland parts of Kenya. It shares the "trap" concept with peatland liverwort *Pleurozia purpurea*.

The species *Colura apiculata* syn. *C. leratii* contains frullanolide, which has been found to have strong anticancer activity against MDA-MB-468 and 231 breast cancer cell lines, and weak cytotoxicity against MCF-7 breast cancer cell lines. The anticancer mechanism occurs via cellular apoptosis by p53-dependence (Chimplee et al. 2019). Frullanolide suppresses ornithine decarboxylase, suggesting inhibition of Epstein Barr virus–associated early antigen (Okamoto et al. 1983).

CONOCEPHALUM

Great-Scented Liverwort Snake Liverwort

Geographic Range: North America, Europe, and East Asia
Habitat: moist and shady rocks and cliffs; sandy riverbanks
Practical Uses: cosmetics, insecticide
Medicinal Applications: antibiotic, anticancer, antifungal, antiviral, cardioprotective, immunomodulatory, skin, snakebite, vulnerary

Italian naturalist and biologist Fabio Colonna (1567–1640) first named this liverwort *lichen primus plinii pileatus*, meaning Pliny's hat lichen. His contemporary, Italian botanist Pier Antonio Micheli (1639–1737), renamed it *hepatica vulgaris major vel officinarum Italiae*, which basically translates as "Italian liverwort." Somewhat later, Italian botanist Giuseppe Raddi (1770–1829) suggested the binomial *Fegatella officinalis*, where *fegatella* translates as "liver," suggesting its value as a liver medicine. And then further down the line, botanist Vittore Benedetto Antonio Trevisan de Saint-Léon (1818–1897) suggested *Conocephalus officinalis*. This alludes to its early use in Italy for medicine, as *officinalis* pertains to material stored in apothecaries, the drugstores of those days. English biologist John Lightfoot (1735–1788) compared its use to *Marchantia polymorpha*, "but to a higher degree. Used to treat or prevent scurvy and to thin the blood."

Conocephalum conicum goes by the names common snakeskin liverwort, great-scented liverwort, and common mushroom-headed liverwort. The male thallus has a pronounced mushroomlike odor. The fragrance is due to a mixture of simple monoterpenoids and some special mushroom compounds: (+)-bornyl acetate, sabinene, trans-methyl cinnamate, and 1-octen-3-ol and its

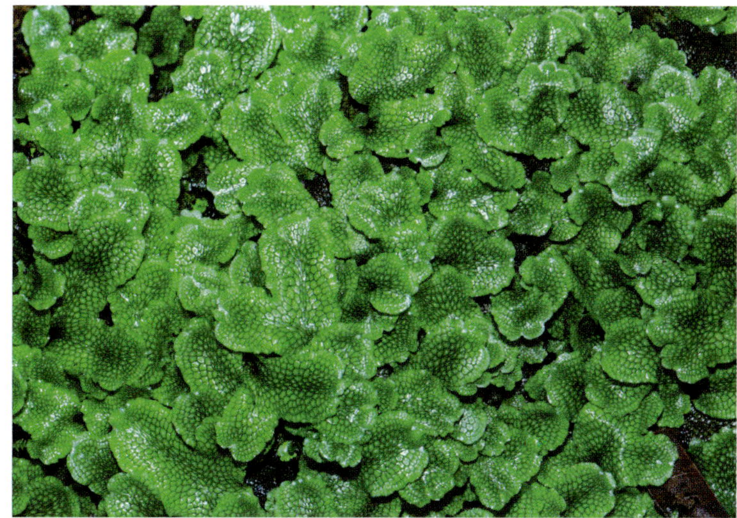

Conocephalum conicum (Great-Scented Liverwort)
Photo by Drew T. Henderson

acetate. These compounds produce the flavors found in the most prized matsutake mushrooms from Japan.

The constituents of *Conocephalum conicum* include riccardin C, tulipinolide, zaluzanin, bicyclogermacrenal, norpiguisone, various guaianolides, eudesmanolides, and germacranolides. Tulipinolide and zaluzanin are anticancer substances that require further investigation. Bicyclogermacrenal inhibits superoxide release from guinea pig peritoneal macrophage. Essential oils containing bicyclogermacrenal have been researched for their antioxidant, antibacterial, antifungal, and cytotoxic properties (Xavier et al. 2020). This may be of some importance, since an excess of superoxide anion radicals causes various angiopathies, including cardiac infarction and arterial sclerosis. Norpiguisone is a potent antimicrobial. Various guaianolides from *Conocephalum conicum* have shown cytotoxic activity against murine leukemia (P-388) cell lines.

Other constituents isolated from this liverwort are isolepidozen-14-al; (1Z,4E)-lepidoza-1(10); 4-dien-14-ol; rel-(1(10)Z,4S,5E,7R)-germacra-1(10), diene-11,14-diol; rel-(1(10)Z,4S,5E,7R)-humula-1(10),5-diene-7,14-diol; conocephalenol; methyl cinnamate; bornyl acetate; sabinene; 2α; and 5β-dihydroxybornane-2-cinnamate. The monoterpene esters 2α and 5β-dihydroxybornane-2-cinnamate exhibit cytotoxicity against human hepatoma (HepG2) cancer cell lines (Lu et al. 2006).

The liverwort was a traditional remedy for cuts, wounds, and burns. Work by Singh et al. (2011) studied the antibacterial activity for treatment of burn infections. The alcohol conocephalenol is used in the cosmetics industry.

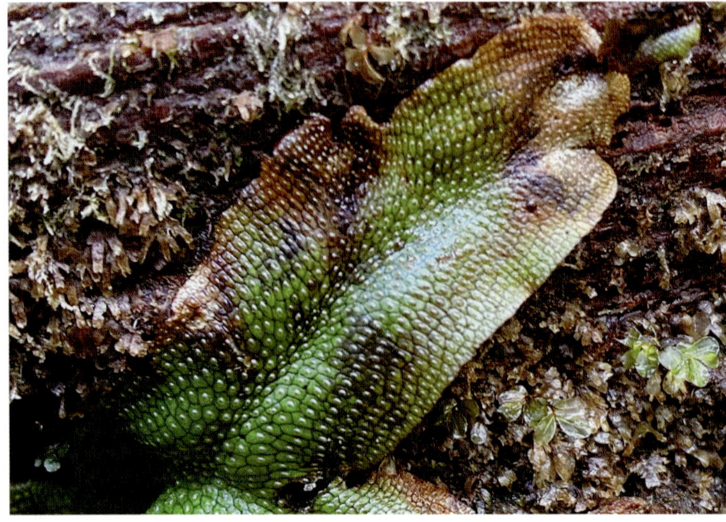

Conocephalum conicum (Snake Liverwort)
Photo by Alan Rockefeller

One common name of *Conocephalum conicum*, great-scented liverwort, is fitting: it has a strong mushroomlike smell when crushed. It can be mixed with a carrier oil to make an ointment for cuts and burns that inhibits the growth of microorganisms. Traditional Chinese Medicine uses it for eczema, cuts, and snakebite (Ando and Matsuo 1984). In North America, the Kwakiutl of British Columbia rub this liverwort on skin rashes for itching and chew it for mouth sores (Boas 1966).

In studies of British Columbia medicinal plants conducted by McCutcheon et al. (1995), great-scented liverwort was found to exhibit antiviral activity against bovine herpes virus type 1. Later studies revealed activity against herpes simplex type 1, the virus related to cold sores. (Lopez et al. 2001).

Tulipinolide is a tumor growth inhibitor found in a number of liverworts, including *Sandea japonica* syn. *Conocephalum supradecompositum*, *Frullania monocera*, *F. tamarisci*, *Marchantia polymorpha*, *Porella japonica*, *Wiesnerella denudata*, *Lepidozia vitrea*, *Plagiochila semidecurrens*, and *P. ovalifolia*.

Work by Radulovic et al. (2020) identified three new sesquiterpenes from the *Conocephalum conicum*, and these, along with conocephalenol, were evaluated with an in vitro model for possible immune modulation effects. In both non-stimulated and mitogen-stimulated splenocytes, varying degrees of cytotoxicity were noted. Two sesquiterpenes exerted immunosuppressive effects on concanavalin-A-stimulated splenocytes, while not being cytotoxic at the same concentration.

Work by Singh et al. (2011) found this liverwort and other bryophytes were more active against gram-negative bacteria when extracted with chloroform, while those subjected to butanol were more active against gram-positive bacteria, especially *Staphylococcus aureus*. Acetone, but not water extracts, have antimicrobial activity against *Escherichia coli*, *Salmonella typhi*, *Aspergillus niger*, and *Candida albicans* (Vashistha et al. 2007). Work by Madsen and Pates (1952) found this liverwort extract active against *Candida albicans*.

There are three distinct chemotypes of this liverwort—those exhibiting sabinene, bornyl acetate, or methyl cinnamate as their major component (Toyota 2000). In Japan, this liverwort produces sabinene as well as limonene, bornyl acetate, camphene, β-pinene, germacrene D 1(10), 4-germacradien-11-ol. Some of the other compounds, such as myristic, palmitic, and lauric acids, exhibit insecticidal activity against the wheat weevil (*Sitophilus granarius*) (Abay et al. 2013).

The related species *Sandea japonica* syn. *Conocephalum japonicum* is the only other species of *Conocephalum* after *C. conicum* that occurs in eastern Asia and Japan. It differs from *Conocephalum conicum* in producing abundant gemmiferous attenuate branches of the thallus. It contains a variety of aromatic compounds: cis- and trans-1,2-bis(3,4-dimethoxyphenyl) cyclobutene; 2α,5β-dihydroxybornane-2-cis-cinnamate; 2α,5β-dihydroxybornane-2-trans-cinnamate; perrottetin E; isoriccardin C; marchantin A; marchantin E; marchantin C; and isomarchantin C. The last eight show cytotoxicity against the epithelial (KB) human cancer cell lines (Liu et al. 2011).

SNAKE LIVERWORT ESSENCE

This essence from *Conocephalum conicum* is associated with the concept of regeneration, cell division, and transmutation. It can be helpful for those who feel vulnerable to parasites, including "energy vampires" in social or workplace environments. Some women feel that a fetus during pregnancy is parasitically feeding off of her, and this essence will help calm both mother and unborn child. The concept of the soul as parasitic is frightening to some people. Some symptoms include lifeless, dry skin; compartmentalizing emotions and will; an interest in sickness; a tendency to wear dark colors or goth clothing; a dislike of anything bright; and language filled with scatological words. Overall, there is a preference for the images of death over life. Rogers (2016). It is available from my company, Self Heal Distributing listed under Mushroom Essences, which contain two lichens and this liverwort.

CORSINIA

Chequerwort

Chequerwort (*Corsinia coriandrina*) is widespread on calcareous soils in North and South America, north Africa, and Mediterranean islands. The species name refers to the fresh leaf scent reminiscent of coriander.

An in vivo study found this liverwort exhibits significant inhibition of carrageenan-induced paw edema as well as promising suppressive effects on p-benzoquinone–induced abdominal constriction in animal models (Tosun et al. 2013).

This liverwort contains corsifuran A, two similar derivatives, two related stilbenoids, and a bibenzyl (von Reuss and König 2004). Extracts significantly inhibit mouse lymphoma induced by the leukemia virus (YAC-I) and mouse myeloma (Sp2) cell lines (Onder and Ozenoglu 2019).

CUSPIDATULA

Many of the genus have been moved to *Jamesoniella* and *Jungermannia*.

Cuspidatula kirkii syn. *Jamesoniella kirkii* contains three known kaurenes and two isopimarane diterpenoids. (Nagashima, Toyota et al. 2006).

CYATHODIUM

The genus *Cyathodium* is represented by nine taxa in India. They are *Cyathodium indicum*, *C. tuberosum*, *C. mehranum*, *C. aureonitens*, *C. tuberculatum*, *C. cavernarum*, *C. smaragdinum*, *C. denticulatum*, and *C. acrotrichum*.

The genus is mainly characterized by thin, delicate, hyaline, spongy, dichotomously branched thallus. It is found in lowland areas along the ground, on clay soil with humus, and on cement walls, rocks, and ladders of temples.

Glime (2022) speculates that the cave-dwelling *Cyathodium cavernarum* and *Cyathodium tuberosum* possess poor to no antimicrobial activity. This may be correct, as where this liverwort lives the environment cannot support most bacterial or fungal growth.

The Tahitian liverwort (*C. foetidissimum*) contains volatile oils including skatole (15.9%), which gives a very strong feces or urine odor (Sakurai et al. 2018).

CYLINDROCOLEA

Cylindrical-Leaved Liverwort

Cylindrocolea recurvifolia contains a novel gymnomitrane-type alcohol. Research by Wang et al. (2006) found very little bacterial inhibition, possibly due to the lack of oil bodies in this liverwort as compared to *Pleurozia subinflata*.

Ethanol extracts of *Cylindrocolea kiaeri* syn. *Cephaloziella kiaeri* syn. *Jungermannia kiaeri* syn. *Cephaloziella pentagona* contain sixteen new clerodane diterpenoids (cephaloziellins A–P) and two known analogs (Li, Zhu et al. 2013). Clerodane diterpenes are widely present in a number of plant families. For example, the major active clerodanes of *Salvia divinorium*, a member of the sage genus, are novel opioid receptor molecules.

DENDROMASTIGOPHORA

Whip Bearing Tree Liverwort

Dendromastigophora flagellifera syn. *Herbertus flagellifer* contains herbertane sesquiterpenes, including the major components herbertenone A and B. These two compounds are also found in *Herbertus dicranus* syn. *H. sakuraii*. Herbatane sesquiterpenes found in Tahitian liverwort *Mastigophora diclados* (see below) exhibit cytotoxicity against acute promyelocytic leukemia (HL-60) and epidermoid (KB) cancer cell lines (Komala et al. 2010, "Zierane").

DIPLOPHYLLUM

Common Fold-Leaf Liverwort White Earwort

The genus name may derive from the Greek *diploos*, meaning "double" or "twofold," and *phylon*, referring to a plant division. The taxonomic rank of phylum is below that of kingdom and above that of class. There are about 30 species.

Common fold-leaf liverwort or white earwort (*Diplophyllum albicans*) contains diplophylline, a compound that exhibits cytotoxic activity against epidermoid carcinoma (KB) cells (Saxena and Harinder 2004). *Diplophyllum* species also contain ent-eudesmanolide. The liverwort taste is pungent, containing the same eudesmanolides as *Chiloscyphus polyanthos*.

This liverwort has antifungal action against *Botrytis cinerea*, *Alternaria solani*, as well as *Phytophthora infestans* in tomatoes (Mekuria et al. 2005).

The essential oils of *Diplophyllum albicans* and *Diplophyllum taxifolium* contains diplophyllin, 9α-acetoxydiplophyllin, beta-patchoulene, beta-santalene, cubebol, beta-himachalene, and albicanol (Celik et al. 2023).

In the same study, methanol extracts exhibited antioxidant and powerful urease inhibition comparable to acetohydroxamic acid. Urease inhibitors may be useful in treating *Helicobacter pylori*, a urease-producing bacteria, related to gastric and duodenal ulcers (Modolo et al. 2015).

Work by Ohta et al. (1977) found that *Diplophyllum taxifolium* and the isolated constituent diplophylline to be cytotoxic against the human epithelial carcinoma cell line. Due to laboratory confusion this may be the same as, or related to, the cervical/epithelial (HeLa) cell line, previously reported as an ovarian carcinoma cell line but now considered an epithelial line. Hong et al. (1980) reported extracts active against the HeLa cell lines.

Diplotaxifols A and B and various ent-eudesmanolides were extracted with ethanol and investigated for their quinone reductase–inducing activity (Wang, Zhang et al. 2016). As well, the induction of quinone reductase is a primary screen for natural product anticarcinogens (Kang and Pezzuto 2004). It is one of the phase 2 drug-metabolizing enzymes that plays a key role in cancer chemoprevention. Quinone reductase plays a role in cell signaling and may be a molecular target of melatonin and resveratrol (red wine). Hsieh et al. (2006) found resveratrol increased quinone reductase in K562 (chronic myelogenous leukemia) cancer cell lines by 2.5-fold.

DOUINIA

The genus was named in 1928 in honor of the French bryologist Charles Isadore Douin (1858–1944). There are three species.

Douinia plicata syn. *Diplophyllum plicatum* contains the secondary metabolites clerodane diterpenoids. Extracts exhibit antifungal activity against *Coniophora cerebella*, *Trametes versicolor*, *Botrytis allii*, *Fusarium bulbigenum*, and *Magnaporthe grisea* (Wolters et al. 1966).

DREPANOLEJEUNEA

Pouncewort

The long-winded name of one of these liverworts is *Drepanolejeunea madagascariensis*. It was collected from the cloud forests of Reunion Island by

Gauvin-Bialecki et al. (2010). *Drepanolejeunea madagascariensis* has a pleasant warm, woody-spicy and herbaceous fragrance reminiscent of dill. Upon distillation, 34 compounds were isolated, including p-menth-1-en-9-ol (28–43.5%), limonene (10.5-14.7%), β phellandrene (8.8–11.6%), and a dill-scented ether (8.5–16.6%). P-meth-1-en-9-ol is a monoterpene alcohol which exhibits sedative effect in mice (de Sousa et al. 2007).

DUMORTIERA

Dumortier's Liverwort

Dumortier's liverwort (*Dumortiera hirsuta*) is widespread, and in North America it is found in the southeastern United States. This liverwort is rich in dumortane-type sesquiterpenoids. It contains the cyclic bisbibenzyls riccardin C and D, marchantin C, lunularin, 7-hydroxycalamenene, and 5,7-dihydroxycalamenene.

Riccardin C induces apoptosis on prostate cancer (PC-3) cells in a manner similar to marchantin C, marchantin M, and plagiochin E (Xu et al. 2010). The researchers observed apoptosis via the caspase signaling pathway.

Riccardin D induces apoptosis through the caspase signal pathway, DNA topoisomerase II inhibition, and NF-kB inhibition. Work by Xue, Qu et al. (2012) found inhibition of human leukemia (HL-60, K562 and MDR K562/A02) cell lines. The compound shows both in vivo and in vitro antiproliferative activity against human non-small lung cancer (H460 and A549) cells (Xue, Sun et al. 2012). Induction of apoptosis was noted.

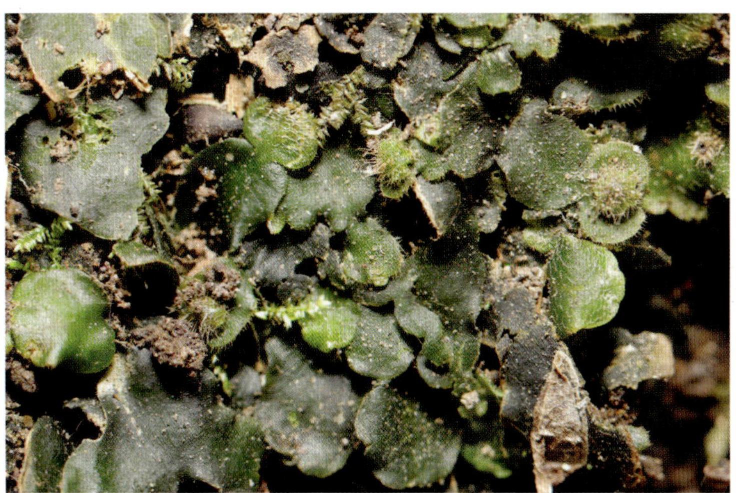

Dumortiera hirsuta (Dumortier's Liverwort)

Riccardin D inhibits angiogenesis in xenografts of human lung carcinoma (H460) in mice (Sun et al. 2011). Injections decreased the vascular density of tumors and downregulated the angiogenesis-related genes VEGF, EGF, and MMP-2 in HUVEC cells. In a later 2017 study, Sun et al. found adding a nitrogen group to riccardin D increases cytotoxicity and exhibits potent anticancer activity against lung (A549), breast (MCF-7), and myelogenous leukemia (K562) cell lines. For example, lung cancer cells reduced from 28.14 from parent molecule down to 0.51.

Riccardin D derived from *Dumortiera hirsuta* inhibited intestinal adenoma formation in a mice study (Liu, Gao et al. 2012). It also suppressed the NF-kappaB signaling pathway in colon cancer cells (Liu et al. 2018).

Isomarchantin C and isoriccardin C derived from *Dumortiera hirsuta* show cytotoxicity against human leukemia (HL 60) and epithelial (KB) cancer cell lines (Toyota et al. 2013).

Work by Madsen and Pates (1952) found the liverwort active against *Candida albicans*. Riccardin D interferes with the biofilm of this common fungus through downregulating the expression of hyphae-specific genes and inhibiting their formation (Chang et al. 2009). This was confirmed by Li et al. (2012), who identified riccardin D as both a prophylactic and a therapeutic inhibitor of *Candida albicans* biofilm. Increased efficacy or synergistic activity was noted when combined with the antifungal drug fluconazole.

Lunularin, isolated from this liverwort, exhibits moderate cytotoxicity against human hepatoma (HepG2) cancer cell lines (Lu et al. 2006) and exhibits inhibition of the bacterium *Pseudomonas aeruginosa*. The liverwort's ethyl acetate extracts exhibit weak antibacterial activity (Luthfiah et al. 2021).

The compound 7-hydroxycalamenene is responsible for activity against various *Candida* species, including *C. albicans*, *C. dubliniensis*, and *C. parapsilosis*, although its ability to inhibit *C. albicans* biofilm is poor (Azevedo et al. 2016). The same compound, isolated from the essential oil of the heartwood of the ornamental tree *Zelkova serrata* has potential as an antioxidant or in the treatment of Alzheimer's disease (Yen et al. 2016).

FOSSOMBRONIA

Frillworts

The arctic/Alaska liverwort *Fossombronia alaskana* contains 7,17-sacculatadiene-11,12-dial (sacculatal), triterpene 22-(30)-hopene-29-acid, and 5-oxo-neoverrucos-(13)-ene (Hertewich et al. 2001).

When grown in culture, frillwort or cheap frillwort (*Fossombronia pusilla*) produces the well-known perrottetianals A and B, as well as (-)-santonin. Seven terpenes have been identified, and both the ether extract and isolated terpenes exhibit antibacterial activity (Sauerwein and Becker 1990).

Axenic cultures of acid frillwort, *Fossombronia wondraczekii*, contain sacculatal, sacculatanolide, and five sacculatane diterpenoids.

FRULLANIA

Hanging Millipede Liverwort Scaleworts

Geographic Range: worldwide

Habitat: humid, shaded environments; on tree bark, rocks, and soil

Practical Uses: cosmetics

Medicinal Applications: antiallergic, antibacterial, anticancer, antidiabetic, antifungal, anti-inflammatory, antioxidant, antipyretic, bone-remodeling, hair growth, neuroprotective, urinry tract issues

Warning: *Frullania* species can cause contact dermatitis, so caution is advised while harvesting and using it.

There are an estimated 300–375 *Frullania* species worldwide, with 98 investigated for their constituents to date. Ludwiczuk and Asakawa (2021) have published a very detailed list of their secondary metabolite chemistry. The genus honors the Italian politician l. Frullani (1756–1824).

The characteristic compounds in this genus are sesquiterpene lactones, with eudesamnolides as the most diverse group, and some aromatic molecules belonging to bibenzyls. Sesquiterpenoids may play a highly significant role in human health, both as part of a balanced diet and as pharmaceutical agents, due to their potential for the treatment of cardiovascular disease and cancer. Eudesmane-type sesquiterpenoids in particular are widespread in nature, with multifaceted biological activities such as anti-inflammatory, anticancer, antimicrobial, antimalarial, and insecticidal activities, thus they are gaining interest in life science research.

The *Frullania*, *Porella*, *Lepidozia*, and *Plagiochila* liverwort genera, as well as the moss *Marchantia polymorpha*, contain the tumor-inhibiting sesquiterpenoid compounds tulipinolide and costunolide. In cell cultures these substances show activity against carcinoma of the naso-pharnyx. Early work by Doskotch and el-Feraly (1969) identified both tulipinolide and costunolide as antitumor agents. The tulip poplar tree (*Liriodendron tulipifera*) also contains these two cytotoxic compounds. Living in northern Canada, I was unfamiliar with these magnificent trees, and beautiful flowers, until a trip to South Carolina many years ago.

Costunolide's cytotoxic activities are found in other liverworts, notably *Concephalum*. One study of interest by Wei et al. (2020) found the compound induces apoptosis and inhibits migration and invasion in human non-small cell lung cancer (H1299) lines. Another study by Jin et al. (2020) found inhibition of osteosarcoma both in vitro and in vivo.

In India, the pale scalewort (*Frullania monocera* var. *acutiloba*) is crushed and combined with cumin seeds to treat burning urination. It is combined with cumin seeds and sugar for pus oozing in the ears. One other traditional use is to prepare a paste by crushing it with turmeric root and salt and fermenting it for 12 hours in rum or other alcohol. This is taken for short-lived fevers. Note the term *ephemeral* is derived from the Greek *hemeral*, meaning "day." Trained herbalists and naturopaths understand the occurrence and duration of fevers indicate various body system dysfunctions. That is, is the fever worse day or night? Does it occur every day, every second, or every third or fourth second? These are subtle but very effective diagnostic tools that served me well while in clinical practice.

Frullania monocera was collected and studied for volatile compounds by Koid et al. (2022). It contains 22.7% pentanoic acid; 2,2,4-trimethyl-3-carboxyisopropyl; isobutyl ester; 13.3% limonene; 11.6% 1-tetradecene; and minor amounts of linalool, menthol, and methyl salicylate.

Bardón et al. (2002) undertook a study of Brazilian scalewort (*Frullania brasiliensis*) and found it contains a number of eudesmane-type sesquiterpene lactones, including nepalensolide A and B; (+)-frullanolide; (+)-dihydrofrullanolide; 5-epidilatanolides A and B; zeorin; as well as four sterols and a small amount of atraric acid. Zeorin is found in a few liverworts and fungi. The compound exhibits strong inhibition of bacteria and fungi and significantly inhibits histamine release from mast cells, showing a 40% decrease. As well, zeorin shows promising potential as an antidiabetic and antioxidant (Thadhani and Karunaratne 2017).

This liverwort has been distilled by Valarezo et al. (2020), who found the essential oil is composed mainly of gamma-muurolol (32.4%) and germacrene D (11.98%). These terpenoids and aromatic compounds exhibit diverse biological properties related to antitumor, antimicrobial, antifungal,

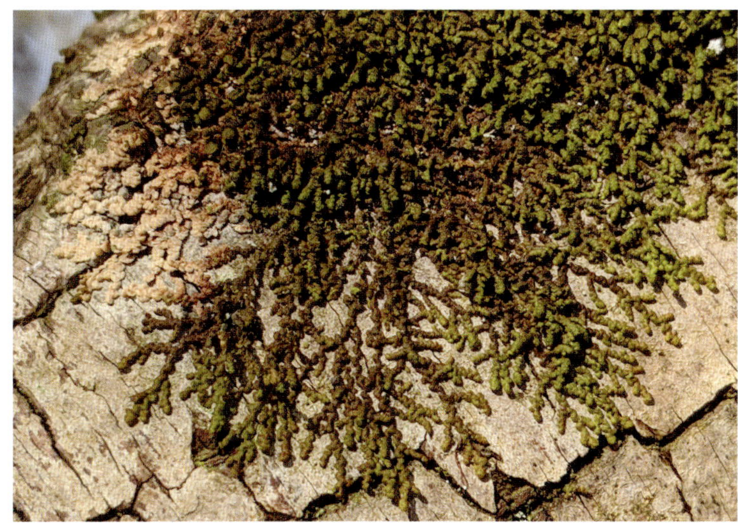

Frullania dilatata
(Dilated Scalewort)

antioxidative, and insecticidal activities, as well as being cytotoxic and insect-antifeedant. Germacrene D, for example, exhibits anti-candida properties (Azimi et al. 2011).

Water and ethanol extracts of *Frullania dilatata* were tested against *Staphylococcus aureus* by Nikolajeva et al. (2012). Antimicrobial activity was found for two of the liverwort species included in this investigation, *Frullania dilatata* and *Lophocolea heterophylla*.

Antibacterial activity of *Frullania dilatata* was also noted in recent work by Simsek et al. (2023): an ethanol extract exhibited activity against *Enterococcus faecalis*, *E. faecium*, *Listeria monocytogenes*, *Staphylococcus aureus*, and *Providencia rustigianii*. The latter bacterium is responsible for urinary tract infections accompanied by fever, tachycardia, and hypotension (low blood pressure). It presently responds to several antibiotics but is nevertheless poorly diagnosed by family physicians. Antioxidant activity was also noted, and various compounds were identified, including frullanolide (19.08%), 2,3-methylanisole (15.21%), linoleic acid, palmitic acid, and valerenic acid (5.3%). Frullanolide exhibits strong activity against breast cancer cell lines MDA-MB-468 and 231, and weak cytotoxicity against the MCF-7 breast cancer cell line. The anticancer mechanism occurs via cellular apoptosis, by p53-dependence (Chimplee et al. 2019).

Valerenic acid suppresses the progression of glioblastoma multiforme, inhibiting cell proliferation, migration, and invasion by increasing innate immune signals such as enhancing ROS levels and activating the AMPK pathway

(Lu et al. 2020). It should be noted that inhibition of ROS by N-acetylcysteine (NAC) is contraindicated and could block valerenic acid–induced apoptosis, or cell death. Herbalists will recognize the compound as a key constituent in valerian (*Valeriana officinalis*) rhizomes. They also know that fresh tinctures contain the optimal amount of valerenic acids compared to the dry rhizomes, which degrade by temperature and oxidation.

The liverwort *Frullania ericoides* is used to improve the hair and scalp in India, as it nourishes the hair and gets rid of head lice (Chandra et al. 2017; Remesh and Manju 2009). It is made into a paste, roasted with coconut oil, and applied to the hair and scalp on alternate days. In Virginia the liverwort is known as New York scalewort (*Frullania squarrosa*).

Another species, rufous scalewort (*Frullania falciloba*), contains α-bazzanene and cyclocolorenone, a bibenzyl and phthalide derivative (Asakawa et al. 2003, "Cytotoxic and Antiviral"). Later work by Nagashima, Toyota et al. (2006) isolated two new bazzanane-type sesquiterpenoids from this liverwort.

Frullanians A–F (labdane diterpenoids) were isolated from hooked frullania (*Frullania hamatiloba*) by Qiao et al. (2019). Frullanian D displayed antioxidant activity, and it ameliorated hydrogen peroxide–induced oxidative insults without toxicity by increasing cell viability, attenuating morphological changes, and reducing intracellular ROS production. It promoted the nuclear translocation of Nrf2, a master regulator of cellular antioxidant potential, and upregulated the expressions of antioxidant proteins NQO1 (a quinone oxidoreductase) and gamma-glutamyl cysteine synthetase, which reduce the free radical load in cells and supports the detoxification of xenobiotics. Hamachilobenes A–E and gamma-cyclocostunolide were isolated by Toyota et al. (1988).

The liverwort *Frullania inouei* contains brittonin A and B. Work by Guo et al. (2010) investigated both compounds. After 24 hours of treatment, synergistic activity with the chemotherapy drug vincristine increased cytotoxicity in KB/VCR oral cancer cells threefold, and nearly doubled when combined with adriamycin, another cancer drug. In the same study, chrysotobibenzyl exhibited the most potent multidrug resistant reversal activity. Chrysotobibenzyl inhibits lung cancer (H460 and H292) cell migration and sensitizes them to cisplatin-mediated apoptosis (Petpiroon et al. 2019).

Frullania muscicola contains 3-hydroxy-4'-methoxybibenzyl 7,4-dimethylapigenin; and muscicolone. Muscicolone is an *ent*-labdane type diterpenoid, found along with two bibenzyls and four flavonoids in *Frullania muscicola*. Muscicolone exhibits cytotoxicity against some human cancer cell lines (Lou

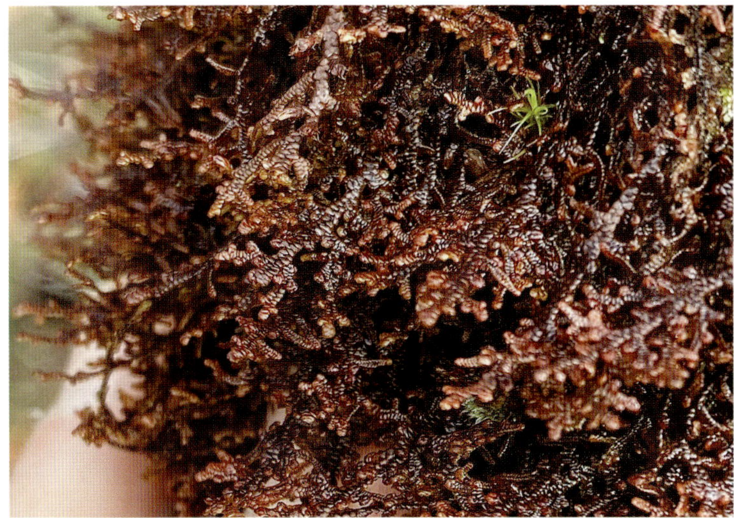

Frullania nisquallensis (Hanging Millipede Liverwort)
Photo by Drew T. Henderson

et al. 2002) and inhibits the fungi *Candida albicans*, *Trichophyton rubrum*, and *Microsporum gypseum*. The latter, a soil fungus, can cause human skin diseases in the *Tinea* genus such as ringworm. Tinea pedis (athlete's foot) is also common. More severe forms can occur on the scalp (*Tinea capitis*) or thighs (*Tinea manuum*), sometimes with severe inflammatory pain.

Costunolide is a moderate DNA-damaging sesquiterpene derived from *Frullania nisquallensis* that shows inhibition against the human lung carcinoma (A549) cell line. Frullanolide and tenuiorin are also present in this species (Kim et al. 1996). In later preclinical studies, costunolide shows antioxidant, anti-inflammatory, antiallergic, bone-remodeling, neuroprotective, hair-growth promotion, anticancer, and antidiabetic properties (Kim and Choi 2019).

There are over 330 studies listed in PubMed on costunolide's benefits for a number of chronic health conditions, including numerous in vitro research articles on various cancer cell lines. These include melanoma and lung, gastric, and bone sarcomas, as well as ulcerative colitis. Here are a few of the more recent, interesting studies:

- Costunolide is a dual inhibitor of MEK1 and AKT1/2, which when synergistically combined with osimertinib (a cancer drug), overcomes any resistance in lung cancer cell lines (Tian et al. 2022).
- Costunolide ameliorates intestinal dysfunction and depressive behavior in mice with stress-induced irritable bowel syndrome via colonic mast cell activation and central 5-hydroxytryptamine metabolism (Li et al. 2021).

- It ameliorates colitis via specific inhibition of HIF1*a*/glycolysis-mediated Th17 differentiation (Lv et al. 2021).
- It suppresses skin cancer (A431) cell lines via induction of apoptosis and blockage of cell proliferation (Lee et al. 2021).
- It induces apoptosis of human chronic myeloid leukemia in adriamycin-resistant (K562/ADR) cell lines (Cai and Hu 2021).

Tenuiorin is found in several *Frullania* species, as well as in common kettlewort (*Blasia pusilla*). This compound is weakly antioxidant but shows moderate to weak reduction of human pancreas (PANC-1) and colon (WIDR) cancer cell lines (Ingólfsdóttir et al. 2002).

Frullanic acid, frullanic acid methyl ester, brittonin B, and other known bibenzyl derivatives have been isolated in *Frullania serrata* (Li, Zhu et al. 2014).

Squarrose scalewort (*Frullania squarrosula*) contains bazannane sesquiterpenoids, a fusicoccane diterpenoid, a lupine triterpenoid, a flavone, methyl 3-methoxy-orsellinate, methyl 3-hydroxyorsellinate, dimethyl everninic acid, everninic acid, and methyl lecanorate. Bazzanane sesquiterpenoids are important chemical markers also found in the *Bazzania* genus, yet there is no morphological similarity between *Frullania* and *Bazzania* liverworts. Dimethyl everninic acid and everninnc acid are medicinal compounds also found in various lichen species, including *Roccella montagnei*.

Hanging millipede liverwort or tamarisk scalewort (*Frullania tamarisci*) contains antiseptic compounds. *Frullania tamarisci* subsp. *tamarisci* has a carrot-like odor. The phytocompound tamariscol is responsible for its distinct aroma, which also expresses hints of the woody, green notes of oakmoss, hay, violet leaves, and seaweed. There is commercial interest in this compound for use in perfumes and cosmetics of the floral, oriental, chypre, and fancy violet and white rose type. A synthetic compound with a sweet, mossy aroma similar to tamariscol is now used by the perfume industry. It is 1-hydroxy-1-(2-methyl-1-propenyl)-cyclohexane, produced through a thirteen- step process (Conart and Simonsen 2025). Hanging millipede liverwort exhibits modest activity against *Bacillus subtilis* (Russell 2010).

In China, this liverwort is used to treat pulmonary tuberculosis (Harris 2008). Tamariscene and pacifigornianes were isolated from the essential oil of *Frullani tamarisci* in a 2001 study comparing the oil constituents with the medicinal herb *Valeriana officinalis* (Paul et al.). Compounds in the oils were enantiomeric to each other, meaning they are mirror images, but different in three dimensions. Other examples in the essential oil world include the enantiomeric structure of spearmint and caraway, or aspen poplar bud oil and German chamomile. Tamariscol is a tertiary alcohol that is prone to transformation when dissolved in deuterated chloroform (Pannequin et al. 2020).

Frullania species from Indonesia show activity against human leukemia (HL-60) and epidermoid (KB) cancer cell lines (Komala et al. 2010, "Volatile"). This unspecified liverwort from Indonesia contains (+)-3α-(4'-methoxybenzyl)-5,7-dimethoxyphthalide; (-)-3α-(3'-methoxy-4',5'-methylenedioxybenzyl)-5,7-dimethoxyphthalide; 3-methoxy-3',4'-methylenedioxybibenzyl; 2,3,5-trimethoxy-9,10-dihydrophenanthrene; and atranorin. The latter compound is also plentiful in lichens and possesses a number of health benefits. These include anti-inflammatory, analgesic, wound healing, antibacterial, antifungal, cytotoxic, antioxidant, antiviral, antianxiety/antidepressant, and immune modulating properties. In my book *Medicinal Lichens* (Rogers 2025), I cover this compound extensively. The Tahitian sample contains costunolide and tulipinolide, both of which possess antitumor activity (Doskotch and El-Feraly 1969).

GACKSTROEMIA

Deceptive Liverwort

Gackstroemia decipiens has six rosanes, along with the enantiomer of 11-β-hydroxy-rosa-5,15-diene; 5-β-hydroxy-ros-15-ene; and the sesquiterpenes 3-acetoxy-7,11-dihydroxy-farnesa-1,5,9-triene and 1β; and 10 β-epoxy-nardosin-7,11-diene (Geis and Becker 2000). The sesquiterpenes supply a noticeable scent. Other compounds identified to date are β-photosantalol A and B; two β-santalanes, 9-hydroxy-santala02(14),11-diene and 11-hydroxy-santala-2(14),8-diene; and a bergamotane derivative, (-)-13-hydroxy-bergamota-2,11-diene (Geis and Becker 2001). Beta-photosantalol is a sesquiterpene comprising about 20% of sandalwood essential oil. More than 230 constituents, mainly terpenoids, have been identified to date in the heartwood of sandalwood. Pure sandalwood (*Santalum album*) essential oil is rare and costly, due to overharvest and adulteration.

GOTTSCHELIA

Cup Liverwort

The genus name is in honor of Carl Moritz Gottsche (1808–1892), a German physician and bryologist. In his day he was a leading expert on Hepaticae and co-authored *Synopsis Hepaticarum*, a landmark work in the field of hepaticology, the study of liverworts.

There are now two species worldwide: *Gottschelia maxima* and *G. schizopleura*. Others have been moved to the genus *Solenostoma*.

Cis-clerodane diterpenoids isolated from *Gottschelia schizopleura* moderately inhibit breast (MDA-MB-435) and colon adenocarcinoma (LOVO) cancer cell lines (Liu et al. 2009). Nine years later, in 2018, Ng et al. tested some new and known clerodane-type diterpenoids from this liverwort against human promyelocytic leukemia (HL-60) and melanoma (B16-F10) cancer cell lines. Two of the compounds showed active inhibition.

GYMNOCOLEA

Inflated Notchwort

Inflated notchwort (*Gymnocolea inflata* syn. *Jungermannia inflata*) is incredibly bitter and will induce vomiting when a few gametophyte fragments are chewed for only a few seconds. The bitterness will last for eight hours due to gymnocolin A, a cis-furanoclerodane diterpene (Connolly 1982; Huneck et al. 1983). This liverwort is widespread in North America and elsewhere.

GYMNOMITRION

Frostworts

The genus name may derive from ancient Greek *gymno*, meaning "bare," "nude," or "naked," and *mitrion*, "turban." There are about 35 species.

An ethanol extract of *Gymnomitrion revolutum* syn. *Acolea revolta* syn. *Apomarsupella revolta* syn. *Sarcocyphos delavayi* was found to contain five eudesmane-type sesquiterpenoids, two of which are tri-norsesquiterpenoids. Work by Liu, Zhang et al. (2012) evaluated their antifungal and cytotoxic activity and concluded that there was synergistic antifungal activity against *Candida albicans* when combined with the standard drug fluconazole.

White frostwort (*Gymnomitrion obtusum*) contains gymnomitrol, also found in the liverwort *Bazzania trilobata*. This compound exhibits antifungal activity against *Phytophthora infestans*, *Pyricularia oryzae*, and *Zymoseptoria tritici* (Scher et al. 2004). The former fungus is responsible for the Irish potato famine and is today a major issue with Solanaceae crops, including potatoes, tomatoes, eggplants, and other crops. The latter fungus is the most destructive known agent to wheat grown in temperate climates.

Alpine rushwort (*Gymnomitrion alpinum* syn. *Marsupella alpina*) is a dark, reddish-brown liverwort widely distributed throughout the world. It contains marsupellins A–F and three ent-longipinane-type sesquiterpenoids. All compounds exhibit moderate to weak acetylcholinesterase inhibition. Marsupellins A and B showed the best activity. Both compounds showed moderate acetylcholinesterase inhibition (Zhang et al. 2014). This suggests more research should be done to address various neurological diseases.

When hydrodistilled, this liverwort yields eudesmane sesquiterpenoids, ent-diplophylloide, as well as (-)-alpina (-)-trans-seina-4(15),11-dien-5-ol; (+)-8,9-epoxyselina-4,11-diene; and (+)-cis-selina-4(15),11-dien-5-ol (Adio et al. 2002).

HEPATOSTOLONOPHORA

Hepatostolonophora paucistipula contains (-)-ent-arbusculin and (-)-ent-costunolide. Both compounds exhibit cytotoxicity against murine leukemia (P-388) cell lines (Baek et al. 2003).

HERBERTUS

Juniper Scissorleaf Prongworts

Various species of *Herbertus* have been traditionally used in India as a filter for smoking. They were also used as antiseptics, antidiarrheal agents, expectorants, and astringent agents (Alam 2012; Chandra et al. 2017; Azuelo et al. 2011).

Northern prongwort (*Herbertus borealis*) was first described by British bryologist Alan Crundwell (1923–2000) in 1970. It is endemic to Scotland and was formerly confused with another species, Viking prongwort, *Herbertus norenus*. The genus honors science patron Thomas Herbert (1766–1828).

Herbertus dicranus contains two cyclic bisbibenzyls and isoplagiochin C. All three compounds were tested for in vitro inhibition against human lung (A549), colon (HCT116), breast (MDA-MB-23), and liver (BEL7404) cancer cell lines (Xu et al. 2016). The results exhibited moderately inhibitory activity, offering promise for application in cancer therapy. *Herbertus dicranus* also contains herbertenone A and B, five other herbertane-type sesquiterpenoids, as well as ent-pimara-8(14),15-dien-19-oic acid (Irita et al. 2000). The related *Herbertus herpocladioides* contains endophytic fungi and secondary metabolites that exhibit antifungal activity. One compound identified by Zhu et al. (2023) is a potent antifungal that disrupts fungal mitochondrial respiration through inhibition of mitochondrial complexes I and IV, resulting in intracellular ATP content of the fungi being significantly reduced. In vivo results found the compound effective against the human pathogen *Candida albicans* and, in vitro, against the citrus tree fungal pathogen *Alternaria citriarbusti*.

The essential oil of juniper scissorleaf (*Herbertus juniperoideus*) contains bicyclogermacrene D (18.23%) and caryophyllene oxide (15.29%) (Valarezo et al. 2020.). This species is not to be confused with juniper prongwort (*Herbertus aduncus* subsp. *aduncus*) or with bent scissorleaf prongwort, also called common scissorleaf prongwort (*Herbertus aduncus*). Common scissorleaf prongwort contains (-)-α-herbertenol, (-)-β-herbertol, and (-)-α-formylherbertenol. Work by Matsuo et al. (1982) found it inhibited the fungi *Botrytis cinerea*, *Rhizoctonia solani*, and *Pythium debaryanum*.

HETEROSCYPHUS

Crestwort

The *Heteroscyphus* genus lists 87 species as of 2019. The name derives from the Greek *heteros*, meaning "different" or "other," and *scyphus*, referring to a two-handled, flat-bottomed mug or cup.

Terpenoids isolated from crestwort (*Heteroscyphus coalitus*) include the rare heteroscyphsic acid A and heteroscyphin D (a diterpenoid). The latter compound suppresses the ability of *Candida albicans* to adhere to lung cancer cells and form biofilms (Wang et al. 2020). This Southern Hemisphere liverwort was collected and studied for volatile compounds by Koid et al. (2022). The oil contains 18.4% pentanoic acid, 2,2,4-trimethyl-3-carboxyisopropyl; isobutyl ester; limonene (12.4%); 1-tetradecene (11.7%); and minor amounts of linalool, menthol, tetradecane, hexadecane, 1-dodecanol, decanal, and naphthalene.

Another species, *Heteroscyphus planus* contains plagiochilins C, L, and M. Plagiochilin C exhibits antiproliferative activity against culture cancer cells (Bailly 2023).

The secondary metabolite isomanool, isolated from *Heteroscyphus tener*, induced apoptosis in the prostate cancer cell lines PC-3 and DU145 (Lin et al. 2014). Isomanool can arrest the cell cycle in the G0/G1 phase and induce apoptosis via caspase-3 and -9 activation. Cyclin D1, cyclin E, and cyclin-dependent kinase 4 were reduced after treatment with isomanool. The p21 was upregulated in both cells. Reactive oxygen species accumulation was noted in both prostate cancer cell lines. The heteroscyphins C and E exhibited modest activity against seven cancer cell lines. Heteroscyphin E showed inhibition of prostate cancer (PCa) cell lines and caused cell growth arrest at the G0/G1 phase and induced apoptosis.

An endophytic fungus/mold, *Aspergillus fumigatus*, was isolated by Xie et al. (2015) from *Heteroscyphus tener*. Twenty-one compounds have also been found, including asperfumigatin, isochaetominine, and 8'-O-methylasterric acid. Cytotoxicity of these isolates were tested against four human cancer cell lines. *A. fumigatus* can infect the sinus and lungs of immune-compromised humans.

Aspergillus niger was identified as another endophyte associated with this liverwort. Among the compounds identified in *A. niger* by Li et al. (2013) were rubrofusarin-6-O-α-D-ribofuranoside; (R)-10-(3-succinimidyl)-TMC-256A1; asperpyrone E; and isoaurasperones A and F. In addition, dianhydroaurasperone, aurasperone D, and asperpyrone A and D have also been isolated, along with the cytotoxic malformin A1. The latter is a cyclic pentapeptide widely used in the supplement industry to produce plant-based enzymes. Malformin A1 is cytotoxic to human breast (MCF-7) cancer cells and sensitizes cisplatin-sensitive and resistant ovarian (A2789S and A2780CP) cancer cell lines (Abdullah et al. 2021). The synergistic effect is confirmed, as respectively only 13% of MCF-7 and 7% of A2789S and A2780CP cells were alive after 24 hours of treatment with malforming A1 and cisplatin. Malformin A1 induces apoptosis, necrosis, and autophagy in prostate (PC-3 and LNcaP) cancer cell lines as well (Liu et al. 2016). Malformin A1 is also antibacterial and shows potent cytotoxicity on human colorectal (SW480, DKO1) cancer cell lines. It appears to induce apoptosis by activating PARP, caspase 3-7 and 9, and by stimulating the p38 signaling pathway (Park et al. 2017).

Another compound derived from the endophyte *Aspergillus niger* is asperpyrone A, which attenuates RANKL-induced osteoclast formation, suggesting possible benefit in preventing and treating osteoporosis (Chen et al. 2019). Aurasperone A exhibits potent, in vitro, anti-SARS-CoV-2 activity by targeting the main protease (Frediansyah et al. 2022).

HYMENOPHYTON

Fan Liverwort

The genus name is a combination of the Green *hymen*, "membrane," and *phyton*, from the Greek *phuton*, meaning "plant." The hymen located between the labia minor and vagina has been renamed the "vaginal corona" by a Swedish sexual rights group. Further back, *hymen* derives from the ancient Greek *humen*, referring to Hymenaios (or Hymenaeus), the god of marriage ceremonies, the son of Apollo, and a muse who inspired feasts and song. He vanished on his own wedding day but was sought after for other marriages. It was believed if he did not attend, the marriage would not survive. *Hymen* derives even earlier on from the Proto-Indo-European *syuh-men*, meaning "to sew together" or "join." Borrowing from this ancient etymological legacy, William Shakespeare created the character Hymen, who married four couples, in his comedy *As You Like It*.

Shiny Film Liverwort (*Hymenophyton flabellatum*) has a pungent hot taste when sampled fresh. This is probably due to a phenyl butanone, most likely polygodial. *Hymenophyton flabellatum* contains the pungent substance 1-(2,4,6-trimethoxyphenyl) but-2-en-1-one (Toyota et al. 2009), and flavone C-glycosides. The hot-tasting, pungent substance is released immediately when chewed, probably a strategy to discourage herbivores. Maybe. The pungent taste acts as an antifeedant to the larvae of the yellow butterfly (*Eurema hecabe* subsp. *mandarina*). *Hymenophyton flabellatum* also contains phenyl butanone, used in cosmetics and perfumes.

Asakawa (2007) identified the numerous uses of this and other liverworts in New Zealand, including their fragrant odors and hot and bitter tastes.

Work by Classen et al. (2019) reported the presence of arabinogalactan-proteins in the cell walls of this liverwort. In the extracellular matrix these proteins are rich in hydroxyproline. This compound is necessary for collagen stability, helping support the sharp twisting of the triple-helix. Common in animal protein, the richest source for vegans and vegetarians is alfalfa sprouts.

JACKIELLA

Java Pennywort

Jackiella javanica is widespread in Southeast Asia, where it is used in Traditional Chinese Medicine. It contains numerous ent-verticilliane diterpenoids and sesquiterpenoids, as well as three ent-kaurenes. Verticillol is a biosynthetic precursor of taxane diterpenoids. Verticillol might be responsible for antioxidant and antimicrobial activity against gram-positive bacteria (Shadid et al. 2023).

JAMESONIELLA

The genus is named in honor of Scottish-Ecuadorian botanist William "Gulielmo" Jameson (1796–1873), who was born in Edinburgh, studied at the Royal College of Surgeons, and made voyages to Baffin Bay and South America as a ship's surgeon, eventually settling in Quito, Ecuador. He was appointed professor of chemistry and botany at Universidad Central del Ecuador in Quito, where he spent his final days. I spent time in this beautiful city in 1983. Quito is one of my favorite cities in the world, and I can understand his attachment to the geography, the climate, and the people of Ecuador.

Most of the species, except *Jamesoniella convoluta*, have been reclassified as *Syzygiella*.

JUNGERMANNIA

Ludwig Jungermann (1572–1653), after whom this genus is named, was a German botanist and physician who served as professor of anatomy and botany

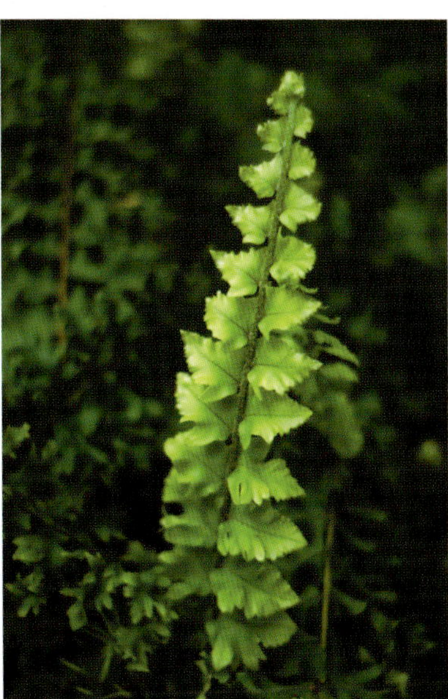

Jungermannia lycopodiodes (Clubmoss Liverwort)

in Giessen from 1614 to 1625. He refused the prestigious position of Chair of Botany in London as a successor to the Flemish physician and plant enthusiast Matthias Lobelius. He laid out Germany's oldest botanical garden in Giessen and published two books on flora that no longer exist. Jungermann famously said he would only marry when brought a plant he could not identify, and so he died a bachelor. The genus contains approximately 120–125 species.

Various ent-kauranes and kauranes isolated from *Jungermannia* species exhibit cytotoxicity and apoptosis against human leukemia (HL-60) cell lines (Suzuki et al. 2004).

Cordate flapwort (*Jungermannia exsertifolia* ssp. *cordifolia*) contains fourteen trachylobane diterpenoids (*ent*-trachylobane-17-al). The activity of trachylobanes against *Mycobacterium tuberculosis* was noted in work by Scher et al. (2010).

LEJEUNEA

Yellow Pouncewort

Lejeuneaceae is the largest family of liverworts in the world, comprising 592 species as of October 2022. Many members contain frullanolides. The genus name honors Alexandre Louis Simon Lejeune (1779–1858), a Belgian physician and botanist. He entered medical school in Paris in 1801, but his studies were interrupted by military service. He is the co-author, with Richard Courtois, of *Compendium florae belgicae* ("Compendium of Belgian Flora").

Lejeunea aquatica contains the sesquiterpenoids aquaticenol; 1-4-cuparenediol; 1,2-cuparenediol; 2-cuparenol; cuparene-1,4-quinone; 1-cuparenol; deoxy-helicobasidin; and ß-barbatene (Yoyota et al. 1997).

Yellow pouncewort (*Lejeunea flava*) is found worldwide. In North America it grows from the Gulf Coast to Florida and as far north as south-eastern Virginia. It is also found in Great Britain, the West Indies, Central and South America, Japan, and in Australia and New Zealand. It contains cupranene-1,4-quinone and 1,2-cuparenediol (Yoyota et al. 1997). Work by Zhu et al. (2022, "Unprecedented") isolated 4,9-seco-oplopanane, two drimane epimers, and five drimane sesquiterpenoids from this liverwort. Inhibition of nitric oxide production in LPS-induced RAW 264.7 murine macrophages, indicating anti-inflammatory activity, and cytotoxicity against lung (549) and human liver (HepG-2) cancer cell lines is discussed.

The related *Lejeunea japonica* contains 1,2-cuparenediol; 1,4-cuparenediol; and (-)-cuparene (Yoyota et al. 1997).

LEIOMITRA

Leiomitra genus contains 16 species at present time, mainly confined to Central America, southern United States; East Asia and Indonesia; Australia and New Zealand. The name may derive from the Greek *leio* meaning "smooth" and *mitra,* a "headband or turban," and earlier from the Proto-Indo-European root meaning "to bind." This alludes to the non-plicate calyptra.

Leiomitra tomentosa syn. *Trichocolea tomentosa* inhibits methicillin-resistant *Staphylococcus aureus* (MRSA) (Rodriguez-Rodriguez et al. 2012). This liverwort is common throughout Central and South America.

In addition, *Leiomitra lanata* was found to contain 3,3-dimethylallyl ester (Perry, Foster et al. 1996).

LEPICOLEA

The 11 *Lepicolea* genus is found in South America, New Zealand, and Africa. The widespread range of *Lepicolea ochroleuca* syn. *Jungermannia ochroleuca* suggests it existed on Gondwana, a large landmass that split into South America, Africa, Australia, New Zealand, Arabia, and the Indian subcontinent that began 200 million years ago during the late Triassic period.

The tropical *Lepicolea ochroleuca* contains ledol; 13-epi-neoverrucosan-5-β-ol; and minor amounts of ent-4 β-hydroxy-10 α-methoxyaromadendrane; ent-3 β-hydroxyspathulenol; and 1,10-dioxotayloriane (Liu et al. 2000). Ledol, also found in *Rhododendron tomentosum*, Labrador tea, exhibits repellant activity against mosquitoes. The species also contains various lignans, including epiphyllic acid and other lignan conjugates (Cullmann and Becker 1999).

LEPIDOLAENA

Taylor's Scale Sedge

The genus name may derive from the ancient Greek *lepis*, "scale," and *laena*, "cloak" or "wrapper." Not positive. *Leaena* is also the Greek word for "lioness."

Lepidolaena clavigera, found widely in New Zealand, contains atisane diterpenoids, including clavigerins A–D, which are antifeedants but also show cytotoxicity against murine lymphoma (P-388) cell lines (Perry et al. 2001). Clavigerins A–D also show weak cytotoxicity against African green monkey kidney cells. In a later study, Perry et al. (2003) reported that clavigerins B and

C specifically exhibit insecticidal activity against the Australian carpet beetle, *Anthrenocerus australis*, and the common clothes moth, *Tineola bisselliella*.

Another species, *Lepidolaena hodgsoniae*, contains hodgosonox, which has insecticidal activity against the Australian sheep blowfly, *Lucilia cuprina*. It also contains (7R,10R)-calamenene (Ainge et al. 2001).

Another liverwort from Down Under, Taylor's scale sedge, *Lepidolaena taylorii*, contains four cytotoxic 8,9-secokauranes and six related kauren-15-ones. Some of these compounds show cytotoxicity against human cancer cell lines and mouse leukemia (P-388) cell lines (Perry et al. 1996).

The related *Lepidolaena palpebrifolia* contains two 8,9-secokauranes possessing potent cytotoxicity (Perry, Burgess et al. 1999). Cytotoxicity was also noted against mouse leukemia cell lines and five other leukemia cell lines, as well as seven colon cancer cell lines.

LEPIDOZIA

Fingerworts   Little Hands Liverwort

Geographic Range: Australia and New Zealand

Habitat: rotten tree stumps and logs, usually in the shade

Practical Uses: ecological and environmental indicator

Medicinal Applications: antibacterial, anticancer, antifungal, anti-inflammatory

At last count there are over 138 species of *Lepidozia*.

Bakar et al. (2015) investigated the activity of an 80% methanol extract of *Lepidozia borneensis*. At least 35 compounds were identified, and antioxidant activity was noted. The extract induced cytotoxicity against breast (MCF-7) cancer cells, inducing significant arrest within 24 hours, and later apoptosis.

The liverwort *Lepidozia cupressina* syn. *Lepidozia chordulifera* was collected in Argentina by Gilabert et al. (2015) and was found to contain five dammarane-type triterpenoids, five pentacyclic triterpenoids, and two aromadendrane-type sesquiterpenoids. Viridiflorol, an aromadendrane-type sesquiterpene, exhibits potent inhibition of biofilm formation in *Pseudomonas aeruginosua* and *Staphylococcus aureus*. The compounds betulin and urosolic acid (pentacyclic triterpenoids) reduced elastase activity of these gram-negative bacteria by 92% and 96% respectively.

The farnesoid X receptor (FXR) is widely studied for its link to chronic liver disease and hyperglycemia. Lepidozenolide, derived from the liverwort *Lepidozia faurieana*, acts as a FXR agonist (Lin 2015). FXR is also known as a bile acid receptor expressed in the liver and intestines that regulates cholesterol and triglyceride levels. Studies on diabetic mice show improved insulin sensitivity when FXR is activated. In an earlier study by Shu et al. (1994), lepidozenolide from this liverwort as well as from *Lepidozia vitrea* show potent cytotoxicity against the lymphocytic leukemia (P-388) cell line, as well as inhibition of methicillin-resistant *Staphylococcus aureus*. The researchers note that *Lepidozia fauriana* is divided into three chemotypes: amorphane, chiloscphane, and eudesmane, while *L. vitrea* is mainly composed of eudesmane-type sesquiterpenoids, including eudesm-4-en-7α-ol, eudesm-4(15)-en-7α-ol, and eudesm-3-en-7α-ol. In an early study by Matsuo et al. (1981), lepidozenal, a sesquiterpenoid isolated from *Lepidozia vitrea*, exhibited activity against nasopharynx cancer cell lines.

Secondary metabolites serve diverse survival functions in nature, as well as being very important for the health, nutrition, and economics of human societies. The liverwort *Lepidozia incurvata* was found to be a rich source of various types of secondary metabolites by Scher at al. (2023, "Bazzanins"). The species contains seven chlorinated bisbibenzyls (bazzanins L–R), as well as isoplagiochin C. The metabolite isoplagiochin D, also found in the liverwort *Bazzania trilobata*, exhibits activity against *Zymoseptoria tritici* (Yongabi 2016), a destructive fungal agent in wheat grown in temperate climates.

Little hands liverwort, also called creeping fingerwort (*Lepidozia reptans*), is widespread and plentiful in my part of northern Alberta. Its nickname is a result of the appearance of its leaves, which resemble a small, club-shaped hand with three fingers curled down. It is found on rotten tree stumps and logs, usually in the shade. It contains dolabellane- and ent-kaurane-type diterpenoids, which exhibit anti-inflammatory activity (Li, Niu et al. 2018). Work by Russell (2010) found that this liverwort exhibits modest activity against *Bacillus subtilis*.

Work by Zhang, Chu et al. (2021) isolated lepidozin G from *Lepidozia reptans* and found it caused apoptosis and reactive oxygen species accumulation, and mitochondrial dysfunction in prostate (PC-3) cancer cell lines. Lepidozin A and F are cytotoxic to lung (PC-3 and A549) cancer cell lines and large cell lung (H446) cancer lines but were inactive against non-small cell lung (H3255) cancer cell lines.

The essential oil contains α-and β-barbatene and α-longipinene. The latter compound inhibits biofilm and hyphal growth of *Candida albicans* (Manoharan et al. 2017).

Sesquiterpenoids play a highly significant role in human health, both as part of a balanced diet and as pharmaceutical agents. The New Zealand liverwort *Lepidozia spinosissima* contains four sesquiterpenoids, including 1,5-cyclo-3,6-gorgonadien-15,11-olide (Nagashima et al. 2005).

LEPTOLEJEUNEA

Small-Leaved Liverwort

The genus name derives from the Greek *lepto*, "slender," and *lejeunea*, after Alexander Louis Simon Lejeune (1779–1858), a Belgian physician and botanist. There are 47–74 species. Note that *Lejeunea* is also a genus of liverworts.

Leptolejeunea balansae was collected from the leaves of an endangered tree in India and analyzed for its fragrant components, with implications for the perfume industry. Anisole p-ethyl was identified as the main contributor to its unique, sweet scent (Subin et al. 2021). The leaves of the Asian evergreen tree *Atuna indica* also possess this same pleasant odor.

Another species, *Leptolejeunea elliptica*, is a subtropical liverwort found in Florida, New Zealand, and elsewhere. It produces an intensely fragrant odor due to a mixture of 1-ethyl-4-methoxy-, 1-ethyl-4-hydroxy-, and 1-ethyl-4-acetoxybenzene (Toyota et al. 1997).

Recent work by Sakurai et al. (2020) identified additional volatile compounds found in *Leptolejeunea elliptica* growing on the leaves of *Camellia sinensis*, the common tea plant. They include 1,2-dimethoxy-4-ethylbenzene; 4-ethyl guaiacol; α and β-selinene; β-elemene; β-caryophyllene; linalool; acetic acid; isovaleric acid; trans-methyl cinnamate; and trans-4,5-epoxy-(2E)-decanal.

LEPTOSCYPHUS

Wedge Flapwort

The genus name may derive from the Greek *lepto*, "slender," and *scyphus*, referring to a large drinking cup with two handles and a flat bottom. The species name *hexagonus* is Latin, meaning "with six angles." From 17–35 species.

Leptoscyphus hexagonus essential oil is composed mainly of cabreuva oxide D (33.77%) and elemol (18.55%), as found by Carroll et al. (2010). Elemol exhibits repellant activity against the black-legged tick and the lone star tick, with similar effectiveness to DEET against the latter. Elemol may also have therapeutic potential in the treatment of atopic dermatitis (AD) due to its immunosuppressive effects. Elemol attenuates the onset of AD-like skin lesions, reduces serum IgE levels, and decreases mast cell infiltration into the dermis and hypodermis. In addition, elemol downregulates the transcriptional expression of several pro-inflammatory cytokines (Yang et al. 2015).

LIOCHLAENA

Long-Leaved Flapwort

Six species are found in northern parts of North America and Eurasia. Long-leaved flapwort (*Liochlaena lanceolata*) is called *indtrykt rormund* or *tungebladet snabelmund* in Denmark, *kantokorvasammal* in Finland and *vanlig rörsvepemossa* in Sweden.

Liochlaena subulata syn. *Jungermannia subulata* contains the unusual (+)-trans-caffeoyl-D-malic acid, otherwise known as caffeoylmalic acid. The compound subulatin, a caffeic acid derivative, exhibits antioxidant activity comparable to α-tocopherol, an organic compound with vitamin E activity (Tazaki et al. 2002).

LOPHOCOLEA

Crestworts

Bifid crestwort (*Lophocolea bidentata*) contains the highly fragrant compound epoxy-trinoreudesmane sesquiterpene and the cytotoxic compound diplophyllolide. This is also found in the liverworts *Chiloscyphus subporosa* and *Clasmatocolea vermicularis* (Lorimer, Burgess et al. 1997).

Another species, variable-leaved crestwort (*Lophocolea heterophylla*), is often found at the base of trees as well as on leaf litter and the tops of roots. Work by Nikolajeva et al. (2012) found extracts inhibit *Bacillus cereus*, which can cause diarrhea from poorly cooked or stored food. Symptoms usually abate within 24 hours, but in some cases the toxin can cause acute liver failure.

Note: the species name *cereus* derives from the Latin for "waxy," alluding to sticky texture of this bacterium's cell wall. *Bacillus cereus* can also cause obstinate skin infections, including keratitis. Because it is related to *Bacillus anthracis*, it contains some toxic genes that can cause anthrax-like respiratory infections.

The compound subulatin, a caffeic acid derivative, is derived from *Lophocolea heterophylla* and exhibits antioxidant activity comparable to α-tocopherol (Tazaki et al. 2002). This liverwort, when hydro-distilled, produces homo-monoterpene alcohols, including 2-methylisoborneol. This compound is also found in an *n*-hexane extract. The compound's odor is a source of the musty, earthy aroma of some fresh and reservoir water as well as cultured fish.

Other compounds include ent-isoalantolactone and furanoeudesma-4(15),7,11-trien-5α-ol. The former compound inhibits the yeast *Candida albicans* by decreasing ergosterol contents and increasing zymosterol and lanosterol accumulation (Li, Shi et al. 2017).

Lophocolea subporosa syn. *Chiloscyphus subporosus* has been analyzed and reveals an aromadendrane-type sesquiterpenoid, 4(15)-aromadendren-12,5α-olide; and an aromadendrane-guaianolide dimer (Nagashima et al. 2004). A cytotoxic sesquiterpene lactone, diplophyllolide A, has also been identified (Lorimer, Burgess et al. 1997).

LOPHOZIA

Tri-Tip Leafy Liverwort   Tumid Notchwort

Tumid notchwort, also called tri-tip leafy liverwort (*Lophozia ventricosa*) is found in Europe and North America. Methanol and ethyl acetate extracts were tested and found to have antimicrobial activity against *Bacillus cereus*, *Listeria monocytogenes*, *Micrococcus flavus*, and *Staphylococcus aureus*, as well as against four *Aspergillus* species, two *Penicillium* species, and *Trichoderma viride* (Bukvicki et al. 2015).

LUNULARIA

Crescent Cup Liverwort

Geographic Range: Western Europe; Mediterranean countries; introduced to Peru

Habitat: shaded forests and gardens; moist areas near water

Practical Uses: beer-making

Medicinal Applications: antibacterial, anticancer, antifungal

The genus name *Lunularia* is from the Latin, meaning "bent like a small half-moon," in reference to this liverwort's crescent-shaped gemma cups.

Crescent cup liverwort, *Lunularia cruciata*, is widespread and is the only species of this genus. The species name *cruciata* is from the Latin for "like a cross," referring to the stalk shape of the sporophyte. The people of Chinchero in southern Peru make a tea of *Lunularia cruciata* to treat kidney disease (Franquemont et al. 1990). The preparation of chicha (corn beer) requires the addition of this liverwort, as well as the liverwort *Plagiochasma appendiculatum*. Originally, the corn was chewed by women, and when thick with saliva, they would spit it into a container to start fermentation. Chicha has been illegal in Columbia since 1949 due to the belief it causes a loss of energy and the desire to work. It was a good thing I drank it while in Peru. Or was it? I had arrived by plane into Cusco and initially did not notice the effects of altitude after drinking a few cups of coco leaf tea. That evening I left my hotel to drink a few beers and listen to music. I was offered chicha and thought *why not?* I was the last patron out of the bar, well after midnight, and could not remember the name or location of my hotel. Standing under a streetlight, I laughed to myself about the old joke told of scientists looking for new discoveries, but only under a streetlight so they could see.

Lunularia cruciata exhibits modest activity against *Bacillus subtilis* (Russell 2010).

The constituents and properties of this liverwort have been investigated by Mukhia et al (2019). The wild and cultivated liverworts have more or less the same constituents. These are lunularin, lunularic acid, bisbibenzyls, derivatives of perrottetin F and riccardins, quercetin, and luteolin-7-O-glucoside. The compound perrottetin F, when biotransformed by *Aspergillus niger*, exhibits activity against *Staphylococcus aureus* and *Pseudomonas aeruginosa* (Bukvicki et al. 2021).

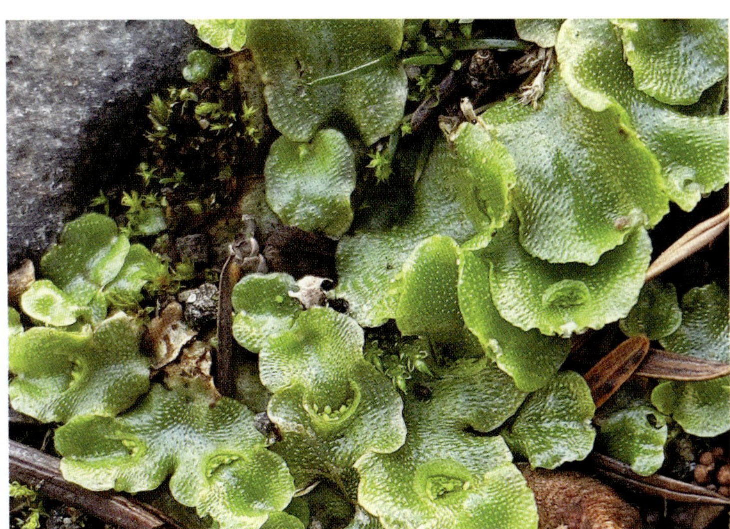

Crescent Cup Liverwort (*Lunularia cruciata*)
Photo by Drew T. Henderson

Mukhia et al. (2019) found the presence of antioxidants α-amylase and α-glucosidase from in vitro grown plants, of possible benefit in blood sugar dysfunction.

Lunularic acid, found in most aging liverworts as a minor component, has anti-hyaluronidase activity (prevents the degradation of hyaluronic acid, found in connective, epithelial, and neural tissues) that is stronger than the antiallergic drug tranilast. Lunularic acid is an aging hormone found in liverworts (but not mosses) that possesses antifungal activity. Liverworts are rarely or never attacked by fungi!

Work by Basile, Giordano et al. (1998) found acetone extracts showed significant antibacterial activity against *Staphylococcus aureus*, *Shigella epidermidis*, *Streptococcus faecalis*, *Proteus mirabilis*, *P. vulgaris*, *Pseudomonas aeruginosa*, *Salmonella typhi*, *Klebsiella pneumoniae*, *Enterobacter cloacae*, *E. aerogenes*, and *Citrobacter diversus*. The latter bacterium, now known as *Citrobacter koseri*, is implicated in urinary tract infections and is well-known for causing sepsis and meningitis in young babies. In fact, 20–30% will die, and the 75% who survive will suffer lifelong neurological issues.

Work by Dhondiyal et al. (2013) found ethanol extracts inhibited *Agrobacterium tumefaciens*, *Xanthomonas phoseoli*, *Escherichia coli*, *Bacillus subtilis*, and *Erwinia chrysanthemi*.

Riccardin and perrottetin derivatives were extracted and identified by Novakovic et al. (2019). These include the unusual phenanthrene, dihydrophenanthrene, and quinone moieties rarely found in nature. The compounds, including riccardin G, exhibit cytotoxicity against lung (A549) cancer cell lines.

Resveratrol is metabolized in the human gut into two metabotypes by gut microbiota. In one of these, lunarin is produced, but not in the other type. Research by Iglesias-Aguirre et al. (2022) found the lunarin nonproducers were more prevalent in females. Other research by Li, Han et al. (2022) found an absence of lunarin in antibiotic-treated mice. The researchers found that lunarin exhibits stronger anti-inflammatory and anticancer effects than resveratrol. Lunarin is also a constituent of fresh celery.

Homeopathy

The homeopathic remedy crescent cup liverwort, from *Lunularia cruciata*, is for those who are shy and afraid to express themselves. They feel diminished, humiliated, or worthless and submissive. They tend to give and serve, and may therefore be exploited by others. They desperately need to feel part of a group.

This remedy is often indicated after a trauma, when there is no desire to recall the triggering event. And because the person wants to maintain their previous perfection and finds it difficult to accept change, they may become rigid or retreat to what they view as a rural paradise. They may convert to puritanical ideaologies or religious fanaticism and express a desire to relive the past. The mind has difficulty with concentration or attention, and there is susceptibility to brain injury.

The recommended dose is 200c.*

MANNIA

Fragrant Macewort Narrow Mushroom-Headed Liverwort

Narrow mushroom-headed liverwort, *Mannia androgyna*, exhibited significant in vivo inhibition on carrageenan-induced paw edema and promising suppressive effects on p-benzoquinone-induced abdominal constriction in animal models (Tosun et al. 2013).

Extracts inhibit mouse lymphoma induced by the feline leukemia virus and mouse myeloma cell lines (Önder and Özenoglu 2019).

Fragrant macewort (*Mannia fragrans*) is common throughout northern North America. Pakyonol, isolated from this species, inhibits proliferation and promotes cell death in human prostate (PC-3) cancer cell lines (Xu et al. 2010). This compound is synergistic with the chemotherapy drug adriamycin in drug-resistant leukemia (K562/A02) cells (Ji et al. 2011).

MARCHANTIA

Common Liverwort
Lung Liverwort
Mountain Liverwort
Plumier's Ducks Foot
Star-Headed Liverwort

Geographic Range: every continent except Antarctica

Habitat: moist, shaded stream banks; bogs and fens; recent burn sites

Practical Uses: agricultural fungicide, food preservative, perfume

Medicinal Applications: antibacterial, anticancer, antifungal, anti-inflammatory, antipyretic, asthma, hepaprotective, immune modulator, kidney stones, neuroprotective, skin conditions, tuberculosis, vulnerary

*Proving by Michal Yakir and Paul Theriault, 2020.

Worldwide, there are about 65 species of *Marchantia* liverworts. Most are tropical to subtropical, with a few exceptions.

The New Zealand liverwort *Marchantia berteroana* exhibits moderate activity against *Staphylococcus aureus* (Calder et al. 1986).

The tropical and subtropical Plumier's ducks foot, *Marchantia chenopoda*, contains chenopodene, as well as marchantin P and riccardin G, beneficial macrocyclic bis-bibenzyls that are rare natural products of the plant kingdom (Tori et al. 1994). *Marchantia chenopoda* has traditionally been used as a diuretic to treat edema (de la Maza 1889). Riccardin G exhibits cytotoxicity against lung (A549) cancer cell lines (Novakovic et al. 2019). This valuable compound is also found in *Lunularia cruciata*.

Marchantia emarginata subsp. *cuneiloba* syn. *Marchantia convoluta* is used in India for jaundice, hepatitis, and other liver complaints (Chandra et al. 2017). This illustrates the doctrine of signatures, as a cross-section of this species appears liver-like and the taste is bitter, like bile, hence the various hepatic applications (Bland 1971). In China, the traditional uses of this species are similar, including treatment of hepatitis, fever, and gastric disorders.

Cao et al. (2007) found that an ethyl acetate extract of *Marchantia convoluta* contains phytol (23.42%); 1,2,4-tripropylbenzene (13.09%); 9-cedranone (12.75%); ledene oxide (7.22%); caryophyllene (1.82%); and caryophyllene oxide (1.15%). Other work identified 3-(4,5-dimethylthiazol-2-yl)-2,5-diphenyltetrazolium bromide.

In a 2005 study (Jian-Bo et al.) it was found that flavonoids from *Marchantia convoluta* inhibit clone cells derived from hepatic (HepG2) cells and reduce the activity of liver enzymes in the blood serum of rats with acute hepatic injury. Total protein and alkaline phosphatase improved as a result. The flavonoids were seen to inhibit the auricle tympanites in mice caused by dimethylbenzene, a petrochemical compound. As well, Xiao et al. (2006) found that the flavonoids also strongly inhibited *Staphylococcus aureus*, *Bacillus enteritidis*, *Hemolytic streptococci* type B, and *Streptococcus pneumoniae*, and an extract showed significant cytotoxicity against human non-small cell lung (H1299) and liver (HepG2) cancer cell lines. Antibacterial activity was also noted against *Escherichia coli*, *Staphylococcus aureus*, *Salmonella typhimurium*, and *Bacillus enteritidis*.

The African liverwort *Marchantia debilis* has been extracted with methanol and yields marchantinquinone-1'-methyl ether, marchantin C, marchantinoquinone, and perrottetin E (Yongabi et al. 2016, "Bis-bibenzyls"). Bacterial infections in the feet of diabetics is a growing concern. Cultures of 30 infected patients were swabbed and grown out, revealing the presence of *Staphylococcus aureus*, *Pseudomonas aeruginosa*, *Escherichia coli*, *Proteus mirabilis*, and several *Bacillus* species (Yongabi et al. 2016, "Management"). In vitro inhibition was observed with extracts of *Marchantia debilis*, and then a light petroleum-oil based cream called BryoCream was formulated from the extract. This was administered to 20 patients, resulting in a 90% cure rate in a three-week period. The compounds responsible are lepidozene and β-barbatene, as well as stigmasterol and β-sitosterol.

Isomarchantin C and isoriccardin C have been isolated from *Marchantia emarginata* syn. *Marchantia palmata*. In India and China this liverwort is applied externally to skin tumors as well as to burns, boils, blisters, and abscesses caused by hot water or burns (Tag et al. 2007). It is taken as a tea for liver disorders, pulmonary tuberculosis, and other conditions, in much the same manner as *Marchantia polymorpha*. It inhibits *Staphylococcus aureus* (Pant and Tiwari 1989) and MRSA (Kandpal et al. 2016) and exhibits antioxidant activity (Siregar et al. 2021) as well. Marchantin A isolated from *Marchantia emarginata* subsp. *tosana* induces apoptosis in breast cancer (MCF-7) cells (Huang et al. 2010).

Ether extracts isolated (3S,10R) 1,6-humuladien-10-ol from the *Marchantia emerginata* subsp. *tosana* liverwort (Toyota et al. 2004).

Marchantia papillata subsp. *grossibarba* syn. *Marchantia tosana*, exhibits antitumor, antifungal, and antimicrobial inhibition, as well as inhibition of superoxide anion release, inhibition of thrombin activity, and relaxation of muscles (Lahlou et al 2000). This liverwort contains marchantin A, which induces cell growth inhibition leading to apoptosis in breast (MCF-7) cancer cells (Huang et al. 2010).

Marchantia paleacea has traditionally been used to reduce swelling and fever (Sabovlijevic et al. 2011). This species contains marchantin A, which inhibits nasopharyngeal cancer cell lines (Asakawa 1982). *Marchantia paleacea* subsp. *diptera* contains paleatin B, which exhibits activity against HIV-1 (Suzuki et al. 2008). This liverwort species, found worldwide, is used to treat hepatitis, skin swelling, and fever in India (Chandra et al. 2017; Sabovljevic et al. 2011). Ethanol extracts given to male mice showed immunostimulant activity (Purkon et al. 2021). While showing increased innate immune response and increased IL-2 levels, immune stimulation can, over time, create autoimmune dysfunction, so the term *immune modulator* is more appropriate when it comes to most natural products.

The essential oil of *Marchantia paleacea* subsp. *diptera* contains about 50% perillaldehyde (a monoterpene aldehyde), as well as minor amounts of β-pinene, limonene, β-caryophyllene, and α- and β-selinene (Sakurai et al. 2016). Perillaldehyde is a very important medicinal compound. It is cytotoxic to both leukemia (HL-60) and acute myeloid leukemia cell lines, as recently revealed via human biopsy (Catanzaro et al. 2022). It inhibits bone metastasis and osteoclastogenesis in prostate cancer (PCa) cell lines (Lin et al. 2022).

Work by Qiu et al. (2021) found it significantly improved learning and memory in rats. It improves the number and activity of brain neurons, increases the length and number of dendrites in the hippocampus, and generally improves cognitive function in studies of rats with vascular dementia. It is a rich antioxidant and acts as a preservative and antifungal for organic fruit and food preservation. It is used in perfume creations and is certified as GRAS (generally recognized as safe). Perillaldehyde shows a protective effect on epilepsy, insomnia, and other central nervous system conditions.

It inhibits *Pseudomonas aeruginosa* biofilm formation and virulence factor by hampering the quorum sensing systems (Benny et al. 2022). This bacterium and others are increasingly drug-resistant, and they are directly related to increased infections and deaths, particularly in hospital-acquired settings.

A 2016 study (Linde et al.) found that another species, *Marchantia pappeana*, exhibits activity against *E. coli*, while Negi at al. (2018) confirmed that *Marchantia papillata* inhibits *Staphylococcus aureus*.

Common liverwort, *Marchantia polymorpha*, is probably the largest and most common of the *Marchantia* species; it goes by a few names: mountain liverwort, star-headed liverwort, and common liverwort. This species contains marchantins A–E; neomarchantin A and M; riccardin C, D, and H; plagiochin E; volatile cyclic dipeptides; perrottetin F; paleatin B; peroxidase phenols; flavonoids; saponins; tannins; and glycosides. Liverworts do not contain anthocyanins, but the presence of auronidins give this liverwort its pigmentation (Harinantenaina et al. 2005).

Marchantin A tri-methyl ether has been isolated from this interesting liverwort (Nowaczynski et al. 2025). The molecule possesses both convex and concave surfaces, with a central hole on the concave surface. Marchantin A is found not only in *Marchantia polymorpha*, but in other *Marchantia* species as well: *M. chenopoda*, *M. paleacea*, *M. plicata*, *M. tosana*, and others.

Marchantin A exhibits significant inhibition of the soil bacterium *Acinetobacter calcoaceticus*. Multidrug-resistant strains of the *Acinetobacter*

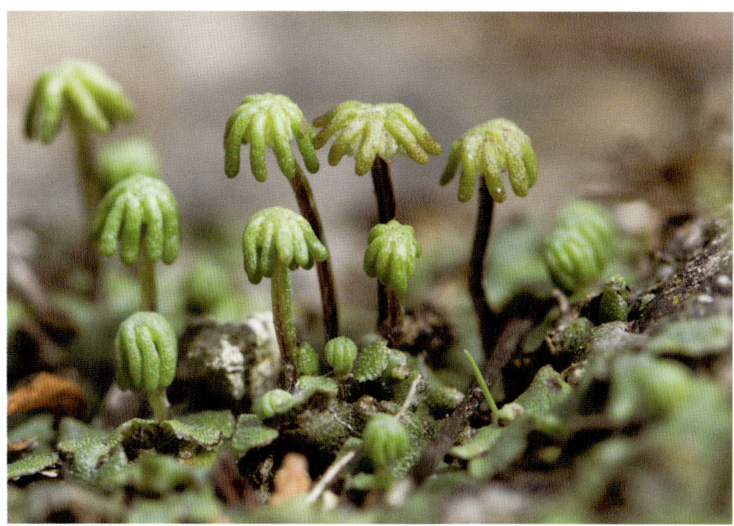

Marchantia polymorpha (Common Liverwort)
Photo by Alan Rockefeller

calcoaceticus and *A. baumannii* complex are a growing concern and a cause of pneumonia, bacteremia, and infections of the urinary tract and skin. Dogs and cats are prone to infection in veterinary hospitals, with fatal results for these difficult-to-eradicate drug-resistant bacteria. There are also reports in the literature of community-acquired necrotizing fasciitis in immunocompromised patients.

Marchantins are of great interest in that like the chemotherapy medication paclitaxel, derived originally from the Pacific yew, they interfere with the degradation of microtubules when cancer cells divide. Paclitaxel has been chemically converted into the breast cancer medication tamoxifen, widely used for hormone-sensitive cancers. And while Pacific yew needles are not recommended as a tea, the leaves, stem, and husks of hazelnuts contain paclitaxel (Hoffman and Shahidi 2009). This suggests possible benefit as a prophylactic beverage or tea for women with familial genetic history of hormone-sensitive cancers.

Common liverwort, *Marchantia polymorpha*, is used in China to treat jaundice, hepatitis, and pneumonia, and is used externally to reduce inflammation, to set broken bones, and to treat insect bites and burns. In the Himalayas it is used for boils and abscesses and mixed with vegetable oil for boils, cuts, wounds, eczema, and burns. In the Brazilian Amazon it is used for tuberculosis and dissolving kidney stones (Pinheiro et al. 1989).

Early Mesoamerican cultures found medicinal benefits from 36 byrophyte species and used them as well in ceremonies and for making crafts. A few of these uses are mentioned in *Libellus de Medicinalibus Indorum Herbis* (1552),

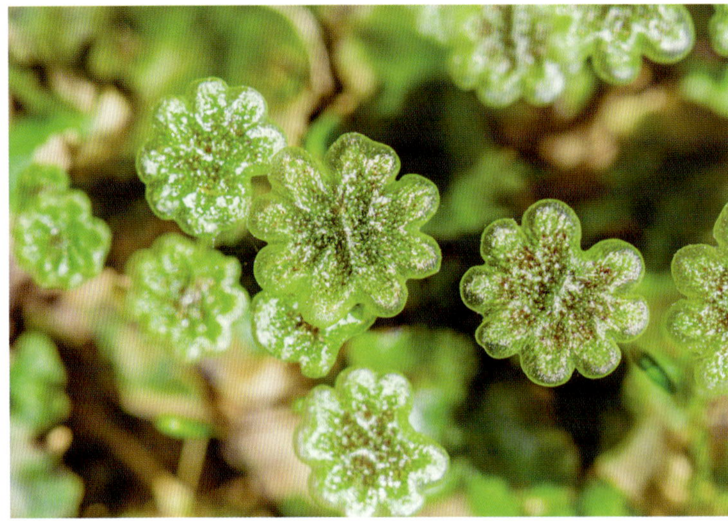

Marchantia polymorpha (Common Liverwort)

the oldest record of the medicinal uses of bryophytes in Mesoamerica (de la Cruz et al. 1939). The thalli of common liverwort, *Marchantia polymorpha*, was a traditional remedy for pulmonary tuberculosis (Bland 1971).

In Mesoamerica *Marchantia polymorpha* was combined with *Begonia* species and *Lithachne pauciflora*, an herbaceous bamboo, to treat mouth sores and fever (Alcorn 1984). In Germany, a thick decoction of this liverwort was used as an analgesic and poultice for swollen tissues and in Germany and France it was used as a diuretic and to dissolve both kidney and gallbladder stones. The fresh plant was soaked in white liquor, which was then taken as a medicine (Bowman 2016).

In the Shetland Islands, where it is used to treat asthma, *Marchantia polymorpha* goes by the name dead man's liver. In Berwickshire, England, it was traditionally used for colds and consumption, as a diuretic in cases of dropsy, and as "a binding at the heart" (Allen and Hatfield 2004). The similar texture and appearance to human lungs led to its use in pulmonary tuberculosis in accordance with the doctrine of signatures.

Marchantia polymorpha contains a range of flavonoids that exert hepatoprotective effects via antioxidant and gene-regulatory mechanisms (Zhang, Cao et al. 2022). It has been tested for its activity against various bacteria and fungi; a methanol extract and a free flavonoid extract exhibited good inhibitory activity against most pathogens tested (Mewari and Kumar 2008; Gahtori and Chaturvedi 2011). The species has also been found to exhibit modest activity against *Bacillus subtilis* (Russell 2010).

Recent work by Stelmasiewicz et al. (2023, "Chemical and Biological Studies") identified several metabolites produced by endophytes of *Marchantia polymorpha*. Isolated compounds show a potential selective activity against all cancer cell lines tested—cervical/epithelial (HeLa), colon (RKO), and hypopharyngeal (FaDu). The antiviral potential was examined, and the endophyte and fraction noticeably diminished the formation of the herpes simplex type 1. Previously the same team identified significant cytotoxicity from an ethyl acetate extract of the endophytes on the above-mentioned cervical/epithelial and pharyngeal cancer cell lines, as well as showing cytotoxicity against cervical carcinoma cells (Stelmasiewicz et al. 2021).

Work by Wang, Cao et al. (2016) examined the flavonoid content and the archegoniophore (female sex organ) of *Marchantia polymorpha*. The latter has a flavonoid content ten times higher than the gametophyte and showed significant inhibition of acetylcholinesterase, which catalyzes the breakdown of esters that function as neurotransmitters, suggesting neuroprotective potential.

A pharmacological study by Taira et al. (1994) showed that the skeletal muscle relaxation activity of marchantin A trimethyl ether is about 3.5 times less potent than that of the more toxic d-tubocurarine, formerly used during surgeries to provide skeletal muscle relaxation. The mode of action is not fully understood, but it is interesting to note that the cyclic bis-bibenzyls contain no nitrogen atoms. Both marchantin A and its trimethyl ether show in vivo muscle relaxation in rats. Marchantin A, as mentioned, is structurally similar to d-tubocurarine and has been shown to increase coronary blood flow and may

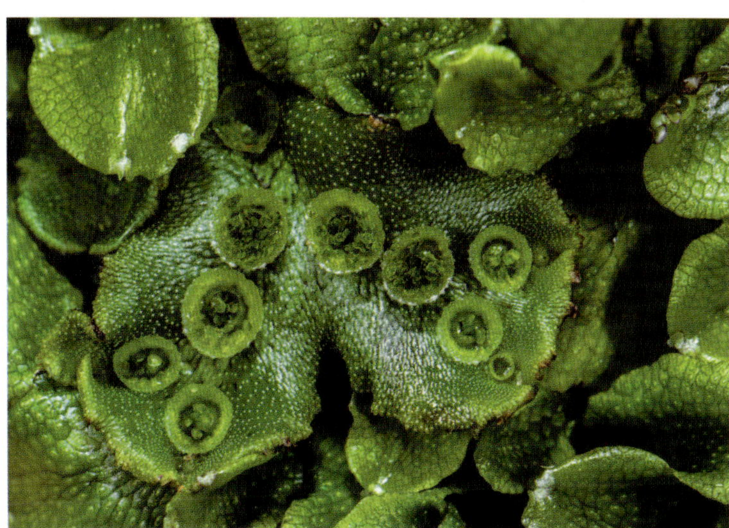

Marchantia polymorpha (Common Liverwort)

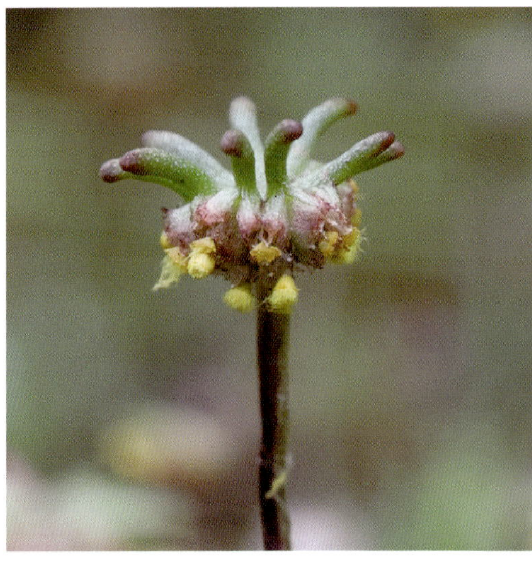

Marchantia polymorpha (Common Liverwort)

turn out to be a valuable coronary vasodilator as well as being cytotoxic against various bacteria and fungi.

Marchantin A derived from *Marchantia polymorpha* is cytotoxic to breast cancer cell lines (MCF-7, A256, and T47D) (Jensen et al. 2012). Work by Gawel-Beben et al. (2019) found the compound cytotoxic to melanoma (A375) cells as well. Marchantin A induces cell growth arrest and apoptosis in human prostate (PC-3) cancer cell lines (Xu et al. 2010). It shows antibacterial activity against a wide range of pathogens: *Acinetobacter calcoaceticus*, *Alcaligenes faecalis*, *Bacillus cereus*, *B. megaterium*, *B. subtilis*, *Cryptococcus neoformans*, *Enterobacter cloacae*, *Proteus mirabilis*, *Pseudomonas aeruginosa*, *Salmonella typhimurium*, and *Escherichia coli* (Asakawa 1990). Kamory et al. (1995) investigated marchantin A isolated from *M. polymorpha* and identified colony propagation activity against gram-positive bacteria, including *Streptococcus viridans*, *S. pyogenes*, *S. faecalis*, and *Staphylococcus aureus*, as well as activity against the gram-negative bacteria *Escherichia coli*, *Pseudomonas aeruginosa*, *Pasteurella multocida*, *Proteus mirabilis*, *Neisseria meningitidis*, and *Haemophilus influenzae*. Activity against the latter two was relatively moderate, however it should be noted that they can cause serious infection of the meninges, the membranes covering the brain and spinal cord, hence meningitis. This is a serious and often devastating disease. *Pasteurella multocida* is a common cause of soft tissue infection following licks, bites, or scratches from dogs and cats. Respiratory disease can result, in some cases, in pneumonia, central nervous system involvement, and endocarditis, with a mortality rate of approximately 30%.

Marchantin A is antifungal and shows activity against *Alternaria kikuchiana*, *Aspergillus fumigatus*, *A. niger*, *Candida albicans*, *Microsporum gypseum*, *Penicillium chrysogenum*, *Piricularia oryzae*, *Rhizoctonia solani*, *Saccharomyces cerevisiae*, and *Sporothrix schenckii* (Asakawa 1999). The latter is the cause of sporotrichosis, which affects both immunocompromised and immunocompetent people. Current antifungal treatments are prolonged, with significant mortality in immune-suppressed populations (Lin et al. 2023).

Marchantin A is cytotoxic to human melanoma (A375) cancer cells (Gawel-Beben et al. 2019). It increases coronary blood flow (Asakawa 2007), however, application for humans is unknown.

Marchantin A and plagiochin A show in vitro cytotoxicity against the protozoan parasite *Trypanosoma brucei*, which causes the deadly vector-borne disease African trypanosomiasis, or sleeping sickness, in humans and in animals (Otoguro et al. 2012). Activity is comparable to the standard therapeutic drugs eflornithine and suramin. Infection by this parasite is transmitted by the tsetse fly. Once a serious, even fatal disease, the numbers in sub-Saharan Africa have dropped to only 600 people diagnosed with this infection in 2020.

Marchantin A and E are farnesoid X receptor agonists. This receptor controls the expression of critical genes involved in bile acid and cholesterol homeostasis, suggesting possible application for hyperlipidemia (Asakawa et al. 2007).

Marchantin B, also isolated from *Marchantia polymorpha*, inhibits the biosynthesis of 5-lipoxygenase products and the release of arachidonic acid in Ca2+ ionophore A23I8–stimulated human granulocytes. The compound also shows significant cyclooxygenase inhibitory activity (Panossian et al 1996). This suggests powerful anti-inflammatory potential.

Marchantin C is found in *Marchantia polymorpha*, *M. paelacea*, and *M. tosana*, as well as in the liverworts *Dumortiera hirsuta* and *Reboulia hemisphaerica*. It shows promising antitumor activity, including angiogenesis, cell migration, and microtubule polymerization inhibition (Shi et al. 2009). Apoptosis on human glioblastoma (A172) cells was noted. The researchers also noted Bax expression was up-regulated, and Bcl-2 was down-regulated, which indicates a positive step forward in cancer treatment. The same authors used marchantin C on xenografted nude mice, suggesting in vivo inhibition of cervical cancer (A172 and HeLa) cell lines. Lv et al. (2012) have established that this compound inhibits angiogenesis, wherein cancer tumors produce blood vessels to feed themselves. Tube formation associated with glioblastoma (T98G) was inhibited, but not so much in human leukemia (THP1) cells. A macrocyclic bisbibenzyl, marchantin C inhibits the migration of glioma cancer (T98G and U87) cell lines and induces apoptosis of human glioma A172 cells (Shi, Liao et al. 2008).

Marchantin C and its derivatives may be useful in chemotherapy multidrug resistance, increasing the toxicity in vincristine-resistant human oral epithelial (KB/VCR) cells (Xi et al. 2010). The structure of marchantin C is distinctly different than other microtubule inhibitors such as colchicine, paclitaxel, vinblastine, and vincristine. But it does inhibit microtubule polymerization, with potential antitumor activity as a result.

Induction of apoptosis in human prostate cancer (PC-3) cells by marchantin M was noted by Zhang, Xing et al. (2015).

Marchantin A, B, D, perrottetin F, and paleatin B all show anti-HIV activity. Paleatin B is also found in *Marchantia paleacea* var. *diptera* (Asakawa 2008).

The H1N1 and H5N1 influenza viruses have caused pandemics around the world. Marchantins A, B, and E, as well as plagiochin A and perrottetin F all exhibit anti-influenza activity (Iwai et al. 2011; Asakawa et al. 2013, "Cytotoxic and Antiviral"). Marchantin E may inhibit the SARS-Cov-2 virus as well (Prateeksha et al. 2021).

Jiang et al. (2013) found marchantin M inhibited P13K activity responsible for controlling cell growth and downregulated the pathway that activates autophagy in prostate cancer cells. This anticancer activity has been noted in other studies as well. Marchantin M inhibits proliferation and promotes cell death in human prostate PC-3 cancer cell lines (Xu et al. 2010) and LNCaP prostate cancer cell lines (Hu et al. 2016). It induces apoptosis through endoplasmic reticulum stress in prostate cancer (DU145) cell lines as well.

Marchantin M sensitizes prostate (PC-3) cancer cells to the cancer drug docetaxel, inducing apoptosis. This suggests a useful adjuvant to improve standard chemotherapy approaches to this increasingly common cancer (Niu et al. 2014). Marchantin M may play a key role in increasing the efficiency of standard chemotherapy drugs, which are pro-inflammatory. By decreasing and regulating senescence-associated secretory phenotype (SASP), which promotes malignant phenotypes, marchantin M may activate synergistic effects during co-treatment with doxorubicin (Niu et al. 2019). The research team notes that it is critical to regulate the senescence-associated secretory phenotype due to its effect on promoting malignant phenotypes and limiting the efficiency of cancer therapy. Their study found that inactivation of transcription factor EB and nuclear factor-$_k$B by marchantin M significantly contributes to the suppression of SASP.

Cathepsin is a lysosomal cysteine protease enzyme correlated with health issues regarding osteoporosis and allergies. It may also be involved in the processing of antigens in the immune response, hormone activation, and bone turnover. There is evidence that cathepsin B is implicated in the pathology of chronic inflammatory diseases of the airways and joints, and in cancer and pancreatitis. Enzyme inhibitors from natural products to develop chemopreventative drugs for these diseases have led researchers to the marchantin series, including isomarchantin C, found to be the strongest inhibitor of both cathepsin L (95%) and B (93%) (Mort and Buttle 1997).

Cathepsin B produces β-amyloid plaquing in Alzheimer's disease, and cathepsin L helps to generate peptide neurotransmitters (Hook et al. 2012). Scientists note that future research will unveil significant roles of cysteine cathepsins in cellular, physiological, and disease conditions, pointing to the potential of new target strategies, such as compounds found in bryophytes, to address neurodegenerative diseases.

Another compound found in liverworts, perrottetin D, has been studied extensively by Schwartner et al. (1996). This compound gave proof to the verifiably superior radical-scavenging capability of the aroxyl radical derived from the phenolic antioxidant.

Perrottetin E exhibits inhibitory activity for thrombin, which is associated with blood coagulation (Asakawa et al. 1987).

Common liverwort, *Marchantia polymorpha*, has been found to be an aromatase inhibitor useful in the prevention and treatment of hormone-sensitive cancers such as breast and prostate (Hegazy et al. 2012). The endogenous plant hormone idole-3-acetic acid was isolated from this liverwort. This lectin has been shown to agglutinate erthrocytes of different mammals and exhibits carbohydrate specificity against complex carbohydrate structures. Common liverwort also contains α-tocopherol, vitamin K, plastoquinone, plasto-hydroquinone, and α-tocoquinone, as well as prelunaric acid and (S)-2-hydroxycuparene.

Various antifungal bisbibenzyls found in *Marchantia polymorpha* exhibit activity against *Candida albicans*, including marchantin A, B, E; plagiochin E, 13,13'-O-isoproylidenericcardin D; and neomarchantin (Niu et al. 2006). Plagiochin E helps reverse fungal resistance to fluconazole by inhibiting cell wall chitin synthesis in *Candida albicans* (Wu et al. 2008). And reverses fungal resistance via the efflux pump (Guo, Leng et al. 2008). Plagiochin E induces apoptosis in *Candida albicans* through a metacaspase-dependent apoptotic pathway (Wu et al. 2010). This secondary metabolite is cytotoxic to murine leukemia (P-388) cell lines, and it increases the cytotoxicity of the cancer medication adriamycin in multidrug-resistant leukemia (K562/A02) cancer cell lines (Shi, Qu et al. 2008).

Marchantins O and P have been synthesized. It is hoped the resulting drugs from these highly bioactive compounds will retain the microtubular inhibition and antitumor activity found in marchantin C and have similar reduced side effects (Speicher et al. 2011). We will see.

A chlorophyll derivative found in *Marchantia polymorpha*, pheophorbide A, is a porphyrin compound similar to animal protoporphyrin IX, which shows extraordinary activity against SARS-CoV-2, preventing infection in cultured monkey and human cells. Work by Jimenez-Aleman et al. (2021) found it targets the viral particle, interfering with its infectivity in a dose and time-dependent manner. Besides SARS-CoV-2, the compound also displays broad-spectrum antiviral activity against enveloped RNA viral pathogens such as human coronavirus, West Nile virus, and other coronaviruses.

Ethanol extracts of *Marchantia polymorpha* induced apoptosis in hepatic (H22) tumor growth in a mouse model and improved their survival rate (Zhou et al. 2021).

MARCHESINIA

MacKay's Pouncewort

MacKay's pouncewort (*Marchesinia mackaii*) forms dense, dark patches that look like graffiti scribbled on rocks. It has been collected and distilled. The essential oil has antibacterial activity against *Bacillus subtilis*, *Escherichia coli*, *Salmonella pullorum*, *S. aureus*, and *Yersinia enterocolitica* (Figueiredo et al. 2002). Pullorum disease caused by *Salmonella pullorum* is a serious infection in the poultry industry, causing high morbidity and mortality from multidrug-resistant infections in young chicks. Yersiniosis infection is mainly caused by eating raw or undercooked pork, causing an estimated 117,000 illnesses, 640 hospitalizations, and 35 deaths annually in the United States alone (Ong et al. 2015).

MARSUPELLA

Rushwort

Marsupella is mainly a northern hemisphere genus containing at least 33 species.

Water rushwort (*Marsupella aquatica*) contains amorphane sesquiterpenoids, including (+)-7ß-hydroxyamorpha-4,11-diene; (-)-9α-hydroxyamorpha-4,7(11)-diene; (-)-3α-hydroxyamorpha-4,7(11)-diene; (-)-3α-acetoxyamorpha-4,7(11)-diene; (-)-amorpha-4,7(11)-dien-3-one; (+)-2,8-epoxyamorpha-4,7(11)-diene; (+)-5,9-epoxyamorpha-3,7(11)-diene; (-)-2α-hydroxyamorpha-4,7(11)-diene; and (-)-2ß-acetoxyamorpha-4,7(11)-diene (Adio et al. 2007). When hydro-distilled, the amorphane sesquiterpenoids dominate, including (-)-myltayl-8(12)-ene; ent-(+)-amorpha-4-11-diene; (-)-amorpha-4,7(11)-diene; and the sesquiterpene alcohols (+)-9-hydroxyselina-4,11-diene and (-)-2-acetoxyamorpha-4,7(11)-diene (Adio et al. 2002).

Notched rushwort, *Marsupella emarginata*, contains marsupellone and acetoxymarsupellone, both of which are cytotoxic against leukemia (P-388) cell lines (Nagashima et al. 1993). When hydro-distilled, the liverwort yielded the longipinanes marsupellone; marsupellol; 5-hydroxymarsupellol acetate; (-)-7-epi-ereophila-1(10),8,11-triene; and the sesquiterpene derivatives (-)-4-epi-marsupellol; (-)-marsupellol acetate; (+)-5-hydroxymarsupellol acetate; and (-)-9-acetoxygymnomitr-8(12)-ene. Crude extracts of the liverwort *Marsupella* show activity against *Staphylococcus aureus* and *Bacillus subtilis* (Adio et al. 2002).

MASTIGOPHORA

Wood's Whipwort

The genus name may derive from the ancient Greek *mastigophoros*, meaning "scourge-bearing," from *mastic*, "whip" or "scourge," and *phoros*, "carrying" or "bearing." The name is also applied to a group of protozoal flagellates from the kingdom Protista. Fifteen species have been identified to date.

Fukuyama and Asakawa (1991a) studied the Malaysian liverwort *Mastigophora diclados* and found it contains various ent-trachylobane diterpenoids, including the novel ent-18-hydroxytrachyloban-19-oic acid. It also contains four dimeric isocuparane-type sesquiterpenes, mastigophorenes A–D. The compounds A, B, and D have been found to accelerate neuritic sprouting in a cell culture. It is proposed by the authors that their biosynthesis is initiated by phenolic oxidation of (-)-herbertenediol. The search for neurotropic natural products includes the activity and synthesis of dimeric isocuparane-type sesquiterpenes derived from this liverwort (Fukuyama et al. 2020).

The compounds (-)-α herbertenediol; (-)-α-herbertenediol; (-)-mastigophorene A; (-)-mastigophorene C–D; and (-)-diplohyllolide A show cytotoxicity against leukemia (HL-60) and human oral epithelial (KB) cancer cell lines (Komala et al. 2010, "Cytotoxic"; Komala et al. 2010, "Volatile"). Antimicrobial activity against *Bacillus subtilis* was also noted.

The presence of herbatane monomers and dimers as well as cuprenes show inhibition of LPS-induced production of nitric oxide. Alpha-herbertenol showed 76% inhibition.

Ng et al. (2017) examined *Mastigophora diclados* and dentified dicladoic acid and the enantiomer of chlorantene G. These herbertane-type sesquiterpenes were identified as the major metabolites and can be regarded as suitable chemotaxonomical markers.

This Southern Hemisphere liverwort was collected and studied for volatile compounds by Koid et al. (2022). It contains 25.2% pentanoic acid; 2,2,4-trimethyl-3-carboxyisopropyl; isobutyl ester; decanal (9.1%); and minor amounts of limonene, linalool, geranyl acetone, methyl salicylate, geranylacetone, nonanal, and decanal.

METZGERIA

Veilworts

The genus is named in honor of Johann Metzger (1789–1852), a German botanist. Maybe.

Rock veilwort, *Metzgeria conjugata*, and nine other bryophytes out of twenty-three studied by Sevim et al. (2017) exhibit good antimicrobial activity

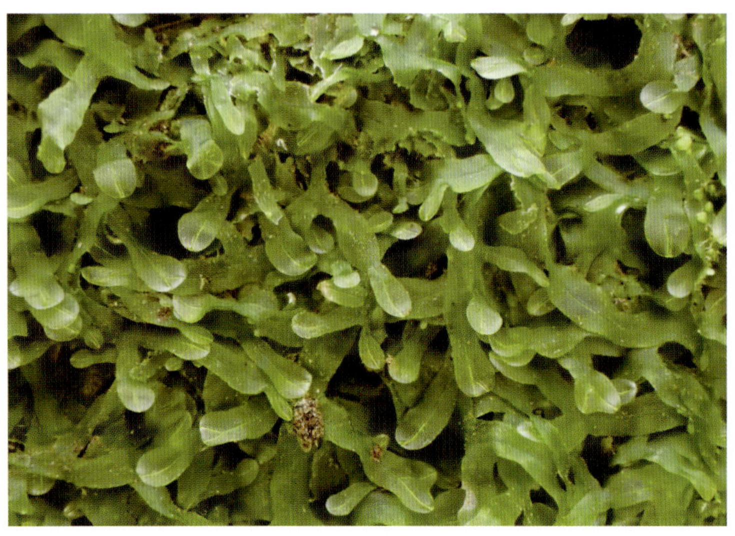

Metzgeria furcata (Forked Veilwort)

against *Paenibacillus* larvae isolates that cause American foulbrood diseases in honeybee larvae. Other bryophytes showing benefit are the mosses *Polytrichum formosum*, *P. commune*, *Calliergonella cuspitada*, *C. lindbergi*, *Isothecium alopecuroides*, *Syntrichia calcicola*, *S. intermedia*, *Tortella densa*, and *Grimmia alpestris*.

Forked veilwort (*Metzgeria furcata*) is a pioneer liverwort, meaning its habitat is being quickly overtaken by stronger mosses.

Homeopathy

The homeopathic remedy forked veilwort, from *Metzgeria furcata*, is for the "locked-in" syndrome. Other people do not understand, thinking there is a mental handicap or an inability to comprehend things. The person feels awkward or naïve, misunderstood by others, and avoids situations where they feel exposed. When irritated or annoyed, the person loses sleep, and when worse, they scream loudly when no one can hear.

The recommended dose is 30c once a week.*

MOERCKIA

Ruffworts

Irish ruffwort, *Moerckia hibernica*, is found in the Northern Hemisphere. Reports of this liverwort may be incorrect, however, and they probably refer to Flotow's ruffwort, *Moerckia flotoviana*.

Another species, *Moerckia erimona*, the former name of *Hattorianthus erimonus*, contains the lignan derivative erimopyrone (Tazaki et al. 1999).

MONOCLEA

The large New Zealand liverwort *Monoclea forsteri* contains the valuable compound riccardin D, also found in *Marchantia polymorpha*. As a result, it exhibits antiproliferative activity on human glioma (A172) cancer cell lines and induction of apoptosis (Asakawa 1995a). Riccardin D also reverses P-glycoprotein-mediated multidrug resistance.

*Case study by Christina Ari, in Narayana Verlag's *Mosses and Ferns* (2021–22), 35–36.

MYLIA

Gray Hard Scale Liverwort Naked Liverwort Taylor's Flapwort

Two main chemotypes are found in the Northern Hemisphere *Mylia* genus. The genus is named in honor the Dutch physician Willem Mylius (1674–1748), and author of *Dissertatio festiva de viribus imagiationis foeminarum praegnantium in suos foetus.*

Taylor's flapwort or gray hard scale liverwort (*Mylia taylorii*) and another species, *Mylia nuda*, dubbed naked liverwort, both yield essential oils containing aromadendranes and *seco*-aromadendranes. The former liverwort is found on rotten wood on cliffs in higher elevations. Work by Von Reuss et al. (2004) revealed 13 new constituents in both species. These include the aromadendranes and *seco*-aromadendranes myli-4(15)-ene; aromadendra-1(10),4(15)-diene; aromadendra-4,10(14)-diene; and aromadenra-4,9-diene. Three oxaspiro-compounds were identified as well: 7-epi-bourbon-3-en-5,11 oxide; guai-4,10(14)-diene-5,11-oxide; and guai-3,9-dien-5,11-oxide. Alpha taylorione, taylocyclane, taylofuran, and taynudol were also identified.

The sesquiterpenes of Taylor's flapwort possess insecticidal and antibacterial activity. Aromadendrene, globulol, and barbatene exhibit activity against a range of bacteria as reported by Yan et al. (2021). Aromadendrene, for example, shows significant inhibition of methicillin-resistant *Staphylococcus aureus* (MRSA) and vancomycin-resistant *Enterococcus* (Mulyaningsih et al. 2010). Aromadendrene is not only antibacterial, but it also possesses insecticidal activity (Giuliani et al. 2020).

The related species *Mylia nuda* contains two diterpenoids, (+)-labda-7,14-dien-13-ol and (+)-manoyl oxide; and one *bis*(bibenzyl) compound, isomarchantin C (Wu and Asakawa 1987).

Manoyl oxide is a major constituent of essential oil derived from the shrubby *Cistus creticus*, or pink rock rose, a shrubby plant that is reported to give considerable pain relief to those infected with Lyme disease (Hutschenreuther et al. 2010). It should be noted the leaf of pink rock rose is widely used as a tea, but in vitro tests found the volatile oil exhibits the strongest inhibition against *Borrelia burgdorferi*, the bacterial species of the spirochete class that causes Lyme disease. Isomarchantin C is also found in the Japanese liverworts *Dumortiera hirsuta* and *Conocephalum japonicum*. It exhibits cytotoxicity against the human epithelial (KB) cancer cell line (Toyota et al. 2013; Liu et al. 2011). *Mylia nuda* also contains nudenoic acid, a novel tricyclic sesquiterpenoid (Liu et al. 1996).

The species *Mylia anomala* and *Mylia verrucosa*, which are secondary chemotypes, produce mainly cyathane-type diterpenoids. The latter liverwort contains a novel diterpene alcohol, (-)-neoverrucosan-5*B*-ol (Matsuo et al. 1980).

NARDIA

Flapworts

Two-lobed flapwort (*Nardia insecta*) is rare or endangered in North America. Its original common name, bug flapwort, is derived from an error, as the Latin *insectum* means "to cut in," in reference to two lobes incised in the leaf.

Nardia subclavata and other *Nardia* species contain typical diterpenoids with a malonate moiety. This liverwort contains ent-kaurene monool, 3 kaurene malonate diterpenoids, ent-clerodane, (-)-kolavelool, ent-kaurene, and perrottetin E (Toyota and Asakawa 1993). The latter compound is also found in the liverwort *Cladoradula perrottetii* syn. *Radula perrottetii.*

NOTOSCYPHUS

Rose Moss

The genus name derives from Greek *notio*, meaning "south," and *scyphus*, "drinking vessel."

The Chinese liverwort *Notoscyphus lutescens* syn. *N. collenchymatosus* contains notolutesins K–P, along with five known dolabrane derivatives and a known pimarane derivative. Notolutesin P shows cytotoxic activity against a small panel of human cancer cell lines, with one compound, notolutesin A, exhibiting activity against the PC-3 prostate cancer cell line (Wu et al. 2016; Wang et al. 2014).

Rose moss (a liverwort), *Notoscyphus lutescens*, is commercially used in freshwater aquariums. The species name is derived from *luteo*, meaning "yellow." It contains dolabrane-type diterpenoids, notoscarins A–J, and a butrylactone derivative. All show weak quinone-reductase-inducing activity in hepatic cancer cells (Han et al. 2021, "Dolabrane"). The extinct *Notoscyphus balticus* was found in Baltic amber.

PALLAVICINA

Questionable Veilwort   Ribbonwort

In the Philippines, various *Pallavicinia* species are used for their antimicrobial properties (Azuelo 2011). The genus honors L. O. Pallavicini (1719–1785).

The antibacterial properties of axenic cultures of various liverworts, including *Pallavicinia lyellii*, show mild inhibition of *Bacillus subtilis* (Millar et al. 2007).

Questionable veilwort, *Pallavicinia ambigua*, contains pallamins A–C. Isolated compounds demonstrate significant anti-inflammatory activity in vivo (Li, Li et al. 2023).

Pallamins A and B, along with pallambins C and D, were tested for cytotoxicity against human cancer cell lines (Wang et al. 2012).

Ribbonwort, also called veilwort (*Pallavicinia lyellii*) is usually found in swampy areas in temperate forests. The species is named in honor of Charles Lyell (1767–1849), the famous Scottish botanist who studied mosses and lichens who was well-known as the English translator of Dante. His son, Scottish geologist Charles Lyell (1797–1875), was an associate of Charles Darwin and a pioneer in explaining the significance of "deep time" for understanding the earth and environment and the concept of what we now think of as "climate change."

Pallavicinia lyellii contains some interesting compounds, including polygodial, sacculatal, pallavicinol, a rare chettaphanin-type diterpenoid, 4-desmethylsterol, and ascorbate peroxidase, which is most active at 40° C. It was found to exhibit antibacterial activity by Belcik and Weigner (1980). Later work by Millar et al. (2007) found an extract from axenic culture showed only slight activity against *Bacillus subtilis*. Linde et al. (2016) found a 1:1 chloroform/methanol extract active against *Escherichia coli*. Its antifungal activity was tested against *Aspergillus niger*, *A. fumigatus*, *Fusarium oxysporum*, and *Candida albicans* by Subhisha and Subranomiam (2006). Various solvents were used, and alcohol extracts exhibited the maximum activity. *Aspergillus fumigatus* was determined the most vulnerable. A mouse study determined the alcohol extracts showed no short-term toxicity.

The species *Pallavicinia levieri* contains the pungent diterpene sacculatal, which has also been identified in *Trichocoleopsis sacculata*, *Pellia endiviifolia*, and *Fossombronia wondraczekii* (Asakawa et al. 1977).

Pallavicinia subciliata contains pallacivinin and its diastereomer, neopallavicinin, as well as pallasubin A and pallasubin-derived dimers B–D. Pallasubin B exhibits strong cytotoxic activity with a 73% inhibition rate of nitric oxide production on LPS-induced murine leukemia (RAW 264.7) macrophages (Liu et al. 2022).

PARASCHISTOCHILA

One Sided Pocketwort

Paraschistochila pinnatifolia is found throughout New Zealand and Tasmania. It contains sacculatane-type diterpenoids which are also found in *Porella perrottetiana*. Lorimer, Perry et al. (1997) identified ent-1α-hydroxykauran-12-one. The compound ent-1β-hydroxykauran-12-one isolated from this liverwort showed cytotoxicity against leukemia (P-388) cell lines, and antifungal inhibition of *Candida albicans* (Lorimer, Perry et al. 1997).

PEDINOPHYLLUM

Craven Featherwort

The genus name encorporates the Latin *ped* and its Greek counterpart, *pedino*, meaning "the ground" and *phylum*, "leaf," probably referring to its prostrate shoots.

Craven featherwort (*Pedinophyllum interruptum* syn. *P. pyrenaicum*) is found in eastern North America, usually among mosses growing under white cedar trees (*Thuja occidentalis*). It is also found near limestone creeks or on dolomitic soil throughout Quebec, with small patches in Massachusetts, Indiana, Ohio, and upstate New York. It is imperiled in Tennessee, but found in forests of northern Europe and Asia.

It contains 10 ent-pimarine-type diterpenoids, pedinophyllols A–J, which inhibit germination of *Arabidopsis thaliana*, a common roadside weed (Liu, Li et al. 2013). Work by Feld et al. (2014) identified two prenylated benzoic acid derivatives and two new chromenes from diethyl ether extracts.

PELLIA

Endive Pellia   Overleaf Pellia

Geographic Range: cool, temperate areas of North America, Europe, and Asia

Habitat: damp, sheltered woodlands with neutral or acidic soil; wet rocks

Practical Uses: perfume

Medicinal Applications: antibacterial, anticancer, antiviral, immune modulation, neuroprotective, pain

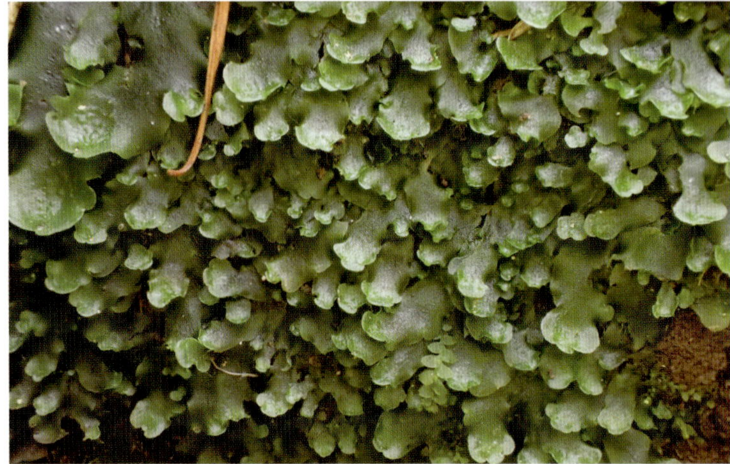

Pellia sp. (Pellia)

The Hesquiat of Vancouver Island would chew or gargle the juice of *Pellia epiphylla* "if a child had a sore mouth or throat that prevented them from eating or drinking. They would either drink the juice or chew the pulp of the liverwort" (Turner and Efrat 1982). The Ditidaht, another First Nations people, used it internally and externally for pain (Dey and de Nath 2011).

Pellia endiviifolia, endive pellia, usually found east of the Rockies near my home, has a sweet mossy odor with a trace of dry, seaweed. It contains the unusual diterpenedial sacculatal, which exhibits antibacterial activity against *Streptococcus mutans* (dental caries) and antiviral activity against HIV-1. Succulatane diterpenedial, the hot-tasting substance found in *Pellia endiviifolia* as well as in *Pellia neesiana*, shows cytotoxicity against lung (Lu-1), squamous mouth, drug-resistant squamous (KB-V), prostate (LNCaP), and ductal breast (ZR-75-1) cancer cell lines (Asakawa et al. 2008).

Ivkovic et al. (2021) found that perrotettin E, derived from *Pellia endiviifolia*, exhibits activity against promyelocytic lymphoma (HL-60), human myeloid leukemia (U-937), myelogenous leukemia (K562), testicular carcinoma (NT2/DI), glioblastoma (A-172), and glioblastoma multiforme (U-251) cancer cell lines. As well, the compounds 10'-hydroxyperrottetin E and 10,10'dihydroxyperrottetin E exhibit cytotoxicity against promyelocytic leukemia (HL-60), testicular (NT2/D1), glioblastoma (A-172), lymphoma (U-937), chronic myelogenous leukemia (K562), and glioblastoma multiforme (U-251) cancer cell lines.

Ivkovic et al. (2021) identified perrottetin E, 10'-hydroxyperrottetin E and 10,10'-dihydroxyperrottetin E in *Pellia endiviifolia*. Modest cytotoxicity was noted for three human leukemia cancer cell lines (HL-60, U-937, and K-562),

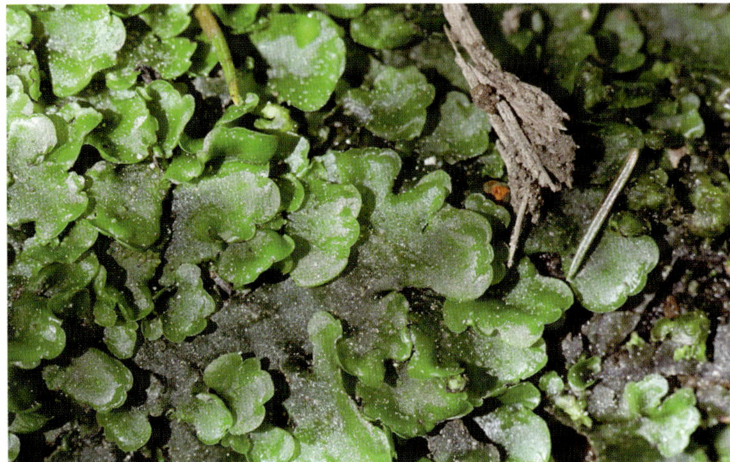

Pellia epiphylla
(Overleaf Pellia)

and significant activity against NT2/D1 (human embryonal teratocarcinoma); and U-251 and A-172 (human glioblastoma) cancer cell lines.

Overleaf pellia, *Pellia epiphylla*, exhibits antimicrobial activity against *Staphylococcus aureus*, *S. epidermidis*, and *Bacillus cereus* (Akatin et al. 2022); following this investigation the researchers created soap and cream formulations that proved efficacious against all three pathogens. This would be a huge improvement over the antibacterial soaps presently on the market, since there is no evidence they are more effective than plain soap for preventing infection in most cases. In fact, lab studies suggest triclosan contributes to making bacteria resistant to antibiotics. It is estimated that one in ten bacteria exposed to triclosan manage to survive the antibiotic. This compound, found in most liquid soaps and one third of bar soaps, moves from the sink where we wash our hands to our river systems. A final ban by the FDA took effect in April 2020.

The whole plant has a unique, seaweed-like aroma that could be useful in perfumery. It has a persistent pungent taste when the fresh plant is chewed, probably due to the presence of sacculatal, 1β-hydroxysacculatal, and various sacculatane-type diterpenoids. The liverworts *Pallavicinia levieri*, *Lobatiriccardia coronopus* syn. *Riccardia lobata*, and *Trichocoleopsis sacculata* contain this sacculatal compound as well. When dried, *Pellia endiviifolia* loses its hot taste. The compound sacculatal exhibits cytotoxicity against human melanoma and lung adenocarcinoma (SK-Lu1), leukemia (KB), androgen-sensitive prostate (LNCaP), and ductal breast carcinoma (ZR-75-1) cell lines (Novakovic et al. 2021). It also exhibits strong activity against dental caries, *Streptococcus mutans*, and kills the tick species *Panonychus citri*.

Overleaf pellia (*Pellia epiphylla*) is also quite common. Italian botanist Fabio Colonna originally named it the cumbersome tome, "*lichen alter minor caule calceato hypodedemenos*" (Colonna 1616). This was before Linnaeus proposed the well-known shortened binomial used today. Epiphyllins A–H are sacculatane diterpenoids found in this liverwort, along with pellianolactone B. The latter compound is protective against hydrogen peroxide–induced oxidation and apoptosis in adrenal-medulloblastoma/pheochromocytoma (PC12) cells (Li et al. 2019). The cells are used in laboratory studies to test for neuronal death. When the cells are subjected to neuron growth factor, they synthesize acetylcholine and form neurite growth. The cell wall contains NMDA receptors that regulate synaptic plasticity, memory, and cognition. They are one of the cellular models for current Alzheimer's disease research. In 2021 it was reported that 6.2 million Americans aged 65 years or older were living with Alzheimer's disease. This number is projected to grow to 8.2 million by 2030, and 15.2 million people by 2050. It is estimated that Alzheimer's and other forms of dementia cost the U.S. economy $355 billion in 2021, and will come to more than $1.1 trillion by 2050.

Pellia neesiana contains α-gurjunene, bicyclogermacrene, calamenene, and gamma-cadinene (Asakawa et al. 2007). Calamenene induces dendritic cells from human monocytes and enhances T cell proliferation to activate anti-inflammatory effects (Takei et al. 2006). Gamma-cadinene inhibits human histamine H2 receptor, which plays a key role in histamine-stimulated gastric acid production. When overstimulated, it can cause excessive production of histamines, which can lead to gastric ulcers (Chaudhary et al. 2017).

PLAGIOCHASMA

Cliff Waxwort Wax Liverwort

Geographic Range: Asia, North and South America

Habitat: moist, shady, and limestone substrates to warm and drier climates

Practical Uses: antioxidant, antimicrobial, detecting heavy metals, skin conditions

Medicinal Applications: antibacterial, anticancer, antifungal, anti-inflammatory, kidneys, muscle relaxant, vulnerary

Plagio means "oblique," and *chasma* has several meanings.

It is Latin for "a wide gap" or "a breach." But it could also derive from the Persian *casma*, meaning "spring," or *casm*, "eye." There are about 16 species.

Plagiochasma appendiculatum syn. *Aytona appendiculata* has been used by traditional healers for cuts, burns, wounds, and various skin disorders. It contains marchantin A–C and neomarchatin A and riccardins C and D. As a result, both water and alcohol extracts of this liverwort show significant activity against a wide range of bacteria and fungi. The bacteria include *Micrococcus luteus*, *Bacillus subtilis*, *B. cereus*, *Staphylococcus aureus*, *Streptococcus pneumoniae*, *Enterobacter aerogenes*, *Escherichia coli*, *Klebsiella pneumoniae*, *Proteus mirabilis*, *Pseudomonas aeruginosa*, and *Salmonella typhimurium* (Singh et al. 2006). Many of these pathogenic bacteria have become drug-resistant.

Fungi inhibited by this liverwort are *Candida albicans*, *Cryptococcus albidus*, *Trichophyton rubrum*, *Aspergillus niger*, *A. flavus*, *A. spinulosus*, *A. terreus*, and *A. nidulans* (Singh et al. 2006). *Cryptococcus albidus* can be fatal in those who are immune-compromised, including children. The soil-borne *Aspergillus spinulosus* was isolated from an immune-competent 22-month-old baby suffering from central nervous system aspergillosis and meningitis. However, a review of 92 cases (1973–2011) of *Aspergillus* meningitis in various age groups by Antinori et al. (2012) suggests it is not that rare and has a fatality rate of 72%.

In work by Singh et al. (2006), extracts of *Plagiochasma appendiculatum* showed wound-healing capability, including wound contraction and increased tensile strength. Antioxidant activity was also noted.

Work by Bodade et al. (2008) found an ethanol extract inhibits *Escherichia coli*, *E. aerogenes*, *Klebsiella pneumoniae*, *Proteus vulgaris*, *P. aeruginosa*, and *Staphylococcus aureus*. Water extracts inhibited *Escherichia coli* better than ethanol extracts. Antifungal inhibition was noted for *Aspergillus niger*, with distilled water extracts as well as acetone, ethanol, and chloroform extracts.

Acetone, but not water extracts, inhibit *Escherichia coli*, *Salmonella typhi*, *Aspergillus niger*, and *Candida albicans* (Vashistha et al. 2007).

Extracts of *Plagiochasma appendiculatum* inhibit *Alternaria alternata*, *Aspergillus niger*, and *A. flavus* in work by Sharma et al. (2014). *Alternaria alternata* is an opportunistic fungus of over 380 plant species that depends on a warm, moist environment to thrive. It causes stem canker in tomatoes as well as leaf spots, blight, and rot in on many plant parts. Planting rows north to south makes plants less susceptible.

Work by Singh et al. (2011) found that *Plagiochasma appendiculatum* and other species were more active against gram-negative bacteria when extracted with chloroform, while those subjected to butanol were more active against gram-positive bacteria, especially *Staphylococcus aureus*. This liverwort shows antioxidant activity against various bacteria and fungi (Joshi, Singh et al. 2022), while water-methanol extracts exhibit antiviral activity (Joshi et al. 2023). When the thallus is cultured in vitro, it possesses the ability to biosynthesize bisbibenzyl, suggesting the possibility of mass-producing certain highly beneficial bisbibenzyls (Zhao et al. 2022).

Riccardins C and D arrest cell cycle and induce apoptosis in prostate (LNCaP) cancer cell lines (Hu et al. 2016). Riccardin D induces cell death and activation of apoptosis and autophagy in osteosarcoma cells (Wang, Ji et al. 2013). Liu, Gao et al. (2012) found that ricardin D induces apoptosis through caspase-3 and topoisomerase II inhibiton, P-gp expression reduction, and angiogenesis inhibition. Riccardin D induces apoptosis of human leukemia cell lines (HL-60 and K562) and multidrug-resistant strains of leukemia cell lines (K562/A02) by targeting DNA topoisomerase II (Xue, Qu et al. 2012). Riccardin D is also found in *Dumortiera hirsuta*.

The synthesized riccardin D-26 shows stronger activity against hepatic carcinoma (SMMC-7721) cells than normal liver cells. When injected into mice, it effectively delays the growth of xenografts without significant toxicity. It activates p53 expression and induces apoptosis in cancer cells via that pathway (Yue, Zhang et al. 2013). Riccardin D-26 inhibits the growth of human oral squamous (KB) carcinoma cells and multidrug-resistant vincristine KB cells both in vitro and in vivo (Yue, Zhao et al. 2013). Riccardin D-26 inhibits cancer growth by inducing apoptosis in the activation of mitochondria-mediated intrinsic pathway (Yue, Zhang et al. 2013).

In North America, *Plagiochasma intermedium* is confined to Georgia, but it is also found in China, parts of South America, and elsewhere. It contains six macrocyclic bis(bibenzyls): pakyonol, neomarchantin A, isoriccardin C, marchantin H, riccardin F, and riccardin C (Xie et al. 2010), as well as plagiochin E. Both riccardin C and plagiochin E are cytotoxic to chemotherapy-resistant human prostate (PC-3) cancer cell lines (Xu et al. 2010). Riccardin F modulates the P-gp protein and significantly increases adriamycin accumulation and toxicity in myelogenous leukemia (A562/A02) cells (Ji et al. 2011). Adriamycin, a chemotherapy drug, is a topoisomerase inhibitor and anthracycline antibiotic originally derived from the *Streptomyces peucetius* bacterium. It is used to treat various cancers, including leukemia, lymphoma, neuroblastoma, Wilms tumor, and some cancers of the lung, breast, stomach, ovaries, thyroid, and bladder. It works by damaging the cancer cells' DNA and blocks an enzyme necessary for cell division and repair. The other compound in this liverwort, pakyonol, also improved adriamycin accumulation. In another study by Xu et al. (2010), pakyonol was found to induce apoptosis in prostate (PC-3) cancer cells, but with a weaker effect than riccardin C, marchantin M, and plagiochin E.

Riccardin C possesses antifungal activity against fluconazole-resistant strains of *Candida albicans*. It has a synergistic or additive activity when combined with this antifungal drug, reducing the minimum inhibitory concentration (MIC) by a highly significant 256-fold (Xie et al. 2010). Riccardin C also induces cell membrane leakage in drug-resistant gram-positive bacteria (Kuroda and Ogawa 2017).

Isoplagiochin C, derived from *Plagiochasma intermedium*, exhibits activity against *Candida albicans* (Yongabi 2016).

Plagiochasma japonicum exhibits antitumor, antifungal, and antimicrobial activity, inhibits release of superoxide, inhibits thrombin activity, and relaxes muscle tissue (Lahlou et al. 2000).

Cliff waxwort (*Plagiochasma rupestre*) extract, when combined with bentonite clay, showed 3 to 3.5-fold higher antibacterial and antifungal activity compared to the individual use of either the liverwort or the bentonite clay (Khan et al. 2022). In Peru, this liverwort is used for fainting spells and kidney disorders (Franquemont 1990). An in vivo study found significant inhibition of carrageenan-induced paw edema and promising suppressive effects on p-benzoquinone–induced abdominal constriction in animal models (Tosun et al. 2013). In China and India, this liverwort is considered antimicrobial and possibly beneficial in leukemia (Asakawa 2007; Azuelo 2011; Alam 2012; Durán-Peña et al. 2015). Extracts significantly inhibit mouse lymphoma induced by leukemia virus (YAC-1) and mouse myeloma (Sp2) cell lines (Önder and Özenoglu 2019).

PLAGIOCHILA

Featherworts

Geographic Range: worldwide

Habitat: fen depressions and calcareous rock crevices, hard limestone, or rocks in coastal districts

Practical Uses: pesticides

Medicinal Applications: antibacterial, anticancer, anti-inflammatory, antiparasitic, menstruation, vulnerary

The genus name may derive from the Greek *plagios*, meaning "slanting," and *cheilos*, "beak" or "rim," for the flattened perianths and wide truncated mouth. Maybe . . .

There may be up to 1,600 species of *Plagiochila* on the planet, many of them tropical or subtropical. More than 950 species, including synonyms and unchecked species, and 633 accepted species. One recent study by Renner et al. (2021) also suggests there are as many as 1,600 validly published species names. They are commonly referred to as featherworts. This is preferable to the former name gurnwort, with *gurn* meaning "grimace" (Edwards 2012).

Various *Plagiochila* species contain natural pesticides, including the sesquiterpenes hemiacetyl and plagiochiline, which are potent poisons of mice. Many species contain plagiochiline A, which when chewed fresh has a hot, pungent taste, and perrottetin E, which is cytotoxic against the KB carcinoma cell line. The compounds most studied, however, are plagiochilin A, first isolated from several species of *Plagiochila* in 1978, and plagiochilin C. Both exhibit antiproliferative activity. Plagiochilin A shows inhibition on prostate (DU145), breast (MCF-7), and leukemia (K562) cell lines (Aponte et al. 2010). In the case of prostate cancer cells, this compound is superior to the chemotherapy drug fludarabine phosphate. Stivers et al. (2018) examined the effects of plagiochilin A on prostate cancer (DU145) cell division, where one cell divides into two daughter cells. The failure of the cells to complete cytokinesis triggers apoptosis. The exact mechanism of action is not fully elucidated but may involve targeting or binding to α-tubulin. It may be that plagiochilin A forms stable complexes with α-tubulin via binding with the pironetin sites.

While plagiochilins are potent on their own, the addition of a methoxy group at position C-3 gives the derivative methoxyplagiochiline A2, which has been shown to be more potent than plagiochilin C against human lung (H460) cancer cell lines (Wang, Ji et al. 2013). In the same study, however, plagiochilin C showed antiproliferative activity against glioblastoma (A172) cancer cells.

In a study of *Plagiochila ovalifolia*, the presence of plagiochilin A exhibited potency against the leukemia (P-388) cell line, but when a octanoyl or dedocadienoate side chain was added, the potency increased by 60 times (Toyota et al. 1998). A metabolite of plagiochilin A was found to inhibit prostate cancer (DU145) cell division by preventing completion of cytokinesis, particularly at the final removal stage, thereby inducing cell death (Stivers et al. 2018).

After *Plagiochila ovalifolia* is chewed for one or two minutes, plagiochilin A is converted by human saliva into hot and pungent plagiochilal B and furanoplagiochilal (Hashimoto et al. 1994). They are formed with a secoaromadendrane skeleton, a type of sesquiterpenoid with anti-inflammatory, antibacterial, antitumor, insecticidal, and antiviral activities.

There are currently 24 derivatives of plagiochilins, taking up nearly the entire alphabet—plagiochilins A–X. They are all related to some degree. Plagiochilin H, for example, is a close analog of C, and plagiochilins G and I are structurally similar to A and B.

Greater featherwort (*Plagiochila adianthoides*) contains plagiochilin S. Arctic Featherwort (*Plagiochila arctica*), when cultured, produces another highly valuable compound, indole-3-acetic acid (Law et al. 1985). Regarding this compound, an interesting observation by Tintelnot et al. (2023) may have implications for patients with pancreatic ductal adenocarcinoma (PDAC), which is projected to be the second most deadly human cancer by 2040 due to its high incidence of metastatic disease and limited treatment options. The microbiota-derived tryptophan metabolite indole-3-acetic acid (3-IAA) is enriched in patients who then better respond to chemotherapy. A combination of short-term dietary manipulation of tryptophan and oral 3-IAA administration was found to increase the efficacy of chemotherapy in mouse models of PDAC. This results in the accumulation of ROS and downregulation of autophagy in cancer cells, which compromises their metabolic health and ultimately causes their death. In two independent PDAC cohorts, the researchers observed a significant correlation between the levels of 3-IAA and the efficacy of chemotherapy.

Greater featherwort (*Plagiochila asplenioides*) and lesser featherwort (*Plagiochila porelloides*) are found in fen depressions and calcareous rock crevices.

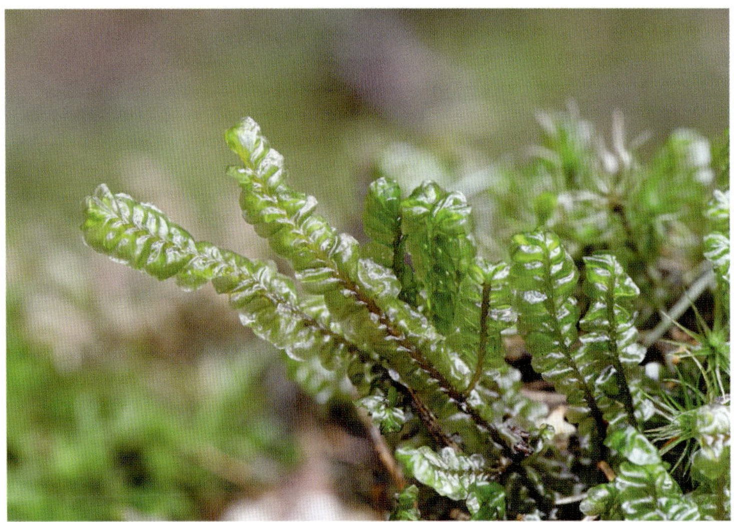

Plagiochila asplenioides (Greater Featherwort)

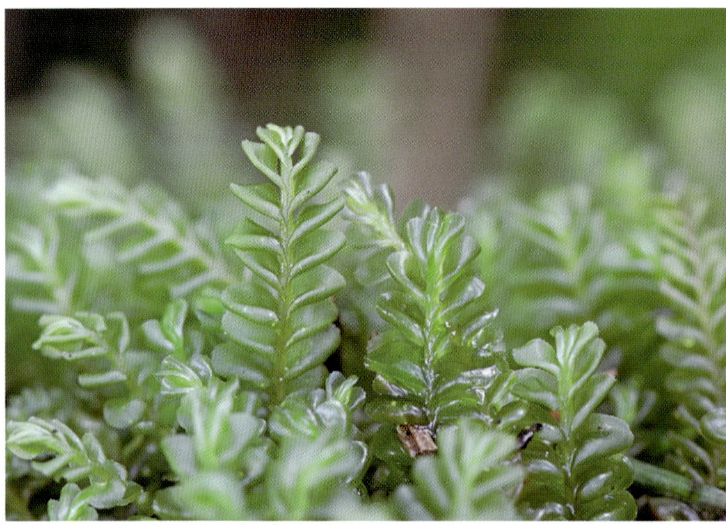

Plagiochila porelloides (Lesser Featherwort)

They are easy to identify, as they have toothed leaf margins and leaves on the top that extend downward along the stem. These species contain plagiochilins C–F, H, P, and W–X, as well as furanoplagiochilal, plagiochilal A–B, anadensin, and plagiochilide P. (Anadensin is also found in *Chandonanthus* species.)

Lesser featherwort, *Plagiochila porelloides*, is common throughout North America. In Quebec it is known as *plumette infléchie*, "inflected feather." It contains various volatile metabolites. Essential oil and ethanol extracts both show moderate activity against *Trypanosoma brucei*, the parasitic kinetoplastid transmitted by the tsetse fly in sub-Saharan Africa that causes sleeping sickness. The essential oil extract shows moderate activity against *Trypanosoma brucei* as well as against the parasite *Leishmania mexicana mexicana* (Pannequin et al. 2023). A diethyl oxide extract of this liverwort exhibits moderate anticancer activity and cytotoxicity against normal human fibroblasts.

In western Scotland is found *Plagiochila macra* syn. *P. atlantica*, which contains plagiochilin C and the structurally similar compound atlanticol.

The Southern Hemisphere liverwort *Plagiochila bantamensis* was collected and studied for volatile compounds (Koid et al. 2022). It contains limonene (17.4%), β-elemene (17.7%), germacrene B (10.4%), 1-dodecanol (9.2%), and minor constituents.

Plagiochila beddomei has been used traditionally to treat skin wounds in parts of India. A study by Manoj and Murugan (2012b) involving water and methanol extracts found both forms helped heal excision wounds and promoted the formation of granulation tissue, collagen production, and angiogenesis.

Results were superior to the standard ointment Madecassol, which contains an extract of gotu kola (*Centella asiatica*). Notably, after the third day of treatment, the methanol extract formed a micro vessel density and vascular endothelial growth factor expression. This suggests not only potent wound healing, but angiogenic activity as well.

In parts of India, *Plagiochila beddomei* is dried and used in a paste to treat different skin diseases. This liverwort contains various phenolic acids such as coumaric, ferulic, gallic, ferulic, protocatechol, cinnamic, sinapate, chlorogenate, and hydroxyl benzoate. Methanol extracts exhibit activity against various bacteria and fungi and possess antioxidant potential as well (Manoj and Murugan 2012a). Antimicrobial activity was noted against *Salmonella* species, *Escherichia coli*, *Staphylococcus aureus*, and *Candida albicans*. Further work by Manoj et al. (2016) examined the antibacterial potential of this liverwort. Methanol extracts strongly inhibited a number of pathogens, including *Salmonella typhimurium*, *S. aureus*, *Klebsiella pneumoniae*, *E. coli*, *Bacillus cereus*, *B. subtilis*, *Proteus vulgaris*, and *Pseudomonas aeruginosa*.

Killarney featherwort (*Plagiochila bifaria* syn. *P. killarniensis*) produces an essential oil containing three eudesmane-type sesquiterpenes: ent-eudesm-3-en-6-one; ent-eudesm-4(15)-en-6-one; and ent-7-hydroxyeudesm-4-en-6-one (Hackl et al. 2006). Extracts contain everninic acid methyl ester, 9.10-dihydrophenanthrenes, and methyl benzoates.

Plagiochila aerea syn. *P. bursata* possesses the insecticidal compounds plagiochilines A and M; fusicogigantone A; 1,4-dimethylazulene; and 2,3-secoaromadendrane. Several of these compounds are effective against the fall armyworm (*Spodoptera frugiperda*) particularly plagiochiline A, which produces abdomen and wing malformation in adults that makes mating impossible (Ramírez et al. 2010). This agricultural pest does the most damage to crops in the late summer in the southern United States and in the early fall in northern states. As the common name suggests, this insect moves through commercial corn, millet, sorghum, rice, and sugarcane crops like a ruthless army.

Plagiochila circinalis are simply C-13 oxidated products derived from plagiochilin C. This liverwort species is widely distributed in Scotland and Ireland and is also found in New Zealand. It contains fatty acid esters and sterols or triterpenoids, including cycloart-24-en-3ß-yl α linolenate; arachidonate; eicosapentaenoate; stigmasteryl gamma-linolenate; and 4α,14α-dimethyl-8,24(28)-ergostadien-3ß-yl arachidonate.

Plagiochila cristata, a Columbian liverwort, contains riccardin D, one of the most investigated macrocyclic bis-bibenzyls isolated from byrophytes (Valcic et al. 1997). Riccardin D induces apoptosis through the caspase signal pathway, DNA topoisomerase II inhibition, and NF-kB inhibition. Work by Xue, Qu et al. (2012) found inhibition of human leukemia (HL-60, K562, and MDR K562/A02) cell lines. It also contains plagiochilins C, H, and O–S.

While living in Peru in the early 1980s, I found dried *Plagiochila disticha* available at street markets. This liverwort is traditionally used externally for rheumatic pain and internally to normalize menstruation (Aponte et al. 2010). It contains plagiochilines A, B, I, and R. An ethanol extract was tested against a panel of human cancer cell lines. Plagiochiline A was tested for in vitro anti-leishmanial and trypanocidal inhibition, and multidrug-resistant strains of *Mycobacterium tuberculosis* (Aponte et al. 2010).

The Chinese liverwort *Plagiochila duthiana* contains plagiochianins A and B. Their inhibition of acetylcholinesterase was tested by Han, Zhang et al. 2018).

Plagiochila elegans contains plagiochilin A and isoplagiochilide.

Plagiochila ericicola contains plagiochilins C, H, O, P, and R. Plagiochilins C and H are closely related to plagiochilin O, whereas plagiochilin R is more closely related to plagiochilin B.

The New Zealand liverwort *Plagiochila fasciculata* inhibits the human leukemia (P-388) cancer cell line (Asakawa 1982). This liverwort contains antifungal hydroxy-acetophenones (Lorimer and Perry 1994), including 2-hydroxy-3,4,6-trimethoxyacetopnenone and 2-hydroxy-4,6-dimethoxyacetophenone. Activity was noted against herpes simplex type 1 and polio type 1 viruses and the fungi *Trichophyton mentagrophytes* and *Amorphotheca resinae.* The former fungus is a source of ringworm in humans and animals, and the latter is known to thrive in environments containing aviation fuel, hence the moniker "kerosene fungus." It is a microbial contaminant in diesel fuel. Both ethanol and acetone extracts inhibit *Escherichia coli*, *Bacillus cereus*, *Pseudomonas aeruginosa*, and *Dickeya dadantii* syn. *Erwinia chrysanthemi.* The latter bacterium causes soft rot in a number of flowering plants and vegetables and is a major pathogen in potato, banana, and pineapple crops. It has both a dark side and a bright side, however.

Work by Duarté et al. (2000) found it can adhere to and cause oxidative stress and kill cultured human adenocarcinoma cell lines. This bacterium expresses a surface protein similar to intimin, a protein necessary for full virulence of enterohemorrhagic and enteropathogenic *Escherichia coli.* It also contains asparaginase, an enzyme used along with chemotherapy drugs for acute lymphoblastic leukemia and non-Hodgkin's lymphoma. Some patients have allergic reactions to the *Escherichia coli*-derived leukemia drugs asparaginse or pegaspargase. I have direct knowledge of this. A dear friend lived with acute lymphoblastic leukemia for many years. It reached a point of crises, and so he made the decision to undergo chemotherapy, and I took him to the oncology center. Within two minutes of the injection he suffered a near-fatal anaphylactic episode, which was quickly neutralized. I drove him home, and for the next four days and nights he suffered from high fever, which finally resolved. Two months later, blood was drawn, and his oncologist phoned him to arrange an appointment. He excitedly told my friend that he was cured, that no abnormal cells showed in his blood serum, and it was all due to the chemotherapy. I was in the office and disrespectfully reminded the good doctor that it was the four days of raging fever, not the chemotherapy, that achieved this amazing result. His belief system, unfortunately, would not allow him to even consider such an outcome.

Cancer cells cannot live above 105.8° F / 41° C. I observed a similar benefit from thermal baths in a clinic in northeastern Peru. The herb-infused baths began at 98.6° F / 37° C, and patients moved up to hotter temperatures over time. Hippocrates noted the benefit of hot- and cold-water therapies over two millennia ago. Perhaps it is time to revisit some ancient medical wisdom.

Plagiochila fruticosa contains various terpenoids (plagicosins A–N), plagiochilal B, isoplagiochin A and B, plagiochilide, plagiochin A, and plagiochilins J–K. Both plagiochilal B and plagiochilide demonstrate neurite sprouting as well as augmentation of choline acetyl transferase activity in neuronal cell culture. Plagiochin A also exhibits the same activity (Fukuyama and Asakawa 1991b). Plagicosin F exhibits potent inhibition of *Candida albicans*, including anti-virulence activity against hyphal morphogenesis, adhesion, and biofilm formation (Qiao et al. 2020). The isoplagiochins A–B exhibit in vitro inhibition of tubulin polymerization, an in vitro method used to determine the ability of a compound to interact with tubulin and in many cases to alter one or more of the characteristic phases of polymerization (Morita et al. 2009).

Plagiochila parvifolia syn. *Plagiochila hattorii* also contains plagiochilins A and B.

Plagiochila maderensis contains methyl everninate, a compound usually found in some lichen species. The essential oil contains 4-hydroxy-3'-methoxybibenzyl as the major volatile, as well as terpinolene (33–60%).

The tropical, woody liverwort *Plagiochila rutilans* var. *moritziana* contains plagiospirolides A and B, novel dimeric spiroterpenoids, bicylogermacrane, gymnomitrane, eudesmane, aromadendrane, and secoaroadendrane sesquiterpenoids (Spörle et al. 1989 and 1991). Work by Rycroft and Cole (2001) revised the structure of a Cuban specimen extract as 2-methoxy-6-prenylhydroquinone. The aroma is strongly peppermint-like due to the presence of pulegone, menthone, isomenthone, terpinolene, and limonene. Research found one of the specimens from Costa Rica replaced pulegone with the lactone 3,7-dimethyl-2,5-octadien-1,6-olide. The related *Plagiochila rutilans* var. *standleyi* from that country also possesses a peppermint-like odor. In this case, the menthane monoterpenoids are responsible, as are limonene, β-phellandrene, α-terpinene, and the endoperoxide ascaridole. The latter compound possesses antiparasitic activity and is also found in the essential oils of Labrador tea (*Rhododendron groenlandicum*), tea tree (*Melaleuca*), and the liverwort *Chenopodium*. Notably, Labrador tea essential oil is used in French aromatherapy internally (in small doses) for chronic kidney failure.

Plagiochila ovalifolia and *Plagiochila porelloides* contain plagiochilins A and C. These liverworts are a rich source of secoaromadendrane sesquiterpenes, especially ester derivatives of plagiochilin A, which possesses cytotoxic properties (Toyota et al. 1998). These liverworts are pungent, mainly due to the presence of 2,3-secoaromadendrane hemiacetal with an epoxide.

Plagiochila ovalifolia contains plagiochilins G and N, as well as the derivative acetoxyisoplagiochilide; plagiochiline-A-15-yl octanoate; and 14-hydroxyplagiochiline-A-15-yl 2E,4E-dodecadienoate. The latter two compounds show significant cytotoxicity against murine leukemia (P-388) cell lines (Toyota et al. 1998). This liverwort also contains gorgonane sesquiterpene peroxide, 2α-hydroxy-3α, 14-diacetoxybicyclogermacrene, a labdane diterpenoid, globulol, and two maalianes. Work by Birladeanu (2003) found total synthesis of plagiochilin N from santonin, a well-known and easily available anthelmintic sesquiterpene lactone. It does, however, require sixteen steps to complete extraction. Santonin was formerly listed in pharmacopoeias in both the United States and Britain until the 1950s. It is derived from various *Artemisia* species, likely the unopened flower bud of *A. maritima* or *A. cina*. In 1843, candy lozenges containing santonin were marketed in Germany. Santonin has the peculiar ability to paralyze the anterior part of roundworms and threadworms while stimulating the posterior end, leading to confusion. Combined with a purgative, it does the job. Tapeworms, unfortunately, are not affected.

In clinical practice I only had one elderly women with tapeworm. She survived both Nazi and Russian work camps, and all pharmaceutical applications were unsuccessful. Pomegranate root bark finally succeeded in ridding her of this troublesome parasite after forty years.

As a sidenote, a homeopathic product, Santoninum 3X, is prescribed for worms, eye disease, gastrointestinal disorders, muscle twitching, and various bladder issues, including chronic cystitis, incontinence, and dysuria. The urine may appear greenish if acidic and reddish purple if alkaline, a sign that nephritis may be in an early stage. The eyes may suffer sudden dimness of sight, or there could be color blindness.

Wormwood (*Artemisia absinthium*) is found in absinthe, the famed "green fairy" drink of Parisian socialites. It is often blamed for the "yellow vision" suffered by Van Gogh. It is very likely due to thujone, but worth noting that "yellow vision" is one of the symptoms of santonin poisoning. Note: wormwood should not be given to children with fever or constipation.

Peculiar featherwort (*Plagiochila peculiaris*) contains the oxygenated diterpenes, fusicoccanin and neofusicoccantriepoxide, as well as secoaromadendranes and macrocyclic chorobis-bibenzyls.

Plagiochila pulcherrima contains plagiochilins A and B; 7β,11α-dihdyroxypimara-8(14),15-diene; 1β,11α-dihyroxypimara-8(14),15-diene; 11α-hydroxypimara-8(14),15-diene; ethyoxy-plagiochiline A2; and other 2,3-secoaromadendrane-type sesquiterpenoids. Compounds in this liverwort exhibit moderate inhibition of the human epithelial/cervical (HeLa), glioblastoma (A172), and lung (H460) cancer cell lines (Wang, Liu et al. 2013).

Both *Plagiochila retrorsa* and *Plagiochila stricta* contain several methyl benzoates. The former produces allo-ocimene (4.9–15%), neo-allo-ocimene (4.2–9.6%), and β-phellandrene (3.7–10.5%).

Plagiochila sciophila is found in North America and parts of Asia. It contains fusicosciophins A–E, 8-deacetyl, 9-deacetyl fusicosciophin E, and fusicoccin A. Fusicosciophins B and D, as well as fusicoccin A, exhibit moderate activity against human promyelocytic leukemia (HL-60) and human oral epidermal (KB) carcinoma cell lines (Kenmoku et al. 2014).

Tulipinolide extracted from *Plagiochila semidecurrens* inhibits the growth of nasal-pharyngeal carcinoma. This cytotoxic sesquiterpene is also found in the beautiful tulip poplar (*Liriodendron tulipifera*) a tree common in the southeastern United States (Doskotch and El-Feraly 1970). This liverwort also contains plagiochilins A and C, as well as hanegokedial, ovalifolienal, and ovalifolienalone, compounds worthy of further investigation.

Plagiochila stephensoniana, a New Zealand liverwort, contains a bibenzyl compound with antifungal activity (Lorimer et al. 1993).

A liverwort found in the Andes of South America, *Plagiochila tabinensis*, contains plagiochilin M.

Plagiochila parvifolia syn. *P. yokogurensis* contains predominantly 2,3-secoaromadendranes, as well as fusicoccadiene, ent-kaurene, bicyclegermacrene, plagiochilde, fusicogigantone B, plagiochiline H, 3α-acetoxybicyblogermacrene, plagiochilines B and C, stigmasterol, ent-spathulenol, (+)-globulol, plagiochiline A, and 2α-hydroxy-3α.14-diacetoxybicyclogermacrene. Similar dimers have been found in *Plagiochila rutilans* var. *moritziana* (Spörle et al. 1991). Plagiochiline B exhibits a bitter taste.

PLEUROZIA

Spoonwort

The genus name may derive from the Greek *pleura*, meaning "side" or "ribs"; today in medicine the pleura is known as the membrane surrounding the lungs. *Zia* is interesting in that it has roots in Latin, Italian, Arabic, and Hebrew, all meaning "splendor" or "radiance." In the Bible, *zia* means "sweat" or "swelling." I like the former translation more, but I am no taxonomist. *Ozos* likely means "branch," perhaps referring to lateral branches. The genus includes a dozen species that are found worldwide. A unique feature of this liverwort is the growth of the stem by a two-sided apical cell. In all other genera of leafy liverworts it is three-sided.

Pleurozia subinflata ether and alcohol extracts exhibit activity against six of seven selected bacterial species (Wang et al. 2006). Curiously, this genus is carnivorous much like the *Colura* genus, creating a "trap" with its lower leaves to form a pool of water to drown and extract needed nitrogen from small insects.

Various secondary metabolites including 13-epi-neoverrucosan-5ß-ol, chelodane, E-ß-farnesene, and 5ß-acetoxy-13-epi-neoverucosanic acid were derived from this liverwort by Kamada et al. (2020). The latter compound exhibits antifungal activity against the marine fungus *Lagenidium thermophilum*, a pathogen in the commercial crustacean industry.

PLICANTHUS

The genus name derives from the Latin *plic*, meaning "fold" or "bend," and *anthus* (or *anthos*), from the Greek, meaning "flower" or "blossom." The root word *plic* is found in various English words, such *application*, *duplicate*, *complicate*, *explicit*, *replicate*, and *implicate*. In Greek mythology, the mortal Anthus was transformed into a bird whose song imitated the neighing of a horse, but he would flee from the sight of one. *Anthus* is also a genus of birds.

A Southern Hemisphere liverwort, *Plicanthus hirtellus* syn. *Jungermannia hirtella* is widespread in Africa, Asia, and Australia. The species name means "minuscule hairs." Although extremely rare in North America, it can also be found in the Pacific Northwest and in certain other northern regions. Work by Asakawa and Ludwiczuk (2013) and Sabovljevic et al. (2001) found the liverwort's extracts to exhibit cytotoxicity against leukemia (HL-60) cancer cell lines. *Plicanthus hirtellus* was collected and studied for volatile compounds by Koid et al. (2022). It contains 22.7% pentanoic acid; 2,2,4-trimethyl-3-carboxyisopropyl; isobutyl ester; decanal (10.7%); limonene (9%); and minor amounts of methyl salicylate, geranylacetone, nonanal, and decanal.

The major essential oil compound anastreptene is also found in *Plicanthus hirtellus* syn. *Chandonanthus hirtellus*. B-barbatene exhibits potential for treating diabetic bacterial foot infections.

Plicanthus birmensis syn. *Chandonanthus birmensis* contains the diterpenoids chandonanones B, C, E, and F (Li, Lin et al. 2014). These were tested against seven cancer cell lines (DU145, PC-3, A549, NCI-H292, NCI-H1299, and A172). A few of the diterpenoids showed weak activity.

Research by Wang, Qian et al. (2022) identified five cembrane-type diterpenoids, six known cembrane-type diterpenoids, one fusicoccane-type diterpenoid, and a dolabellane-type diterpenoid. Cytotoxicity tests of some isolated diterpenoids against human ovarian (A2780), lung (A549), large cell lung (H460), resistant-treated (H460RT), and epithelial/cervical (HeLa) cancer cell lines revealed moderate inhibitory effects.

The Tahitian/Bornean liverwort *Plicanthus hirtellus* syn. *Chandonanthus hirtellus* contains a number of bioactive sesquiterpene lactones, as well as cembrane and fusicoccane diterpenoids (Komala et al. 2010, "Zierane"). Chandolide, anadensin, and two iso-chandonanthones exhibit cytotoxicity against the human leukemia (HL-60) cancer cell lines.

Fussicoauritone 6α-methyl ether (6α-methoxyfusicoauritione) exhibits weak cytotoxicity against pharyngeal squamous cell lines.

PORELLA

Scaleworts Tree Ruffle Liverwort

Geographic Range: worldwide

Habitat: temperate climates; often growing on tree bark

Practical Uses: food preservatives, insecticides, pesticides

Medicinal Applications: antibacterial, anticancer, antifungal, anti-inflammatory, hypertension, vasodilator

The *Porella* genus contains 50–60 species according to the Global Biodiversity Information Facility. Most are found growing on tree bark in temperate climates, although at least seven species are found in the relatively cooler and drier climate of Montana. The leaves possess a large upper lobe and a small lower lobe.

Porella species are rich in sesquiterpenes and monoterpenes. Research by Bukvicki, Gottardi et al. (2012) identified microbes that are inhibited by the various *Porella* species. These include the fungi *Saccharomyces cerevisiae, Zygosaccharomyces bailii, Aerobasidium pullulans, Pichia membranaefasciens, Pichia anomala*, and *Yarrowia lipolytica*, and the bacteria *Salmonella enteritidis, Escherichia coli*, and *Listeria monocytogenes. Pichia anomala* is an interesting yeast species in that it has a number of medical, environmental, and industrial applications. It is found in raw milk and cheese, helping to restrict the growth of *Aspergillus flavus*, the fungus that produces aflatoxins. When pistachio trees were treated with this yeast, it reduced growth of *Aspergillus flavus* by 97%. Another species, *Pichia membranaefasciens*, can be found in cream cheese.

The *Porella* liverworts contain norpinquisone; perrottetianal A; porelladiolide; and 11,13-dehydroporella-diolide. Work by Dey and Mukherjee (2015) found several *Porella* species active against leukemia (HL-60) and human pharyngeal squamous (KB) cancer cell lines. *Porella acutifolia* subsp. *tosana* contains 2 pinguisane-type and three dimeric pinquisane sesquiterpenoids, which could be exploited as a natural source of cytotoxic compounds. This liverwort has a hot taste due to its hydroperoxyl-germacranolides content. In fact, many *Porella* species, including bitter scalewort, *Porella arboris-vitae*, contain pungent substances reminiscent of spicy green peas or pepper. This may be due in part to the presence of polygodial and other compounds. The constituents of this Serbian liverwort were extracted by Tyagi et al. (2013), who found the major components from a methanol extract consisted of β-caryophllene (14.7%), α-gurjunene (10.9%), α-selinene (10.8%), β-elemene (5.6%), gamma-muurolene (4.6%), and allo-aromadendrene (4.3%). The ethanol extract revealed ß-caryophyllene (11.8%), α-selinene (9.6%), α-gurjunene (9.4%), isopentyl alcohol (8.8%), 2-hexanol (3.7%), ß-elemene (3.7%), and allo-aromadendrene (3.7%). When extracted with ethyl acetate, undecane (11.3%) was the major constituent. Both ethanol and methanol extracts showed significant activity against *Salmonella enteritidis*, suggesting potential antimicrobial food preservation applications.

Porella chilensis, endemic to Argentina, contains four fusicoccane-type diterpenoids, four pinguisane-type sesquiterpenoids, norpinguisone, norpinguisone methyl ester, and two aromadenrane-type sesquiterpenoids. The individual compounds were tested against biofilm formation of the human pathogen *Pseudomonas aeruginosa* and produced a slight decrease in bacterial growth and interference with the process of quantum sensing (Gilabert et al. 2011).

Scalewort (*Porella cordaeana*) methanol extracts inhibit *Salmonella enteritidis*, *Escherichia coli*, and *Listeria monocytogenes* (Bukvicki, Veljic et al. 2012), while ethanol extracts exhibit modest activity against *Bacillus subtilis* (Russell 2010). Extracts also significantly inhibit mouse lymphoma induced by leukemia virus (YAC-I) and mouse myeloma (Sp2) cell lines (Önder and Özenoglu 2019). The presence of porellacetals A–D exhibit weak cytotoxicity against breast (MCF-7) and colorectal (HT-29) cancer cell lines (Tan et al. 2017).

Porella cordaeana contains drimenin and aristolone, both moderately toxic to DNA repair-deficient mutants of *Saccharomyces cerevisiae*. Drimenin noncompetitively inhibits human α4ß2 nicotinic acetylcholine receptors (Arias et al. 2018). These receptor antagonists have the potential for improving

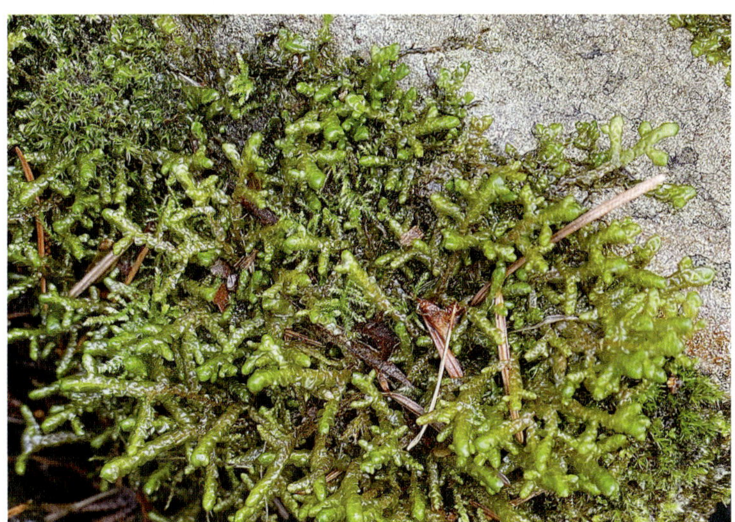

Porella cordaeana (Scalewort)
Photo by Drew T. Henderson

cognitive ability (Jaikhan et al. 2016) and may possibly be useful in treating schizophrenia or schizoaffective disorder (Adams and Stevens 2007). This devastating disease is complex and costly, affecting about 1% of the world's population. Cigarette (nicotine) smoking is one of the strategies used by many sufferers in an attempt to self-medicate. In clinical practice I found the herb *Lobelia inflata* helped many such clients cut down or eliminate tobacco addiction. Both *cis* and *trans* isomers of lobeline are involved and are nonselective antagonists with high affinity for α4β2 and α3β2 nicotinic acetylcholine receptors. Recent studies suggest the possible use of lobeline in various mental addictions and nervous system disorders, such as depression, Alzheimer's disease, and Parkinson's disease (Xu et al. 2022).

In a study of *Porella cordaeana*, activity was tested against various yeast and bacterial strains by Bukvicki, Gottardi et al. (2012). This included the widely used *Saccharomyces cerevisiae*, used in wine, beer, and baking. Antibodies to this yeast have been found in 60–70% of those suffering from Crohn's disease. The test for antibodies is used to distinguish this condition from ulcerative colitis. It may also indicate foods containing this yeast can exacerbate this inflammatory bowel disease. An extract was also found to inhibit the black, yeast-like fungus *Aureobasidium pullulans*, used in biotechnology to produce enzymes such as siderophores and pullulan. It is normally found on various fruits and vegetables, but can create problems in humans with chronic exposure to humidifiers and air conditioners. Known as "humidifier lung" or pneumonitis, this chronic health condition is often proceeded with coughing, dyspnea, fever, and acute respiratory problems. Strains affecting humans have been renamed *Aureobasidium melanogenum*.

Porella cordaeana also contains 7-ketoisodrimenin, 7-ketoisodrimenin-5-ene, and norpinguisanolide. Drimenin and aristolone are moderately toxic towards DNA repair-deficient mutants of *Saccharomyces cerevisiae* (Harrigan et al. 1993). Drimenin is also found in *Porella canariensis*. Aristolone promotes vasorelaxation and alleviates hypertension. Work by Fang et al. (2022) found it reduces both systolic and diastolic blood pressure in spontaneously hypertensive rats.

An in vivo study found *Porella platyphylla* and *P. cordaeana* exhibited significant inhibition of carrageenan-induced paw edema and promising suppressing effects on p-benzoquinone–induced abdominal constriction in animal models (Tosun et al. 2013).

Depending on the solvent, various volatile components are found in *Porella* extracts. Methanol extracts are rich in sesquiterpenes (53.68%) and monoterpenes (22.83%). Ethanol extracts contain sesquiterpenes (51.68%) and monoterpenes (18.9%), and ethyl acetate extracts contain sesquiterpenes (23.16%) and monoterpenes (23.36%). The main compounds are β-phellandrene and β-carophyllene. The former is widely synthesized as a pesticide.

Ether extracts of dense leaf scalewort (*Porella densifolia*) reveal constituents like ent-kauren-15-one, norpinguisone, and norpinguisone methyl ester. Inhibition of nitric oxide production in leukemia macrophage (RAW 264.7) cells, stimulated by lipopolysaccharide, was noted, suggesting anti-inflammatory potential (Quang and Asakawa 2010).

Elegant scalewort (*Porella elegantula*) contains norpinguisone methyl ester, norpinguisanolide, α-pinguisene, norpinguisone, perrottetianal, and methyl 4-oxonorpinguisan-12-oate (Fukuyama et al. 1988). Norpinguisone methyl ester shows 50% inhibition of release of superoxide from macrophages.

Various *Porella* species, including *P. cordaeana*, *P. navicularis*, *P. arborisvitae*, *P. canariensis*, *P. fauriei*, *P. gracillima*, *P. obtusata*, *P. roellii*, and *P. vernicosa*, produce polygodial, also found in the annual herb *Persicaria hydropiper*. *Porella vernicosa* extracts contain 30% polygodial and exhibit cytotoxicity against a human melanoma cell line. Polygodial is cytotoxic, piscicidal, antimicrobial, and a powerful antifungal. The addition of anethole, a compound found in anise seed, increases the antifungal activity of polygodial against *Candida albicans* by 32% (Kubo and Himejima 1991). Polygodial is an agonist of the transient receptor potential vanilloid 1, also known as the capsaicin receptor associated with chronic pain relief, bladder issues, and coughs. It inhibits the enzyme sodium–potassium adenosine triphosphatase (NKA), suggesting that antitumor activity may be linked to this activity (Garcia et al. 2018). Regulation of specific NKA isozymes gives cells the ability to precisely coordinate NKA activity to their physiological requirements. It is the only known receptor for cardiac glycosides used to treat congestive heart failure and cardiac arrhythmias (Suhail 2010).

Prostate cancer is the second leading cause of death in American men. Surgery, radiation, chemotherapy, and androgen deprivation therapies all have poor outcomes, leading to the development of castration-resistant prostate cancer (CRPC). Taxane drugs show poor outcomes in CRPC, however, polygodial activates apoptotic and DNA damage markers in prostate cancer cells and induces apoptosis in CRPC cells (Venkatesan et al. 2022). Natural polygodial also kills mosquitos at concentrations of 40 ppm, and this mosquito repellant activity is stronger than commercial—and toxic—DEET.

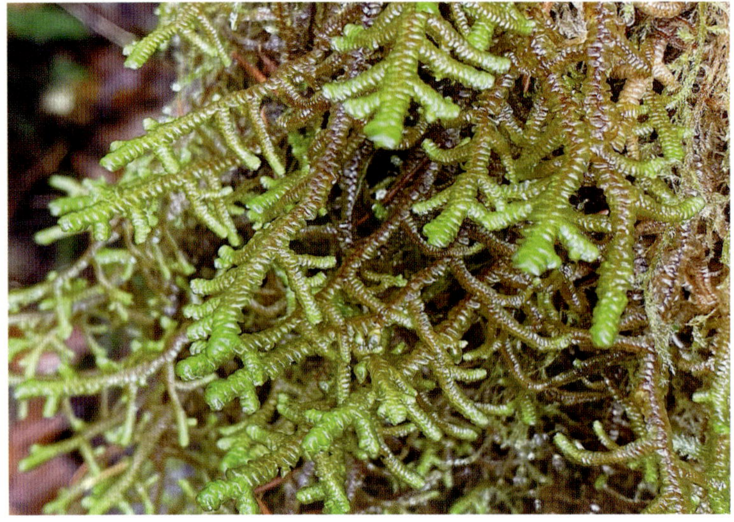

Porella navicularis (Tree Ruffle Liverwort)
Photo by Drew T. Henderson

Porella japonica crude extracts show potent inhibition of cathepsin B and L. Cathepsin B is a lysosomal cysteine protease enzyme that functions in intracellular protein catabolism and may be involved in the processing of antigens in immune response, hormone activation, and osteoporosis. It has been implicated in chronic respiratory and joint inflammation, cancer, and pancreatitis (Mort and Buttle 1997). Cathepsin B produces β-amyloid plaquing in Alzheimer's disease, and cathepsin L generates peptide neurotransmitters (Hook et al. 2012). Inhibition of cathepsin is not strictly an undesired therapy. Cathepsin L plays a key role in SARS-CoV-2 infection in humans and is elevated in the bloodstream following infection (Zhao et al. 2021).

Porella navicularis contains norpinguisone, also found in *Porella densifolia* (see above).

Porella perrottetiana contains the bitter compound perrottetianal B, among other germacrene and pinguisane–type sesquiterpenoids. Work by Nagashima et al. (1996) revised the compound name by means of analysis of nuclear magnetic resonance spectra to 15-hydroxyperrottetianal. Work by Komala et al. (2011) found *Porella perrottetiana* compounds active against human promyelocytic leukemia (HL-60) and human pharyngeal squamous (KB) carcinoma cell lines. An ether extract contains (-)-α eudesmol, a configuration that was found identical to a similar compound found in higher plants (Toyota 2000). Alpha-eudesmol may be useful in the treatment of neurogenic inflammation in the trigeminal-vascular system such as what occurs in migraine headaches, without affecting blood pressure (Asakura et al. 2000). As well, both α- and β-eudesmol display cytotoxicity, the former against melanoma (B16-F10) and myelogenous leukemia (K562) cancer cell lines, and the latter against hepatic (B16-F10 and HepG2) cell lines. An increase in caspase-3 activation in HepG2 cells suggests induction of apoptosis (Bomfim et al. 2013).

Wall scalewort, *Porella platyphylla* syn. *Jungermannia platyphylloidea*, is commonly found on calcareous cliffs in Europe and North America, hence its common name. It is often collected for terrariums. Work by Isoe (1983) uncovered antibacterial activity, while Kumar et al. (2007) reported antifungal activity. Work by Vollár et al. (2018) found various solvent extracts exhibit cytotoxicity against epithelial/cervical (HeLa), ovarian (T47D), and breast (A2780) cancer cell lines. Methanol extracts of this liverwort inhibit the growth of gray mold, *Botrytis cinerea* (Nedeljko et al. 2019).

Bent round scalewort, *Porella chilensis* syn. *P. recurva*, contains norpinguisone; norpinguisone methyl ester; 6, 11-epoxy-15-nor-3,4-dioxo-5,10-pinguisadien-12 acetate; and 6,11-epoxy-15-nor-4-oxo-5,10-pinguisadien-12-acetate (van Klink et al. 2002).

Porella subobtusa contains lepidozane-type sesquiterpenoids, santalane, and two africane-type sesquiterpenoids (Nagashima and Asakawa 2001). Santalane is a constituent of Indian sandalwood, *Santalum album*, an overharvested and now protected tree. It is classified as vulnerable by the IUCN. Most sandalwood essential oil on the market is highly adulterated, and for this reason our essential oil company Scents of Wonder no longer offers it.

Porella swartziana contains several swartzianin-type sesquiterpenoid compounds, including seven africanes, three secoafricanes, and two norsecoafricanes. All were tested for activity against a variety of microbes, but none showed significant activity (Mitre et al. 2004).

Porella viridissima is common in tropical Pacific Ocean countries. It contains various volatile compounds, including 10 santalane and 5 pinguisane-type sesquiterpenes. It also contains the diterpenoid perrotettianal A. Work by Métoyer et al. (2021) found this compound active against the ovarian (A2780) cancer cell line.

PTILIDIUM

Fringeworts Naugehyde Liverworts Pacific Fuzzwort

The genus name may derive from the Latin *ptil*, meaning "down" or "feather," and *dium*, for "blessed" or "divine." Perhaps. In Greek mythology the name

Dius may refer to any number of characters. This genus has only four species.

Ciliated fringewort or northern naugehyde liverwort (*Ptilidium ciliare*) is widespread in northern climates such as Alaska, Canada, Greenland, Iceland, and northern Europe.

Tree fringewort or western naugahyde liverwort, *Ptilidium pulcherrimum*, is one of the few species that live on conifer tree bark. Work by Heinrichs et al. (2015) challenges ideas about this boreal liverwort, which has been found enclosed in warm-temperature Baltic amber dating back to the Eocene, 35 to 50 million years ago. Thirty-five fossil species have been described from this era and were initially thought to be this liverwort. The fossil is morphologically similar to the now rare Pacific fuzzwort, *Ptilidium californicum*, found from southeastern Alaska all the way down the Pacific coast to northern California, and is associated with old-growth Douglas firs and other fir species. It is believed this liverwort species originated 25 to 43 million years ago. Speaking of amber, I gave my beautiful wife, Laurie, amber earrings on the day of our engagement. Ten years later I found an amber perfume vial at the Smithsonian in Washington, D.C. that also found a way back to our home.

Methanol extracts of the most beautiful fringewort, the colorful name of *Ptilidium pulcherrimum*, show antifungal activity against *Aspergillus versicolor*, *A. ochraceus*, *A. flavus*, *A. niger*, *Trichoderma viride*, and *Penicillium funiculosum* (Veljic et al. 2010). In fact, its antifungal activity is comparable to the synthetic drug bifonazole, frequently used in dermal skin ointments. *Penicillium funiculosom*, an endophyte derived from an Antarctic moss, contains penipyridones A–F. Four of the compounds derived from this liverwort elicited lipid-lowering activity in hepatic (HepG2) cancer cell lines (Zhou et al. 2016). The *Penicillium funiculosum* fungus contains chrodrimanins (meroterpenoids), three of which exhibit inhibition against influenza virus A, aka H1N1 (Zhou et al. 2015).

Bifonazole is a potent inhibitor of aromatase. This class of plant-derived drugs is used to prevent and treat various hormone-sensitive cancers. Aromatase inhibition by letrozole and anastrozole is a widely practiced therapy for estrogen-dependent postmenopausal breast cancer.

Several new secondary metabolites were identified in *Penicillium pulcherrimum* by Guo et al. (2009). These include trinortriterpenoid; diospyrolide acetate; a new diphenylmethane derivative, pulcherrimumin; along with ten known pentacyclic triterpenoids and four aromatic compounds. Some of the ursane triterpenoids exhibit moderate cytotoxicity against prostate (PC-3), breast (MDA-MB-231), and epithelial/cervical (HeLa) cancer cell lines (Guo et al. 2009).

RADULA

Scaleworts Radula Liverworts

Geographic Range: worldwide

Habitat: sheltered moist environments; on trees, logs and rocks

Medicinal Applications: antibiotic, anticancer, antifungal, neuroprotective, psychotropic, vasodilator

There are 244 accepted species of *Radula* found worldwide. The horny tooth structure on tongues of molluscs to scrape food is the radula. The word may derive from the Indo-European *rado*, meaning "to scrape," referring to the scaly appearance of this genus, which has no obvious toothlike structure. *Radula* may also derive from the Latin, meaning "little scraper," a term introduced by Russian zoologist and explorer Alexander von Middendorff (1815–1894). Radula is the tonguelike, minutely toothed organ in mollusks to scrape algae.

The *Radula* genus is distinctly different from other liverworts due to the presence of bibenzyl cannabinoids and prenyl bibenzyl derivatives. Many of these compounds show a variety of biological activity, including psychotropic, vasopressin antagonism, antimicrobial, antifungal, inhibition of nitric oxide, muscle relaxation, cytotoxicity against various human cancer cell lines, and influence over twenty different enzymatic pathways.

Work by Asakawa, Nagashima et al. (2022) looked at 679 liverwort species, including *Radula* spp. and found 264 of them contain α-tocopherol, an important antioxidant in the liverworts' fatty oil bodies.

Radula amoena constituents exhibit cytotoxicity against liver (HepG2), hepato-carcinoma (SMMC-7721), and lung (A549) cancer cell lines (Fan et al. 2019). The species name derives from the Latin *amoenus*, meaning "beautiful," "delightful," "lovely," or "pleasant."

Radula acuta syn. *R. apiculata* contains radulapins A–H. Research by Zhang, Gao et al. (2021) found radulapin D induces apoptosis in prostate (PC-3) cancer cells via increased Bax and caspase-9. Radulapins A, C, E, F, G, and H show cytotoxicity against prostate (PC-3), lung (A549), breast (MCF-7), and non-small cell lung (H1299) cancer cell lines. The former species name *apiculata* refers to the liverwort's apiculate (ending abruptly in a small, distinct point) leaves. This species contains three prenylated bibenzyls and seven known congeners. All isolated compounds were tested against several human cancer cell lines, with the chemotherapy drug adriamycin (doxorubicin) as the positive control (Zhang, Zhou et al. 2022). Ethanol extracts show cytotoxic activity against lung cancer (A549) cell lines. Contents include eight radulapins (A-H), four prenylated bibenzyls, and seven previously identified compounds. The radulapins (dimeric prenylated bibenzyls) show significant cytotoxic activity against a panel of human cancer cell lines. In an earlier study, Zhang, Gao et al. (2021) found that radulapin D induces prostate (PC-3) cell death via mitochondrial-derived apoptosis.

The species name *appressa* is from the Latin, meaning "pressed close against." It contains radulannin A and L; 2-geranyl-3,5-dihydroxybibenzyl; 2(S)-2-methyl-2-(4-methyl-3-pentenyl)-7-hydroxy-5-(2-phenyethyl) chromene (o-cannabichromene); 6-hydroxy-4-(2-phenylethyl) benzofuran; and o-cannabicyclol (Harinantenaina, Takahara et al. 2006). All compounds inhibited nitric oxide (NO) production in LPS stimulated RAW 264.7 cells associated with murine leukemia, with the compound 2-geranyl-3,5-dihydroxybibenzyl showing the greatest inhibition.

Brown radula (*Dactyloradula brunnea* syn. *Radula brunnea*) contains 3,5-dihydroxy-2-(3-methyl-2-butenyl) bibenzyl.

Radula complanata, known as flattened radula (the species name means "flattened" in Latin), is found in the eastern Rockies and throughout British Columbia, as well as in parts of Europe. Ecological and environmental influences create variations in secondary metabolites in this liverwort (and in others). Work by Blatt-Janmaat et al. (2023) examined samples from Canada, Germany, and Sweden and found a 39% variation depending on the host tree. The researchers found the metabolic shifts were due mainly to drought response to different humidity levels. The liverwort contains prenyl bibenzyl, shown in early French trials to be a vasopressin antagonist.

Radula constricta contains radstrictins A–I and eleven known congeners (members of the same taxonomic genus). The compound methyl 2,4-dihydroxy-3-(3-methyl-2-butenyl)-6-phenethylbenzoate exhibits significant activity against human lung (A549 and NCI-H1299) cancer cell lines. Cell death was triggered via mitochondria-derived apoptosis (Zhang et al. 2019). Radulanin K, isolated from *Radula javanica*, inhibits the release of superoxide anion radical from guinea pig macrophage (Asakawa et al. 1991a).

Lindenberg's scalewort (*Radula lindenbergiana*) was named in honor of Johann Bernhard Wilhelm Lindenberg (1781–1851), a German bryologist and lawyer who specialized in the research of liverwort. He co-authored *Synopsis Hepaticarum*, a treatise on hepaticology, which refers to the study of Hepaticae,

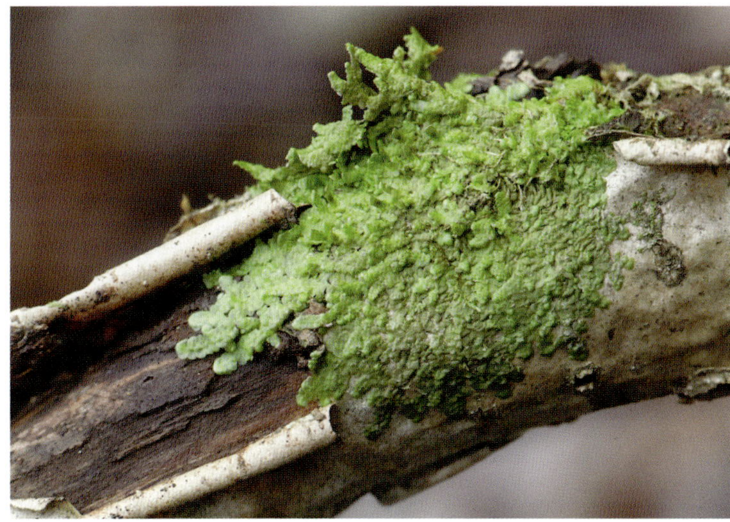

Radula complanata (Flattened Radula)

or liverworts. This species contains an abundance of sesquiterpenes, with (E, E)-α-farnesene/β-curcumene and (Z)-β-bisabolene being the most abundant (Fan et al. 2021).

Another species, *Radula marginata*, contains perrottetinenic acid and perrottetinene (Toyota et al. 2002). This liverwort is endemic to New Zealand, where it is known as *wairuakohu* by the native Maori. It may have been used in traditional medicine, for joint and skin conditions but this is not certain. Its compounds inhibit the growth of *Staphylococcus aureus* at low concentration (Asakawa and Campbell 1982). The same researchers also found perrottetin E from *Cladoradula perrottetii*, formerly known as *Radula perrottetii*, to be cytotoxic against human epithelial (KB) carcinoma cells.

Two species, *Radula laxiramea* and *Radula marginata*, contain the cannabinoid-like (-)-*cis*-perrottetinene and (-)-*cis*-perrottetineic acids. These naturally occurring compounds are similar to the cannabinoid THC (i.e., tetrahydrocannabinol) and have therefore created interest as a pharmaceutical product and for its legal recreational use (Reis et al. 2020). Perrottetinene is a mild to moderately psychoactive activator of CB receptors. This suggests a moderately active—and legal—high for use in countries where cannabis is still illegal (Chicca et al. 2018). The presence of cannabinoid-like substances in plants is still poorly understood, however. Several bryophytes contain anandamide and 2-archidonoyl glycerol that act as receptor agonists or antagonists. They also act as enzyme inhibitors of the endocannabinoid system and can be involved in inflammation, oxidative stress, anticancer, and neuroprotection (Kumar et al. 2019).

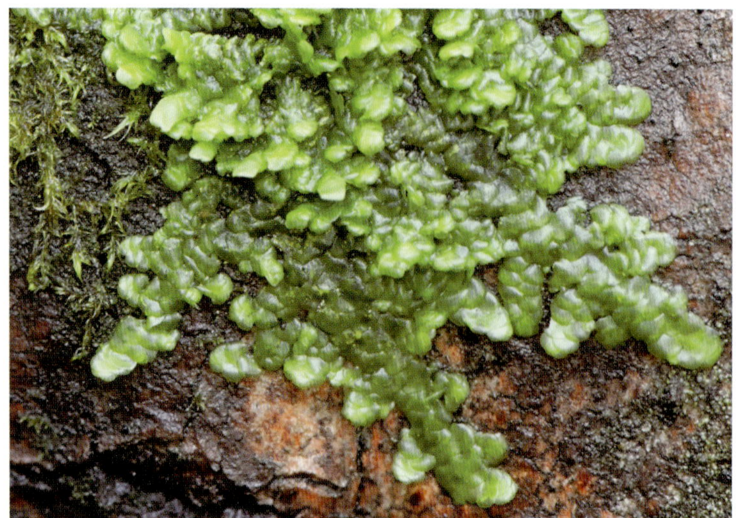

Radula complanata (Flattened Radula)

Other bryophytes produce anandamide and 2-arachidonoyl glycerol, which are endogenous agonists to the endocannabinoid system. The activity of anandamide is limited by cellular uptake through a specific membrane transporter, and then intracellular degradation by fatty acid amide hydrolase (FAAH). Research suggests FAAH inhibitors may be the next exciting target for the treatment of central nervous system pathology (Maccarrone 2006).

Inverted cone scalewort (*Radula obconica*) displays significant antibacterial activity, especially against *Bacillus subtilis* (Millar et al. 2007).

Cladoradula perrottetii syn. *Radula perrottetii* contains perrottetins A, D, and E; perrottetin methyl ester; and the bibenzyl cannabinoid perrottetinene. Unlike most species in this genus that contain low amounts of terpenoids, this species produces large amounts of bisabola-2,6,11-triene. Perrottetin D and perrottetin diacetate were tested on antigen-induced activation of mast cells derived from mice marrow. Both compounds tended to decrease histamine release and inhibited degranulation and/or IL-4 production. This suggests possible benefit for antiallergenic or anti-inflammatory products (Asai et al. 2022). Prenyl bibenzyl derived from this liverwort shows vasopressin antagonistic activity (Asakawa 1990). Perrottetin E is cytotoxic against nasopharyngeal (KB) cancer cells (Asakawa 2008). The essential oil of this liverwort has been analyzed by Tesso et al. (2005). It contains two novel viscidane diterpenes (viscida-2,9,14-triene and viscida-3,11(18),14-triene); four bisabolene sesquitepenes (bisabola-2,6,11-triene; bisabola-1,3,5,7(14),11-pentaene; bisabola-1,3,5,7,11-pentaene; and 6,7-epoxybisabola-2,11-diene); as well as

1-methoxy-4-(2-methylpropenyl) benzene. The oil also contains bisabola-1,3,5,7(14),10-pentaene; ar-tenuifolene; α-helmiscapene; and β-hemiscapene.

The Chinese liverwort *Radula sumatrana* contains (+)-rasumatranin A–D and radulanins M and N. The presence of another compound, 6-hydroxy-3-methyl-8-phenylethylbenzo[b]oxepin-5-one, shows activity against the human breast (MCF-7), prostate (PC-3), and hepatoma (SMMC-7721) cancer cell lines. Induction of the breast cancer cell lines was through a mitochondria-mediated apoptosis pathway (Wang, Li et al. 2017).

REBOULIA

Hemispheric Liverwort   Small Mushroom-Headed Liverwort

The species name *hemisphaerica* means "half a sphere," referring to this liverwort's deep cuplike shape.

Platelet activation is involved in serious pathological situations, including atherosclerosis and constriction of a blood vessel or a heart valve. It is therefore important to find efficient antiplatelet medicines to prevent fatal thrombosis during the course of these diseases. Marchantinquinone, a natural compound isolated from *Reboulia hemisphaerica*, inhibits platelet aggregation. Liao et al. (2000) studied *Reboulia hemisphaerica* and confirmed that this compound exerts antiplatelet effects by inhibiting phosphoinositide turnover.

Small mushroom-headed liverwort, an alternative name for hemisphaeric liverwort, *Reboulia hemisphaerica*, contains four cyclomyltaylane sesquiterpenods,

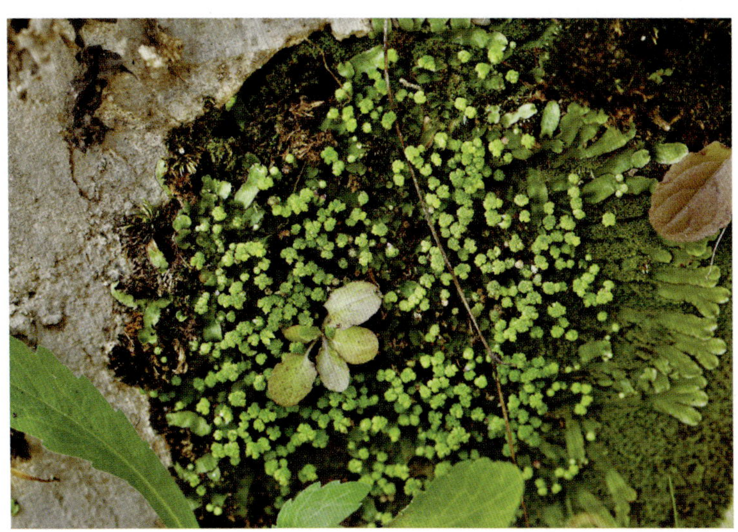

Reboulia hemisphaerica (Small Mushroom-Headed Liverwort)

two ent-chamigrenes, and riccardins C and F (Furusawa et al. 2006). The secondary metabolite riccardin C is found in other liverwort species, including *Marchantia polymorpha*, *M. palmata*, *Mastigophora dyclados*, *Dumortiera hirsuta*, *Concephalum conicum*, *Plagiochasma rupestre*, *P. intermedium*, and *Ricciocarpos natans*. *Reboulia hemisphaerica* expresses at least three chemotypes: atistolane, cyclomyltaylane-bisbibenzyl, and gymnomitrane-cuparane. Xu et al. (2010) confirmed that riccardin C induces apoptosis via the caspase signaling pathway in a manner similar to marchantins C and M, and plagiochin E on prostate cancer (PC-3) cells.

Önder and Özenoglu (2019) found that extracts of this liverwort significantly inhibit mouse lymphoma induced by leukemia virus (YAC-I) and mouse myeloma (Sp2) cell lines. Work by Kuroda and Ogawa (2017) found riccardin C induced drug-resistant bacterial cell membrane leakage, particularly against gram-positive species. Tamehiro et al. (2005) note that riccardins C and F function as liver X receptor alpha agonists and LXR ß antagonists, and that riccardin C effectively enhances cholesterol efflux from THP-1 cells.

In a 1980 study, Belcik and Weigner identified antibacterial activity in *Reboulia hemisphaerica*, while Sharma et al. (2013) found methanol extracts active against various bacteria and two fungi. This liverwort contains marchantinquinone, an inhibitor of lipid peroxidation as a free radical scavenger. Work by Ko et al. (1995) found marchantinquinone an effective antioxidant that protected rat brain homogenate and LDL cholesterol against oxidation.

An in vivo study found this liverwort exhibits significant inhibition of carrageenan-induced paw edema and promising suppressive effects on p-benzoquinone–induced abdominal constriction in animal models; the presence of sesquiterpenes are partly responsible for these activities (Tosun et al. 2013).

The essential oil contains (-)-gymnomitr-3(15),4-diene; (+)-gymnomitrol; (+)gymnomitr-3(15)-en-one, cuparene; (-)-α cuprenone; and (-)-delta-cuprenene (Ludwiczuk and Asakawa 2017). Cuparene has a pine/wood aroma used in desserts and chewing gum. The compound is found in the Japanese *Flammulina velutipes* mushroom, *Juniperus horizontalis* and *Perilla frutescens*.

The TCM decoction *huanglian wendan* modulates gamma-aminobutryic acid (GABA) type A receptors and is used to treat insomnia. When (+)-cuparne was used to potentiate the effect, it increased efficacy by 278% (Li et al. 2024).

RICCARDIA

Comb Liverwort Jagged Germanderwort

Jagged germanderwort (*Riccardia chamedryfolia*) is a terrestrial liverwort that has been adapted for freshwater aquariums. It is sometimes referred to as coral moss, as it looks a tiny bit like coral underwater. It is native to Southeast Asia but now found around the world.

The New Zealand liverwort *Riccardia crassa* contains riccardiphenol C, which possesses mild cytotoxic effects against African green monkey kidney epithelial (BSC-1) cells as well as antibacterial activity (Perry and Foster 1995). The same study found modest activity against *Bacillus subtilis* and the fungi *Candida albicans* and *Trichophyton mentagrophytes.* The latter causes ringworm in humans and companion animals.

Riccardia eriocaula from New Zealand contains 2-hydroxycuparene, spathulenol, cuparene, acoradiene, α-guaiene, and β-gurjunene. Alpha-guaiene is a precursor to rotundone, a grape-derived compound that gives the pepper-like aroma to Syrah varietals (Asakawa et al. 2013, "Chemical Constituents").

Lobatiriccardia coronopus syn. *Riccardia lobata* var. *yakushimensis* contains the hot and pungent compound sacculatal and the phenolic compounds riccardiphenols A and B.

Riccardia marginata contains chlorinated bibenzyls that exhibit antifungal activity against *Bacillus subtilis*, *Candida albicans*, and *Trichophyton mentagrophytes* (Baek et al 2004). The latter fungus is a leading cause of the skin condition tinea in humans and ringworm in companion animals such as cats and dogs. Drug-resistant strains are found in Europe and Asia, with resistance to the antifungal drug terbinafine recorded as high as 11.4% in India. Resistant strains have also been reported in Japan and Denmark.

Comb liverwort, *Riccardia multifida* subsp. *decrescens*, contains riccardins A and B, which are cytotoxic against human epithelial carcinoma (KB) cell lines (Asakawa 1982). Marchantin 1, pusilatin, and egonol 2-methylbutanoate are also present. This liverwort was traditionally prepared in India as a warm leaf juice for rheumatic swellings in cattle and crushed and combined with black pepper and taken internally for stomachache.

Riccardia nagasakiensis contains marchantin C, riccardin A, and sesquiterpenoids such as β-elemene, as well as spathulenol, gamme-cadinene, longifolene, and phytol.

Palmate germanderwort, *Riccardia palmata*, ranges from northwestern

Greenland to Florida in the east, and from Alaska to California in the west. The species name derives from its finger-like lobes. Like many liverworts, it has oil bodies containing terpenoids that protect them from insect attack. "Liverwort-like plants were also the first plants to have evolved from green algal ancestors." (Whiteman 2023). In his fascinating book, he notes that fossilized liverwort plants found in 385 million-year-old rock contains oil body cells that protected them from becoming food for early invertebrates.

Riccardia polyclada syn. *R. umbrosa* syn. *Aneura polyclada* contains two chlorinated bibenzyls: 2,6,30-trichloro-3-hydroxy-40-methoxybibenzyl and 2,4,6,30-tetrachloro-3,40-dihydroxybibenzyl. Both compounds exhibit activity against the cotton leafworm, *Spodoptera littoralis*, the larvae of which attack more than forty plant species, several of commercial importance (Labbé et al. 2007).

RICCIA

Floating Crystalwort

Riccia discolor is prepared into a paste with honey and oil in India and applied to cuts, burns, and wounds, while several *Riccia* species are ground up and made into a paste in the Himalayas to treat ringworm, tinea, and other fungal infections. There are 152 species found mainly in Mediterranean-type climates.

Bryophytes mark the transition from freshwater to land, requiring adaptation for water uptake, gas exchange, and other developed plasticity. Work by Althoff et al. (2022) examined the amphibious floating crystalwort (*Riccia fluitans*) which can live in water or on land. They found the water form initiates air pore formation, but these pores are arrested at early cell stage 4 and do not develop further into open pores. The thallus of the land form develops thicker cell walls and a distinct cuticle, helping the liverwort adapt to its home on earth, and hence its popular use by aquarium enthusiasts.

Early tests on bacteria and yeast by Pates and Madsen (1955) found no inhibition of *Pseudomonas aeruginosa*, *Staphylococcus aureus*, or *Candida albicans*.

An in vivo study found that floating crystalwort exhibits significant inhibition of carrageenan-induced paw edema and promising suppressive effects on p-benzoquinone–induced abdominal constriction in animal models (Tosun et al. 2013).

Extracts significantly inhibit both mouse lymphoma induced by leukemia virus (YAC-I) and mouse myeloma (Sp2) cell lines (Önder and Özenoglu 2019).

Another species, *Riccia nigerica*, was extracted by Ariyo et al. (2011) and found to possess significant antibacterial activity against *Bacillus subtilis*, *Pseudomonas aeruginosa*, *Shigella dysenteriae*, and *Staphylococcus aureus*. The *Rhizopus* species fungi and *Aspergillus flavus*, *A. niger*, and *Penicillium* species were also strongly inhibited.

RICCIOCARPOS

Fringed Heartwort

The aquatic liverwort known as fringed heartwort (*Ricciocarpos natans*) exhibits high tolerance to the standard drug ciprofloxacin (aka Cipro) and can therefore accumulate antibiotic residue at increased rates when temperatures elevate from 68° F / 20° C to 86° F / 30° C. This is the only species in the *Ricciocarpos* genus, which was originally named *Riccia* by Linnaeus in 1759. The species name *natans* means "swimming," as this liverwort loves to float on ponds in calm water. There are two forms of this species, one that grows on land, and the other floating on water. They look so different they were originally assumed to be different species

Since the introduction of this fluoroquinolone antibiotic in early 1960s, it has been widely effective against chronic otorrhea, endocarditis, and lower respiratory, gastrointestinal, skin, and soft tissue and urinary tract infections. Over time, however, an increase in resistance has developed against *Salmonella typhi*, *Staphylococcus aureus*, *Escherichia coli*, and *Pseudomonas aeruginosa*. Increased antibiotic-resistant has been caused in part by overuse by humans, and the resulting accumulation in our water supplies. Drugs flushed down the toilet after urination do not magically disappear but become part of our ecology.

SACCOBASIS

Flush Notchwort

Flush notchwort is found in moist shaded environments in Europe, Asia, and North America. It is collected as an ornamental plant for terrariums.

The essential oil of flush notchwort, or polished saccobasis (*Saccobasis polita* syn. *Tritomaria polita*) is chock-full of valuable sesquiterpenoids that are so essential to human health: (+)-eudesma-3,11-dien-8-one; (+)-eudesma-3,7(11)-dien-8-one; (+)-6,11-epoxy-eudesmane; (-)-6,7-seco-eudesm-7(11)-en-6-al; (+)-6β-hydroxy-eudesm-11-ene; (-)-6α-hydroxy-eudesm-11-ene; and (+)-6,11-epoxy-isodaucane (Adio et al. 2003).

SACCOGYNA

Straggling Pouchwort

Straggling pouchwort, *Saccogyna viticulosa*, is an unusual liverwort in that it has very obliquely inserted leaves that appear opposite but are not. They look similar to *Plagiochia* species, but their leaves are alternate. The species name *viticulosa* was a term used by Pliny the Great to describe Manduria, a village in the bootheel of Italy, as *viticulosa*, "full of vineyards."

An essential oil was produced from *Saccogyna viticulosa* gathered on the island of Madeira and found to be composed of unique sesquiterpenes, especially the rare gorgonane and zierane types, as well as a complex mixture of monoterpenes, oxygenated sesquiterpenoids, and diterpenes.

SCAPANIA

Earworts River Startip Liverwort

Geographic Range: worldwide

Habitat: both wet and dry conditions; from damp acidic clay to sandy soil; wet cliffs; rotting logs; bogs; on living trees

Practical Uses: absorbs metals, coronary benefit, indicator of freshwater quality

Medicinal Applications: antibacterial, anticancer, antifungal, neuroprotective, vasorelaxant

Rough earwort, *Scapania aspera*, contains at least 96 constituents as discovered in an extraction and identification study (Bukvicki et al. 2013). The main compounds in methanol extracts are β-barbatene (25.1%), α-cymene (14%), α barbatene (5.7%), allo-aromadendrene (4.9%), and β-bourbonene. An ethanol extract was composed of α cymene (17.8%), β-barbatene (17.6%), α-thujene (6.7%), octen-1-ol acetate (4.9%), and β-bazzanene (2.4%). And when extracted with ethyl acetate, the compounds discovered include β-barbatene (14.3%), undecane (11.8%), 2-methyldecane (11.2%), decane (10.9%), and α-cymene (3.6%). Testing on various yeast and bacterial strains showed methanol extracts have the highest level of inhibition. Wang et al. (2018) assert that β-bourbonene inhibits the proliferation and induces apoptosis of prostate (PC-3) cancer cell lines.

The various extraction methods reveal a major flaw associated with natural

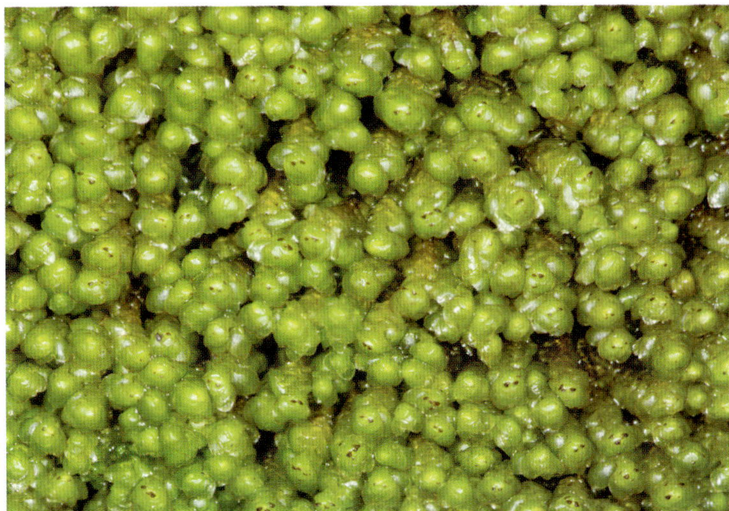

Scapania sp.
(Leafy Liverwort)

product extraction and research. The wide variance of constituents using three different solvents underlies significant variations, and thus different constituent results. The essential oil major constituents of *Scapania aspera* are, anastreptene and asperene. Anastreptene is also found in liverwort *Chandonanthus hirtellus*. Methanol extracts are beta-barbatene (25.1%), cymene (14%), alpha-barbatene, allo-aromadendrene (Bukvicki et al. 2013). Fungal strains were inhibited more than bacterial strains.

The essential oil of lesser rough earwort, *Scapania aequiloba*, contains aequilobene and β-himachalene. The latter compound found in the essential oil of atlas cedarwood (*Cedrus atlantica*) is calming, anti-inflammatory, reduces hypertension, and decongests vein and lymphatic tissue.

Scapania bolanderi contains a clerodane-type diterpenoid that exhibits modest activity against *Bacillus subtilis* (Russell 2010).

Carinthian earwort, *Scapania carinthiaca*, is found in the Northern Hemisphere, mainly in Scandinavia, central Europe, China, and in other regions of Asia. There are two reports from North America, one from southern coast of Alaska or northern British Columbia and another north of Lake Superior. Four diterpenoids, scapanacins A–D, were isolated by Qiao et al. (2018). Several compounds exhibit vasorelaxant activity in vivo. Vasodilatation was mainly produced by inhibiting Ca^{2+}-induced contraction of smooth muscle. This leads to a possible benefit in those suffering from hypertension. In addition, cytotoxicity testing showed inhibitory activities against a small panel of human cancer cell lines.

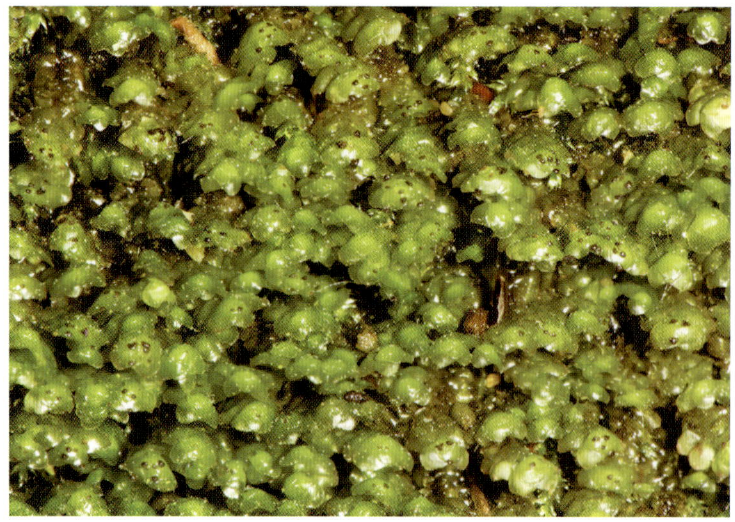

Scapania nemorea (Grove Earwort)

Ciliate earwort, *Scapania ciliata*, contains ciliatolides A–D. The cytotoxicity of these compounds was preliminarily tested against prostate (PC-3) and breast (MCF-7) cancer cell lines (Liu, Zhu et al. 2013).

Heath earwort, *Scapania irrigua*, a Chinese liverwort, contains the ladbane diterpenoids scapairrins A–Q. Work by Zhang, Li et al. (2015) found scapairrins G–J to be cytotoxic against various cancer cell lines, including breast (MDA-MB231), ovarian (A2780), cervicial/epithelial (HeLa), and colorectal adenocarcinoma (HT-29).

Another Chinese liverwort, *Scapania koponenii*, contains scaparins A–C, which exhibit moderate to weak quinone reductase–inducing activity in human hepatocyte (Hepa-1c1c7) cells (Han et al. 2021, "Terpenoids").

A *Scapania ornithopoides* liverwort distillation yields β-barbatene and aequilobene.

Scapania parvitexta contains parvitexins A–E, which are clerodane-type diterpenes. The compound subulatin, a caffeic acid derivative, exhibits antioxidant activity comparable to α-tocopherol (Tazaki et al. 2002). The essential oil contains β-cubebene, calamenene, β-chamigrene, β-selinene, bazzanene, and cuparene.

Strapped earwort, *Scapania stephanii* syn. *S. ligulata* subsp. *stephanii*, contains various stephanialides which significantly inhibit the root elongation of seeds from various plants, suggesting possible benefit in controlling undesirable plants in agricultural crops (Li, Sun et al. 2014).

Water earwort, also called river startip liverwort, *Scapania undulata*, is

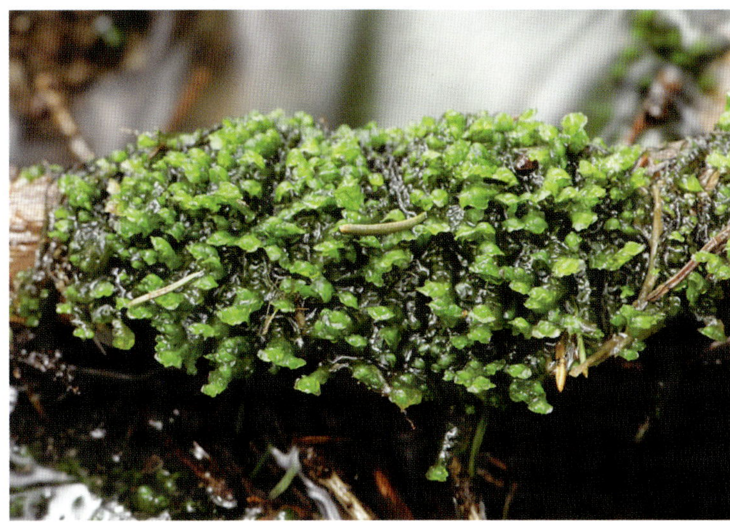

Scapania undulata (Water Earwort)

widespread in North America, from the sub-Arctic to northern Georgia in the east, and New Mexico in the west. This liverwort is also found in Great Britain, North Africa, northern Asia, and Japan. Mention of this liverwort is found in the medieval Welsh manuscript *Meddygon Myddfai* ("The Physicians of Myddfai").

Scapania undulata contains a variety of labdane diterpenoids, including scapaundulin C. Work by Kang et al. (2015) found it cytotoxic against lung (A549), leukemia (K562), and ovarian (A2780) cancer cell lines. The authors of the study also found that the compound inhibits acetylcholinesterase activity, suggesting beneficial applications for brain and other neurological conditions. The essential oil was analyzed by Adio et al. (2004) and new compounds were found, including (+)-helminthogermacrene; the 4Z isomer of germacrene A; (-) cis-β-elemene; and (-)-perfora-1,7-diene. Peroxy muurolane-type sesquiterpenoids and ent-muurolanes, (-)-longiborneol, (-)-longifolene, longipinanol, α- and β-longipinene, longicyclene, anastreptene, β-barbatene, caryophyllene, α- and β-himachalene, and β chamigrene have also been isolated from this liverwort.

Warty earwort, *Scapania verrucosa*, was investigated by Zeng et al. (2011) and found to contain 49 endophytic fungi. Five showed remarkable antioxidant activity, and ethyl acetate extracts of two were comparable to ascorbic acid and BHT (butylated hydroxytoluene). This liverwort's endophytes were examined for antimicrobial and anticancer activity by Wu et al. (2013). The researchers found seven that showed potent toxicity against brine shrimp, in preliminary cytotoxicity work, and one with antibacterial activity against *Staphylococcus aureus*, including two types of methicillin-resistant *S. aureus* (MRSA). One endophytic fungus, *Chaetomium fusiforme*, was ether-extracted and found to contain 49 compounds, including (+) aromadendrene; hexadecenoic acid; 6-isopropenyl-4,8α-dimethyl-1,2,3,5,6,7,8,8α-octahydro-naphthalen-2-ol; s-tetra-chloroethane; and acetic acid (Guo, Wu et al. 2008). The researchers found both antifungal and antitumor activities.

This liverwort contains scaparins D–F, an unknown ent-trachylobane diterpenoid, and three terpenoid derivatives. Four of the compounds exhibit moderate to weak quinone reductase–inducing activity in hepatic (liver) cells (Han et al. 2021, "Terpenoids").

SCHISTOCHILA

Pocketwort

Warning: *Schistochila appendiculata* may cause contact dermatitis.

The tropical liverwort *Schistochila acuminata* contains schistochilic acid D and other known compounds. Two of them exhibit weak cytotoxicity against melanoma (B 16-F10) cancer cell lines (Ng et al. 2016b).

Another compound, one of the minor diterpenoids, is totarol (Wu and Jong 2001). Totarol induces selective antitumor activity in human gastric (SGC-7801) cancer cell lines by triggering apoptosis, cell cycle disruption, and suppression of cancer cell migration (Xu et al. 2019). In addition, an in vitro study by Gao et al. (2015), found that totarol prevented glutamate, oxygen, and glucose deprivation–induced neuronal death in rat granule and cerebral cortical neurons. It also ameliorated brain ischemic injury in a rat model, significantly reduced infarct volume, and improved neurological deficit.

Besides its neurological benefits, totarol also inhibits the growth of the gram-positive bacteria *Bacillus subtilis* and *Mycobacterium tuberculosis* (Jaiswal et al. 2007). The compound exhibits antiproliferative activity on hepatic (HSC-T6) cells, suggesting possible benefit in liver fibrosis (Lee, Yang et al. 2008). And it may have application in dental work as well. Research by Xu et al. (2020) found that a coating of antibacterial totarol on dental implants or abutment surfaces may have potential as a prophylactic approach against peri-implantitis.

Schistochila glaucescens is a distinctive stem leafy liverwort. It contains three macryocyclic bis-bibenzyls, neomarchantin A and B and marchantin C; and glaucescenolide. The latter compound is cytotoxic against leukemia (P-388) cell lines (Scher et al. 2002). In addition, extracts of the whole liverwort exhibit activity against *Bacillus subtilis* and *Trichophyton mentagrophytes*.

Caution: *Schistochila appendiculata* syn. *Jungermannia appendiculata* has been implicated in allergenic contact dermatitis. This liverwort contains several long-chain alkylphenols and alkyl salicylates and their potassium salts, as well as 6-undecyl catechol (Chandra et al. 2016).

SOLENOSTOMA

Flapworts

The *Solenostoma* genus is cosmopolitan and contains, at last count, 143 accepted species. It can be identified by its round, obliquely inserted leaves.

Solenostoma atrobrunneum syn. *Jungermannia atrobrunnea* contains ten ent-kaurane-type diterpenoids (Qu et al. 2008). Ent-kaurane diterpenoids induce apoptosis and ferroptosis in sensitized cisplatin-resistant A549/CDDP (lung) cancer cells both in vitro and in vivo (Sun et al., 2021).

Solenostoma comatum syn. *Jungermannia comata* contains perrottetin E, which exhibits inhibitory activity toward thrombin, a serine protease that plays a physiological role in regulating hemostasis and maintaining blood coagulation (Nagashima et al. 1996). Also found in the liverwort *Apopellia endiviifolia* syn. *Pellia endiviifolia*, this compound, perrottetin E, is cytotoxic to three human leukemia cell lines: acute promyelocytic (HL-60), acute monocytic (U-937,) and chronic myelogenous (K-562). Cytotoxicity was also noted against human glioblastoma (A-172 and U-251) cell lines (Ivkovic et al. 2021). Li et al. (2016) identified nine kaurene-type diterpenoids in this liverwort.

The Chinese liverwort *Solenostoma faurieanum* syn. *Jungermannia faurieana* contains jungermannenone A and B (ent-kaurane diterpenoids). In work by Guo, Lin et al. (2016), both compounds showed high cytotoxicity against several cancer cell lines.

Kondoh et al. (2005) found jungermannenones A–D activated caspase-3 and caspase-8 and induced apoptosis in human leukemia (HL-60) cell lines. Jungermannenones A and D inhibit the activity of nuclear factor-kappaB, which is a transcriptional factor of antiapoptotic factors.

Guo, Lin et al. (2016) found jungermannenones A and B arrested cell cycle, induced apoptosis, and caused mitochondrial damage in prostate (PC-3) cancer cell lines through the caspase-3 signaling pathway.

Infuscaic acid, infuscaside A, infuscaside B, and plagiochilal B isolated from *Solenostoma infusica* syn. *Jungermannia infusca* hindered the release of superoxide anion radicals from rabbit and guinea pig peritoneal macrophage induction. Infuscasides A and B, bitter diterpene glycosides derived from this species, showed neurite bundle formation at 10^{-7} M (Asakawa 2007). This liverwort contains 19 cuparane-type, one acorane-type, one monocyclic-type, one prelacinane-type, and one aromadendrane-type sesquiterpene, as well as two clerodane-type and one halimane type diterpenoid, and labdane and ent-kaurane-type diterpenoids (infuscasides A–E) (Nagashima et al. 2001). The liverwort's intense, bitter taste, which can last up to eight hours, is due to infuscasides A–E.

Tetragon flapwort (*Solenostoma tetragonum* syn. *Jungermannia tetragona*) contains several ent-Kaurane diterpenoids found to bind glutathione and sulfhydryl groups in antioxidant enzymes covalently, leading to destruction of intracellular redox homeostasis. This suggests a possible benefit in cancer therapy. The compound 11β-hydroxy-ent-16-kaurene-15-one exhibits strong inhibitory activity against several cancer cell lines. It also induces apoptosis and ferroptosis in human liver cancer cells and sensitizes cisplatin-resistant lung cancer cell lines (Sun et al. 2021).

The related *Solenostoma truncatum* syn. *Jungermannia truncata* was investigated by Nagashima et al. (2002). The compound ent-11α-hydroxy-16-kauren-15-one (KD), combined with tumor necrosis factor alpha, had a synergistic cytotoxic effect on human leukemia (HL-60) cancer cell lines. Similar effects were noted when KD was combined with camptothecin, an alkaloid isolated from the stem wood of the Chinese tree *Camptotheca acuminata* that selectively inhibits the nuclear enzyme DNA topoisomerase type I. Several semi-synthetic analogs of camptothecin have demonstrated antitumor activity. This suggests the possible use of KD in adjunct chemotherapy, helping increase apoptosis induction. Jungermannenones A–D inhibit tumors through a caspase-dependent pathway (Kondoh et al. 2005).

Acute myeloid leukemia (AML) is a difficult and challenging cancer, characterized by clonal proliferation of myeloid blasts. Work by Yue et al. (2018) found jungermannenone C, a tetracyclic diterpenoid, induces cell differentiation in AML cells. The unnatural enantiomer of jungermannenone was found even more potent at inducing cell differentiation and targets peroxiredoxins I and II by selectively binding to the cysteine residues, leading to cellular reactive oxygen species (ROS) accumulation.

SYMPHYOGYNA

Toothed Liverwort Toothed Ribbonwort

Symphyogyna podophylla syn. *S. hymenophyllum* is common in wetland forests of Australia, New Zealand, South Africa, and South America. Liverwort extracts display antifungal activity against *Cryptococcus neoformans* (Linde et al. 2016). This fungus is the cause of cryptococcosis in humans, often associated with exposure to bird droppings. Symptoms including fever, headache, photosensitivity, and in advanced forms can manifest in a stiff neck and cryptococcal meningitis. Ten years ago, cryptococcosis was responsible for more than 600,000 deaths annually in AIDS patients (Song et al. 2012). The antifungal medication flucytosine is the most commonly used drug for treatment. Around 180,000 cases are reported annually, mainly in sub-Sahara regions; in some areas mortality rates can approach 70%.

Solenostoma obovatum syn. *Jungermannia obovata* has an intense carrot-like odor due to the presence of aromatic compound trinormonoterpene.

SYZYGIELLA

Marsh Flapwort Marsh Earwort

The *Syzygiella* genus contains 33 accepted species ranging from the southern hemisphere to including islands near Antartica. *Súzugos* from Greek means "paired," referring to the opposite stem leaves joined at base.

Autumn flapwort or Jameson's liverwort (*Syzygiella autumnalis* syn. *Jamesoniella autumnalis* syn. *Jungermannia autumnalis*) contains clerodane-type, jamesoniellides M–T, and one *ent*-labdane-type diterpenoid, as well as one known analog. Jamesoniellides Q, R, and S exhibit moderate anti-inflammatory activity (Li, Zhu et al. 2018).

Work by Li et al. (2018) tested for inhibition of LPS-induced nitric oxide production in RAW 264.7 murine macrophages. Jamesoniellides Q, R, and S exhibit moderate anti-inflammatory activity.

Essential oil from *Syzygiella anomala* is composed mainly of silphiperfola-5,7(14)-diene (25.22%) and caryophyllene oxide (8.98%) (Valarezo 2020).

Caryophyllene oxide promotes iron deposition in tumors, killing HCCLMS and HUH7 (liver) cancer cell lines by inducing ferritinophagy (Xiu et al. 2022).

The related liverwort *Syzygiella colorata* syn. *Jamesoniella colorata* contains six labdane type diterpenoids; three seco-clerodane diterpenoids; jamesoniellide

I; two new jamesoniellides, K and L; the sesquiterpene waitziacuminone; and a chlorinated bisbibenzyl (6,6',10,10',12, 12'-hexachloroisoperrottetin A) (Hertewich et al. 2003). Its bitter taste is due to the various furanoclerodane diterpenoids.

TARGIONIA

Orobus-Seed Liverwort

Targionia hypophylla was first described by Italian botanist Fabio Colonna and named *lichen acaulis hypophyllocarpus* in 1616, renamed *lichen petraeus minimus fructu orobi* in 1623, and later *lichen Petraeus minimus acaulis.*

Orobus-seed liverwort, *Targionia hypophylla*, is ground into a paste and mixed with coconut oil in India to treat scabies, itchy skin, and other dermatological conditions (Remesh and Manju 2009). More specifically, a paste is combined with the leaves of the fern *Actiniopteris radiata* in a base of coconut oil and rubbed on the body.

An in vivo study found that orobus-seed liverwort *Targionia hypophylla* exhibits significant inhibition of pain on carrageenan-induced paw edema and promising suppressive effects on p-benzoquinone–induced abdominal constriction animal models (Tosun et al. 2013). Extracts significantly inhibit mouse lymphoma induced by leukemia virus (YAC-I) and mouse myeloma (Sp2) cell lines (Önder and Özenoglu 2019). Water extracts inhibit various fungi, including *Aspergillus niger*, *Botrytis cinerea*, *Penicillium chrysogenum*, *P. expansum*, and *Trichoderma viridae* (Alam et al. 2012), while methanol extracts inhibit *Bacillus subtilis*, *Escherichia coli*, and *Staphylococcus aureus* (Sawant and Karadge 2010).

It should be noted that not all fungi possess negative connotations. *Penicillium chrysogenum*, for example, is a very valuable medicinal fungus. A review by Shaaban et al. (2023) found that in the last ten years, some 277 compounds in this fungus have been identified, leading to new and promising pharmaceutical applications.

THYSANANTHUS

Thysananthus spathulistipus syn. *Jungermannia spathylistipus* syn. *Frullania spathulistipus* contains thysaspathone; 14-clerodadiene; and 2β,4β:15,16-diepoxy-13.

Work by Harinantenaina, Kurata et al. (2006) found the isolated compounds inhibit nitric oxide (NO) production in LPS-stimulated RAW 264.7 cells associated with murine leukemia.

TREUBIA

The genus, containing seven species, honors the Dutch botanist Melchior Treub (1851–1910).

Treubia isignensis var. *isignensis* was extracted with diethyl ether and analyzed. The researchers suggest this liverwort is chemically very primitive as it produced only maaliane, eudesmne, aristolane, and gorgonane sesquiterpenes. No oxygenated terpenoids or aromatic compounds were detected (Coulerie et al. 2014). However, just because they are chemically primitive does not mean these compounds are not valuable.

A review of maaliane, aristolane, and other terpenoids containing the gem-di-methyl cyclopropyl unit was published by Durán-Peña et al. (2015). They found 119 references to their antiviral, antimicrobial, and cytotoxic activities in the literature between 1963 and 2014. The Essential Science Indicators (ESI) database contains tables listing 332 of these terpenoids, their occurrence and biological activity, together with related references.

TRICHOCOLEA

Handsome Woollywort   Wooly Worm Liverwort

Geographic Range: worldwide

Habitat: moist, shaded mineral-rich wetlands particularly with surface water movement, such as mountain streams or seepage on wet rocks

Medicinal Applications: antibacterial, anticancer, antidepressant, antidiabetic, antifungal, anti-osteoporosis, antioxidant, cardioprotective, hepaprotective

The *Trichocolea* genus includes 31 species, most of them endemic to the southern Pacific Ocean, including New Zealand, Tasmania, and South Australia.

Work by Preziuso et al. (2018) reviewed the secondary metabolites of this genus and found anticancer, antibacterial, antifungal, and antioxidant activities.

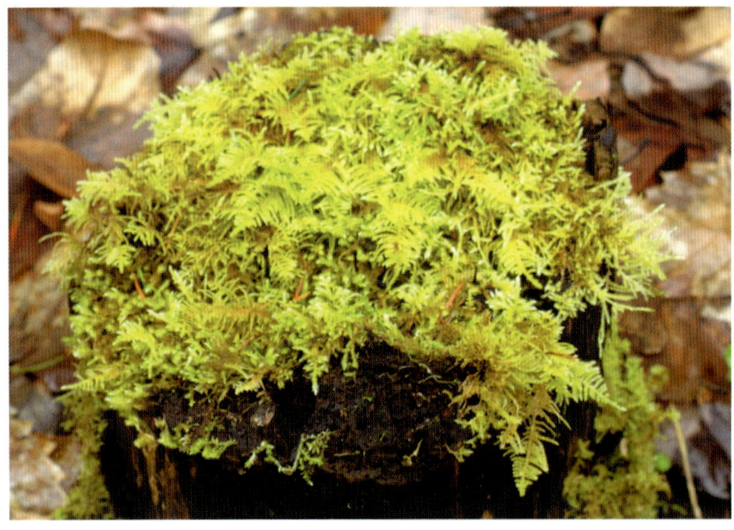

Trichocolea tomentella (Handsome Woollywort)

Woolly worm liverwort (*Trichocolea mollissima*), a New Zealand species, contains 1α-hydroxy-ent-sandaracopimara-8(14),15-diene (Lorimer, Perry et al. 1997). The compound methyl-4-[(5-oxogeranyl) oxy]-3-methoxybenzoate found in this liverwort exhibits cytotoxicity against the leukemia P-388 cell line (Perry, Foster et al. 1996). Tomentellin, the major compound in this liverwort, is active against African green monkey kidney epithelial cells.

Handsome woollywort, *Trichocolea tomentella*, as well as another species, *Leiomitra lanata* syn. *T. lanata*, also produce tomentellin (Perry, Foster et al. 1996).

Handsome woollywort is found in northern Portugal and Spain, Ireland, north to Scandivania, and eastern to western Russia; as well as Asia, North Africa, and eastern North America.

Demethoxy-tomentellin isolated from *Trichocolea tomentella* shows similar inhibitory activity against cancer cells (Novkovic et al. 2021). This liverwort species contains the endophytic fungus *Penicillium concentricum*. Twenty-three compounds were isolated from cultures of this fungal endophyte by Ali et al. (2017). They include 6-chlor-3,8-dihydroxy-1-methylxanthone; 2-bromogentisyl alcohol; a mixture of 6-epimers of 6-dehydroxy-6-bromogabosine C; epoxydon; norlichexanthone; chlorogentisyl alcohol; hydroxychlorogentisyl quinone; 6-dehydroxy-6α-chlorogabosine C; 6-dehydroxyj-6β-chlorogabosine; gentisyl alcohol; gentisyl quinone; (R,S)-1-phenyl-1,2-ethanediol; dehydro-dechlorogriseovulvin; dechlorogriseofulvin; dehydrogriseofulvin; griseofulvin; ethylene glycol benzoate; alternariol; griseoxanthone C; drimiopsin H; griseophenone B and C. The compounds

2-bromo-gentisyl alcohol, 6-epimers of 6-dehydroxy-6-bromogabosine C, and epoxydon display modest cytotoxicity against breast (MCF-7) cancer cell lines, while epoxydon shows selective cytotoxicity against prostate (DU-145) cancer cell lines. In a 2019 study of *Trichocolea tomentella*, Anaya-Eugenio et al. found 2-bromogentisyl alcohol and 3-hydroxy-benzenemethanol exhibited the highest cytotoxic activity against different cancer cell lines, including cervical/epithelial (HeLa), colon (HT-29), breast (MDA-MB-321), and prostate (PC-3 and DU-145) cell lines.

A number of compounds found in this liverwort have been studied for their potential medical uses. Norlichexanthone, for example, reduces *Staphylococcus aureus* toxicity toward human neutrophils and reduces staphylococcal biofilm in MRSA strain USA300 (Baldry et al. 2016). Norlichexanthone is a ligand of estrogen receptor-α and may be useful in postmenopausal osteoporosis. Work by Wang et al. (2021) identified the compound and found it induces osteoblast formation in bone precursor cells. Conversely, it inhibits receptor activator of nuclear factor-kappa B ligand-induced osteoclast formation in both RAW264.7 macrophages and mouse primary monocytes. And most importantly, it exhibits potent anti-osteoporosis efficacy in ovariectomized mice. Compared to estrogen, it is less capable of stimulating endometrial hyperplasia and promoting mammalian cancer cell proliferation.

Moreover, norlichexanthone shows potential to treat or prevent metabolic syndrome type 2 diabetes, atherosclerosis, and cardiovascular disease (Ikeda et al. 2011). The compound is predicted to be active as an antidepressant (an MAO-B inhibitor) as well, based on work by Fatima et al. (2019). The researchers screened thirty-one out of a total of 968 compounds found in African medicinal plants, and norlichexanthone was predicted the most active. This suggests possible benefit in the prevention or treatment of Parkinson's disease and other neurological conditions.

Another compound derived from a fungal endophyte in this liverwort is gentisyl alcohol, known to have antibacterial, antifungal, antiviral, and anticancer effects. Work by Ham et al. (2019) found gentisyl alcohol suppresses proliferation and induces apoptosis in human ovarian (ES2 and OV90) cancer cell lines. Gentisyl alcohol also exhibits selective cytotoxicity against colon (HT-29) cancer cell lines.

Alternariol, another compound in the liverwort, is a strong inhibitor of xanthine oxidase, with activity 12 times higher than the standard drug allopurinol, used to treat gout (Fan et al. 2022). Moreover, alternariol and its derivatives exhibit anticancer activity through several pathways. These include cytotoxic reactive oxygen species (ROS) leading to oxidative stress and mitochondrial dysfunction–linked cytotoxic effects, as well as anti-inflammatory activity, cell cycle arrest, apoptotic cell death, and genotoxic, mutagenic, antiproliferative, autophagy, and estrogenic and clastogenic mechanisms (Islam et al. 2023). It is certainly a cytotoxic compound against cancer.

Griseofulvin is a well-known antifungal metabolite that was developed from related *Penicillium griseofulvum*, into a commercial drug in 1959. It has been widely used to treat dermatophyte skin infections. Recently, it is undergoing interest for its potential to disrupt mitosis and cell division in human cancer cells and arrest hepatitis C virus replication. Work by Aris et al. (2022) and others have found that griseofulvin enhances ACE2 function, contributes to vascular vasodilation, and improves blood flow in capillaries. It also exhibits binding potential with SARS-CoV-2 main protease, suggesting inhibition of viral entry and replication. Since ACE2 is one of the main viral targets, it may be helpful for long-haul respiratory distress associated with viral infection.

TRICHOCOLEOPSIS

Down Liverwort

Warning: May cause contact dermatitis.

Trichocoleopsis sacculata is appropriately named, as it contains the diterpene dialdehydes sacculatal and isosacculatal. Sacculatal is a dialdehyde that can cause contact dermatitis and tastes hot and pungent, giving this liverwort the means by which to protect itself from insects, thereby deterring feeding (Asakawa and Takemoto 1977).

TRITOMARIA

Notchworts

There are presently nine species of notchworts with a cosmopolitan, worldwide distribution. *Tritomaria ferruginea* is an endangered species endemic to the eastern Himalayas, sometimes growing as an epiphyte on *Rhododendron* trees.

Lyon's notchwort (*Tritomaria quinquedentata*) contains another sesquiterpene, ent-isoalantolactone, which inhibits *Candida albicans* by decreasing ergosterol contents and increasing zymosterol and lanosterol accumulation (Li, Shi et al. 2017).

Flushed notchwort (*Tritomaria polita*) has been moved to *Saccobasis polita*. It is found throughout northern North America and Russia.

WETTSTEINIA

The genus is named in honor of Fritz von Wettstein (1895–1945), a Czech-Austrian bryologist and mycologist.

Wettsteinia schusterana contains the naphthalene derivatives wettsteins A and B (Asakawa et al. 1994).

WIESNERELLA

In the western Himalayans, *Wiesnerella denudata* is used to treat gallstones (Kumar et al. 2007). The genus is named in honor of the Austrian botanist Julius Ritter von Wiesner (1838–1916).

Wiesnerella denudata releases an elegant scent when crushed, vastly superior to that of *Conocephalum conicum*, great-scented liverwort. The major constituent is (-)-bornyl acetate, but it also contains germacranolide, guaianolides, limonene, α and gamma-terpinenes, α-terpineol, borneol, 1-octen-3-yl acetate, dehydrocostus lactone, 8β-acetoxycostuslactone, and zaluzanins. Zaluzanins C–D exhibit antibacterial, antifungal, and cytotoxic activity. Guaianolides exhibits cytotoxic activity against lymphocytic leukemia (P-388) cell lines (Asakawa 1990; Lu et al. 2006). The compound 1-octen-3-yl-acetate is responsible for the mushroomy or umami scent of many liverworts. Germacranolide (aka tulipinolide) gives the gametophyte portion of this liverwort a hot and lasting taste on the tongue.

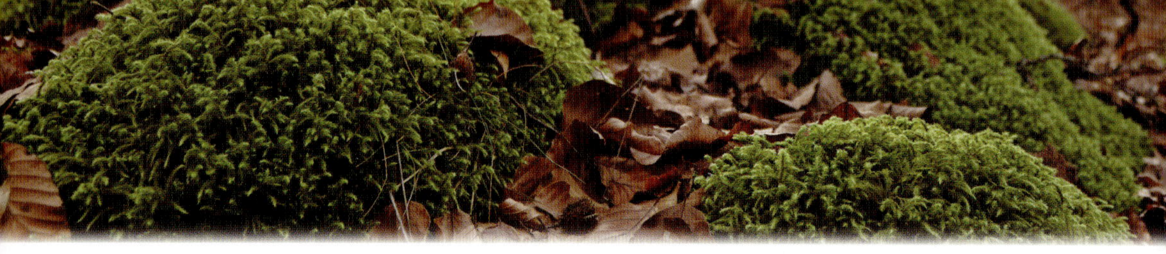

3 Hornworts

Anthocerotophyta

Damp earth's quiet sage,
Hornwort hidden yet profound—
Medicine unpraised.

Robert Dale Rogers (a haiku)

The word *hornwort* is derived from the hornlike shape of the sporophyte (Frangedakis et al. 2022). Hornworts are found on all continents, in a wide range of climates, ranging from deserts to polar regions. Access to moisture is a limiting factor to their growth.

Microbes and their alliances are fundamental to the origin, evolution, and current function of every creature we encounter, from the hornwort to the hippo, says biologist Tom Wakeford in his 2001 book *Liasons of Life: From Hornworts to Hippos, How the Unassuming Microbe Has Driven Evolution*. Hornworts are part of a bryophyte lineage that diverged from other land plants more than 400 million years ago. They have a unique biology, including distinct sporophyte structure, cyanobacterial symbiosis, and a pyrenoid-based carbon-concentrating mechanism. They have but a single chloroplast in each cell. Hornworts are a sister taxa to liverworts.

Work by Li et al. (2020) identified candidate genes involved in cyanobacterial symbiosis and found LCIB, a *Chlamydomonas* (a genus of green algae) carbon-concentrating mechanism gene, is involved in hornworts, but not in other plant lineages. In fact, hornworts share characteristics with algae as well as land plants. For example, the presence of a basal sporophytic meristem and asynchronous meiosis are unique to hornworts. They are among the few plants with a symbiotic relationship with nitrogen-fixing cyanobacteria, including *Nostoc commune*. The presence of structurally different xyloglucans in the cell wall of

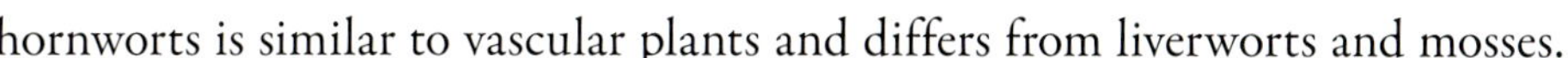

hornworts is similar to vascular plants and differs from liverworts and mosses.

Like all bryophytes, hornworts made the transition from freshwater to land. They share a common ancestor with mosses and liverworts. To survive, a polysaccharide-rich cell wall was necessary to cope with the drastic environmental change. Hydroxyproline-rich glycoprotein backbones are found in hornworts and liverworts, and show differentiation (Pfeifer et al. 2022).

Hornworts are the only land plant lineage harboring a biophysical, carbon-concentrating mechanism. Various scientists are studying the possibilities of engineering this unique feature into crop plants (Li, Villarreal et al. 2017).

CERIUM AND HORNWORTS

Cerium is the 58th element on the periodic table. First discovered in 1803 by two Swedish and one German scientist, it was named after the asteroid Ceres. It is not a rare mineral, as the earth's crust contains 66 ppm compared to copper at 68 ppm. It is formed into ceric acid, ceria, cerium oxide, and cerium dioxide. It is plentiful in allanite, from the western United States, and bastnasite from southern California. Various industrial applications include use in catalytic converters, diesel fuel, solar cells, polishing glass (faster than optician's rouge), fuel cells (instead of zirconium oxide), ferrocerium lighters, carbon-arc lights for motion pictures, and in water-splitting for hydrogen production (the next source of so-called environmentally friendly energy). Nano-ceria is used in sunscreens, replacing zinc and titanium oxide. Nano-ceria also has medical applications, as antibacterial and antioxidant agents; and it is cytotoxic to several human cancer cell lines, including lung (Lin et al. 2006), prostate (Renu et al. 2012), and ovarian (Hijaz et al. 2016.) Cerium nano particles reduce inflammation and autoimmune response to viral infections (Zandi et al. 2022).

However, cerium dioxide nanoparticles also induce apoptosis and autophagy in human peripheral blood monocytes, causing mitochondrial damage (Hussain et al. 2012)—not so good.

So how does all this relate to hornworts?

All the industrial and pharmaceutical usage of cerium, in different forms, eventually finds its way into our water. Work by Zhang et al. (2012) found hornworts possess the ability to bryo-accumulate high levels of ceria nanoparticles, helping to clean up engineered nanoparticle pollution.

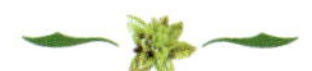

ANTHOCEROS

Hornworts

Geographic Range: worldwide

Habitat: moist and shady; thriving in disturbed environments

Practical Uses: agricultural applications

Medicinal Applications: antiallergenic, antibacterial, anticancer, antidiabetic, antifungal, anti-inflammatory, immune-modulating

The genus name *Anthoceros* derives from the Latin meaning "flower horn." At the present time, the genus has 67 accepted species.

Field hornwort, *Anthoceros agrestis,* was grown in cell suspension cultures containing 2% and 4% sucrose. The cells accumulated up to 5.1% rosmarinic acid and a new derivative of rosmarinic acid, 3'-O-β-D-glucoside (up to 1%) (Vogelsang et al. 2006). The alkaloid anthocerodiazonin has been isolated in cultures of this hornwort (Trennheuser et al. 1994), as was six glutamic acid amides, isorinic acid, and caffeic acid methyl ester. The latter compound induces antiallergic activity by suppressing degranulation of mast cells (Park et al. 2023).

Anthoceros agrestis shares with the liverwort *Conocephalum conicum* various fatty acids, including mono-galactosyldiacylglycerols. When cultured, the presence of cinnamic acid 4-hydroxylase was noted (Petersen 2003). This compound is also found in the moss *Physcomitrella patens* (Wohl and Petersen 2020).

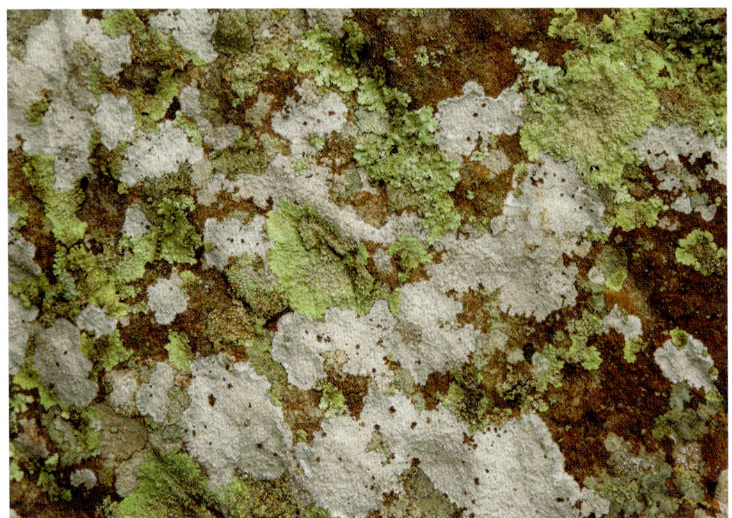

Anthoceros sp. with lichen and moss

Volatiles in *Anthoceros agrestis*, as well as in two other species, *A. caucasicus* and *A. punctatus*, include α- and β-pinene, β-myrcene, terpinolene, camphene, and the most abundant, limonene. Sesquiterpenes include aristolene, anastreptene, β-barbatene, β-bazzanene, delta-cuprenene, maaliol, diplophyllolide, and vetica-dinoxide. Methyl p-coumarate is also found in *Anthoceros agrestis* and *Anthoceros punctatus*. The volatile compound aristolene helps fungus-farming termites selectively bury weedy fungi that smell different than their food crop (Katariya et al. 2017). Anastreptene is also found in liverwort *Chandonanthus hirtellus*.

Maaliol, another compound isolated in *Anthoceros agrestis*, has been identified as one of four cytotoxic compounds in aerial parts of camphor spurflower (*Plectranthus cylindraceus*), a flowering plant in the Lamiaceae family; it shows activity against human breast, skin, and cervical cancers (Amina et al. 2018). Diplophyllolide is a cytotoxic sesquiterpene lactone also found in the liverworts *Clasmatocolea vermicularis* and *Chiloscyphus subporosa* (Lorimer, Burgess et al. 1997).

Another species, *Anthoceros angustus*, has been collected and analyzed for volatile oils (Koid et al. 2022). It contains 34.6% pentanoic acid; 2,2,4-trimethyl-3-carboxyisopropyl; isobutyl ester; and minor amounts of nonanal, decanal, naphthalene, limonene, and geranylacetone. Pentanoate fatty acid, in experimental mice models of colitis and multiple sclerosis, induced regulatory B cells to mediate protection from autoimmune pathology, suggesting this short-chain fatty acid may be useful in treating various inflammatory and autoimmune diseases (Luu et al. 2019).

The related species *Anthoceros caucasicus* contains an unusual disaccharide, α-D-glucuronosyl-(1>3)-l-galactose, which supports the view that a unique compound in an evolutionarily isolated plant (*Anthoceros*) indicates that major steps in plant phylogeny are accompanied by significant changes in cell wall composition (Popper et al. 2003).

Long hornwort (*Anthoceros longii*) inhibits the gram-negative bacterium *Agrobacterium tumefaciens* (Deora and Bhati 2007). This destructive pathogen causes crown gall disease that causes the formation of tumors in many commercial crops, including apples, pears, cherries, raspberries, and roses. A related species, *Anthoceros natalensis*, upon desiccation and rehydration, exhibits oxygen production at a rate 100 times that recorded for the roots of wheat (Minibayeva and Beckett 2001). This suggests the possibility of benefit in space travel.

Dotted hornwort, *Anthoceros punctatus*, contains the powerful antioxidant rosmarinic acid, as well as its glucoside and isorinic acid (Itoh et al. 2000).

CERATOPHYLLUM

Coon Tail Rigid Hornwort

Rigid hornwort or coon tail (*Ceratophyllum demersum*) is aquatic and cultivated for home freshwater aquariums. The genus name derives from the Greek *kerat*, meaning "horn," and *phyllon*, "plant." The species name *demersus* is Latin for "underwater."

Ceratophyllum demersum is used in Traditional Chinese Medicine for cooling and treating illnesses with periodic symptoms. Known as *jīn yú zâo*, it is taken internally for bilious conditions and applied externally to bites and stings of venomous insects and scorpions. However, a look at its contents reveals significant α-glucosidase inhibition. Lupeol was found to have the highest potential. Work by Li, Tu et al. (2020) and Duong et al. (2025) found the $1C_{50}$ of dried coon tail lower than the well-known antidiabetic drug acarbose. Over 80 compounds were found, including 8 organic acids, 11 phenolic acids, 25 flavonoids, and 21 fatty acids, including demersones A–D, acetylvelutins A and B, (+)cyclocolorenone, 1-hydroxycyclocolorenone, 10-hydroxycyclocolorenone, retusin, betulinic acid, and lupeol (Duong et al. 2025).

Work by Maslyk et al. (2024) identified isorhamnetin, sakuranetin, taxifolin, and eriodictyol most likely responsible for cytotoxicity against gastrointestinal cancer cell lines.

Aquaculture is a growing industry, providing protein to a burgeoning planetary population. Due to the tight, enclosed systems associated with raising

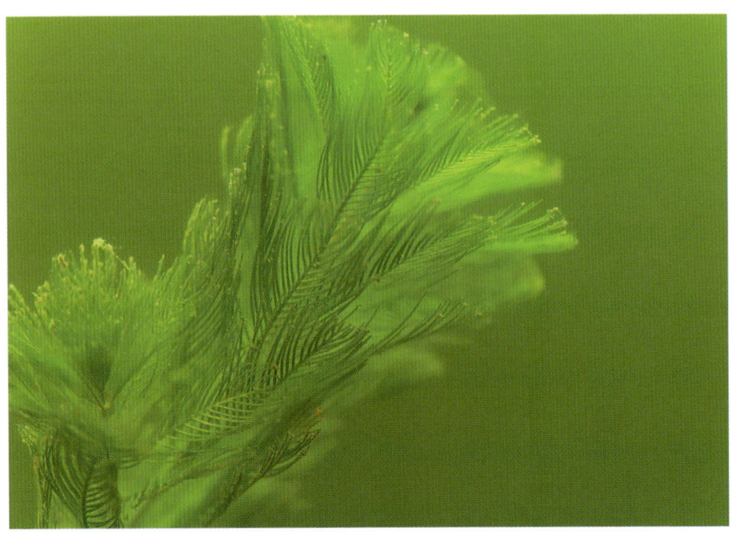

Ceratophyllum demersum (Rigid Hornwort)

fish, disease can easily become a problem. *Aeromonas hydrophila* is one such pathogenic bacteria affecting farmed fish populations. Supplementation with *Ceratophyllum demersum* enhances both cell-mediated and humoral immunity. A 2.5% incorporation into feed could be useful in enhancing fish health by boosting immune response (Verma et al. 2021).

This hornwort exhibits antimicrobial activity. When tested against 17 different gram-positive and gram-negative bacteria and fungi, it was the most effective of four plants tested by Fareed et al. (2008). Water extracts exhibit activity against *Salmonella cholerasuis*. Ethanol extracts showed antibacterial activity against *Bacillus subtilis*, *B. cereus*, *Staphylococcus aureus*, *Escherichia coli*, *Pseudomonas aeruginosa*, *Klebsiella pneumoniae*, *Staphylococcus cholerasius* (*S. enterica*), *Shigella* spp., *Serratia liquefaciens*, *Proteus vulgaris*, and *Brenneria nigrifluens*. *Serratia liquefaciens* is a human pathogen that infects the respiratory and urinary systems. *Brenneria nigrifluens* bacteria infect walnut and horse chestnut saplings and trees. The genus is named after the microbiologist Don J. Brenner.

Ceratophyllum demersum may have potential for phytoremediation of heavy metals. Work by Aasim et al. (2023) found it can efficaciously remediate cadmium-contaminated aquatic environments. Earlier work by Dogan et al. (2018) found the hornwort cell culture can phytoremediate both cadmium and lead contamination in water. As well, this hornwort shows a huge absorptive capacity for the pesticide aminocarb, up to 400 micrograms/gram of fresh weight in the dark, and 1000 micrograms/gram in the light (Weinberger and Greenhaigh 1985).

LEIOSPOROCEROS

Hornwort

The genus name derives from the Greek *leio*, "smooth" or "even," *sporo*, referring to spore, and *ceros*, "horned." This hornwort is placed in a separate family, order, and class for being genetically and morphologically distinct from all other hornwort lineages.

Distillation of the male and female thalli and the sporophyte of *Leiosporoceros dussii*, the only species of this genus, was performed by Garrido et al. (2019). In all, 27 volatile compounds were identified. In the male thalli, the major constituents are hexanol (25.3%), β-ionone (21.1%), benzeneacetaldehyde (17.6%), and β-cyclocitral (14%). Minor constituents are methyl heptanone, nonanal, neoisomenthol, and bornyl acetate. The female thalli are composed mainly of methacamphor (17.8%), hexanol (12.3%), and menthyl acetate (12.3%). Minor volatiles include 3-pentanone, 3-octenol, nonanol, estragole, and menthyl acetate. The sporophytes contain mainly hexanal (19.3%), β-cyclocitral (17.6%), 2-nonenal (15.8%), hexanol (12.5%), and β-ionone (10.2%). Other minor constituents are isomenthol, thymol, isomenthol acetate, and β-methylnaphthalene. Beta-ionone, for example, inhibits the proliferation of RCC (renal) cell carcinoma, induces autophagy via the LKB1/AMPK signaling pathway (Hou et al. 2023).

Bornyl acetate is used to flavor food and aroma in perfumes and in proprietary Chinese medicines. It down-regulates pro-inflammatory cytokines, regulates immune response by up-regulating $CD86^+$, and reduces tau protein phosphorylation, suggesting benefit in inflammation, immune modulation, and prevention/treatment of tau tangles in Alzheimer's disease. It possesses sedative benefit in aromatherapy, and has a more favorable safety profile, compared to traditional NSAIDs (Zhao et al. 2023)

MEGACEROS

Big Hornwort

The genus name derives from the Greek *mega*, "very large" or "huge," and *ceros*, meaning "horned," alluding to the large horn-shaped sporophyte.

The annual hornwort *Megaceros flagellaris* contains rosmarinic acid, two phytyl esters, phaeophytins, sitosterol, and stigmasterol hexacecanoate (Buchanan et al. 1996). The latter antibacterial compound is also found in the liverwort *Plagiochila ovalifolia*.

PHAEOCEROS

Erect Hornwort Smooth Hornwort

Phaeo means "yellow" and of course *ceros* means "horn" refering to the yellow spores produced in the horn-shaped sporophyte whereas *Anthoceros* produces dark brown or black spores.

Erect hornwort (*Phaeoceros erectus* syn. *Anthoceros erectus*) exhibits activity against various bacteria, including *Bacillus subtilis*, *Staphylococcus aureus*, *Escherichia coli*, *Klebsiella pneumoniae*, *Vibrio cholera*, *Pseudomonas aeruginosa*, and *Shigella flexneri* (Sangeetha 2019). Smooth hornwort, *Phaeoceros laevis* syn. *Anthoceros laevis*, contains pockets of the cyanobacteria *Nostoc commune*, which can grow in macroscopic mats and is eaten raw in salads in Indonesia, Japan, China, and the Philippines. The *Nostoc commune* found in pockets of hornworts are microscopic. In Taiwan, smooth hornwort is called *yû lái gû*, meaning "post-rain mushroom." Within this hornwort, *Nostoc commune* helps fix nitrogen from the atmosphere, and because of its photosynthetic pigments it produces energy in the cytoplasm of cells. *Nostoc flagelliforme* is sometimes named as a variety of this species and known in China as *fàcài*. It is used in food traditionally served at Lunar New Year.

It contains pigments that allow it to absorb long and medium wavelength UV radiation, helping it survive in areas of high radiation. This cynobacterium can remain dormant for a long time, and dried colonies are resistant to heat and patterns of freezing and thawing. While dormant, it produces no oxygen.

There is enough literature to write a small book on the health benefits and medicinal properties of *Nostoc commune*. Here are a few recent examples:

- exhibits antioxidant, anti-inflammatory, anticarcinogenic, and immune-modulating properties, suggesting its use as functional food for the amelioration of human diseases (Li and Guo 2017).
- has polysaccharides that suppress the growth and proliferation of breast (MCF-7) and colorectal (DLD1) cancer cell lines (Guo et al. 2015).
- inhibits the growth of small cell lung cancer (NCl-H446 and NCl-H1688) cell lines (Guo, Ding et al. 2016).
- has polysaccharides that are a potent activator of macrophages that contribute to the inhibition of five colorectal cancer cell lines (Guo, Li et al. 2019).
- inhibits colitis-associated colon tumor development in mice and modulates microbiota, suggesting a promising prebiotic for the prevention and treatment of colorectal cancer (Guo and Li 2019).
- has ultrasonic extracts that exhibit antioxidant and hypoglycemic (anti-diabetic) effects in vitro (Wang, Yang et al. 2022).

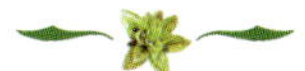

Bryophytes are amongst the first plants to colonize rocks. They prevent soil erosion and retain water, improve soil for agriculture and horticulture and act as bryoindicators of air, water, and soil pollution.

They are edible and medicinal, and peat moss helps produce some of the finest Scotch whiskies on the planet.

They are often overlooked and yet are an integral part of our environment and ecology.

Oh Bryophtyes, so quaint and mossy,
Your healing skills—small yet bossy!
Helping bruises, burns and bites,
Nature's nurses, mossy knights!
Tiny healers under shoes,
Hidden greens—who would choose?
Doctors frowning, quite perplexed—
Bryophytes say, "Our cures are next!"

Robert Dale Rogers

Bryophytes by Common Name

This book is arranged in alphabetical order by genus. The list below is provided for readers who may know a moss, liverwort, or hornwort in their area by its common name but who do not know its Latin genus and species (binomial). The most current Latin binomial is given. Use the first part of the binomial, the genus, to flip to that section in this book. Note that in some cases the genus name has been updated, so the older synonyms reflecting an earlier genus name may also be found in the text. Occasionally you will see that a common name applies to more than one genus-species. My hope is that this list will help you find the information you wish to explore in this book.

Mosses

Acute-leaved bogmoss – *Sphagnum capillifolium*
Akkarghoda lady fern – *Athyrium hohenackerianum*
African carpet moss – *Racopilum* spp.
Air moss – *Aerobryidium* spp., *Aerobryum* spp.
Alpine haircap moss – *Polytrichastrum alpinum*
Alpine watermoss – *Fontinalis squamosa*
Anomalous bristle moss – *Orthotrichum anomalum*
Anomodon moss – *Claopodium rostratum*
Apple mosses – *Bartramia* spp., *Philonotis* spp.
Aquatic apple moss – *Philonotis fontana*
Ariseamos moss – *Rhodobryum roseum*
Armpit moss – *Rosulabryum moravicum*
Baby-tooth moss – *Plagiomnium cuspidatum*
Balding moss – *Oligotrichum hercynicum*
Ball white moss – *Sphagnum palustre*
Bank haircap moss – *Polytrichum formosum*
Beardless mosses – *Anoectangium* spp.
Beard moss – *Barbella pendula*
Beard mosses – *Barbula* spp.
Beautiful branch moss – *Callicladium haldaneanum*
Besser's neckera moss – *Alleniella besseri*
Bicolored bryum – *Gemmabryum dichotomum*
Big red stem moss – *Pleurozium schreberi*
Big shaggy moss – *Hylocomiadelphus triquetrus*
Big star moss – *Atrichum undulatum*
Bird's claw beard moss – *Barbula unguiculata*
Black rockmoss – *Andreaea rupestris*
Bladder mosses – *Physcomitrium* spp.
Blunt-beak moss – *Grimmia pulvinata*
Blunt feather moss – *Homalia trichomanoides*
Blunt-leaved beak moss – *Eurhynchium angustirete*
Blunt-leaved bogmoss – *Sphagnum palustre*
Blunt mousetail moss – *Isothecium myurum*
Bog bead-moss – *Aulacomnium palustre*
Bog grove moss – *Aulacomnium palustre*
Bog haircap moss – *Polytrichum strictum*
Bog mosses – *Sphagnum* spp.

Bonfire moss – *Funaria hygrometrica*
Bordered thyme moss – *Mnium marginatum*
Bottlebrush moss – *Breutelia* spp.
Bowring's pincushion – *Leucobryum bowringii*
Bristle mosses – *Orthotrichum* spp.
Bristly haircap moss – *Polytrichum piliferum*
Bristly hookmoss – *Palustriella falcata*
Broken-leaf curved-tail moss – *Dicranum tauricum*
Brook mosses – *Fontinalis* spp.
Broom fork moss – *Dicranum scoparium*
Broom moss – *Phyllogonium* spp.
Brownish bogmoss – *Sphagnum subnitens*
Bryum mosses – *Bryum* spp.
Bud-headed groovemoss – *Aulacomnium androgynum*
Bun moss – *Octoblepharum albidum*
Capillary thread moss – *Rosulabryum capillare*
Cat's tail moss – *Pseudisothecium* sp.
Cave moss – *Cyclodictyon* spp.
Cedar moss – *Brachythecium rutabulum*
Chalk comb moss – *Ctenidium molluscum*
Charcoal peddler – *Funaria hygrometrica*
Ciliate hoarmoss – *Hedwigia ciliata*
Cinderella moss – *Funaria hygrometrica*
Circle leaf moss – *Sanionia uncinata*
Claw-leaved hookmoss – *Palustriella falcata*
Clear beardless moss – *Anoectangium clarum*
Cloud moss – *Leucobryum martianum*
Coiled-leaf claw moss – *Hypnum cirinale*
Comb mosses – *Ctenidium* spp.
Common apple moss – *Bartramia pomiformis*
Common beard moss – *Barbula unguiculata*
Common cord moss – *Funaria hygrometrica*
Common cotton moss – *Plagiothecium undulatum*
Common feather moss – *Kindbergia praelonga*
Common haircap moss – *Polytrichum commune*
Common hairy-lantern moss – *Rhizomnium punctatum*
Common longevity moss – *Climacium dendroides*
Common octoblepharum moss – *Octoblepharum albidum*
Common striated feather moss – *Eurhynchium striatum*
Common watermoss – *Fontinalis dalecarlica*
Contorted pogonatum moss – *Pogonatum contortum*
Copper moss – *Mielichhoferia mielichhoferiana, M. elongata*
Cord glade moss – *Entodon seductrix*
Cotton mosses – *Plagiothecium* spp.
Cow hair moss – *Ditrichum pallidum*
Cowhorn moss – *Cratoneuron filicinum*
Cowhorn mosses – *Cratoneuron* spp.
Crawling feather moss – *Amblystegium serpens*
Creeping feather moss – *Amblystegium serpens*
Crisped fork moss – *Dicranum bonjeanii*
Crisped neckera moss – *Exsertotheca crispa*
Crispleaf rough moss – *Claopodium crispifolium*
Crispmosses – *Tortella* spp.
Crooked stork – *Campylopus*
Crowned thread moss – *Gemmabryum coronatum*
Crumpled-leaf moss – *Rhytidium rugosum*
Cucumber-scented moss – *Entodon plicatus*
Curled moss – *Palustriella falcata*
Curly hypnum moss – *Stereodon subimponens*
Cushion moss – *Dicranum groenlandicum, Leucobryum* sp.
Cypress-leaved plaitmoss – *Calohypnum cupressiforme*
Dalton's moss – *Daltonia splachnoides*
Delicate fern moss – *Thuidium delicatulum*
Delicate tamarisk moss – *Thuidium delicatulum*
Dense comb moss – *Ctenidium condensatum*
Dense crispmoss – *Tortella densa*
Dense rock moss – *Niphotrichum ericoides*
Dented hydnum moss – *Plagiothecium denticulatum*
Dented mosses – *Plagiothecium* spp.
Dented silk moss – *Plagiothecium denticulatum*
Dog tooth moss – *Cynodontium laxifolia*
Dotted thyme moss – *Rhizomnium punctatum*
Douglas neckera – *Neckera douglasii*

Dragon's gold – *Schistostega pennata*
Dreadlock moss – *Hedwigia ciliata*
Drowned kittens – *Sphagnum palustre*
Dull starry feather moss – *Campylium protensum*
Dusky hoarmoss – *Hedwigia ciliata*
Dwarf larch moss – *Octoblepharum albidum*
Dwarf neckera – *Neckera pumila*
Earthmosses – *Physcomitrium* spp.
Eastern weft moss – *Thuidium cymbifolium*
Elbow-shaped thread moss – *Rosulabryum perlimbatum*
Electric eels moss – *Dicranum polysetum*
Electrified cat's tail moss – *Hylocomiadelphus triquetrus*
Elegant feather moss – *Eurhynchium pulchellum*
Fan moss – *Rhizomnium glabrescens*
Feather-branched watermoss – *Fontinalis hypnoides*
Feather moss – *Amblystegium* spp., *Brachytheciastrum* spp., *Brachythecium* spp., *Calohypnum cupressiforme, Campylium* spp., *Eurhynchium* spp., *Homalia* spp., *Homalothecium* spp., *Hygroamblystegium* spp., *Hylocomium* spp., *Hyophila* spp., *Hypnum* spp., *Isothecium* spp., *Lembophyllum* spp., *Leskea* spp., *Kindbergia* spp., *Neckera* spp., *Oxyrrhynchium* spp., *Rhynchostegium* spp.
Fern feather – *Cratoneuron filicinum*
Fern-leaved hook moss – *Cratoneuron filicinum*
Fern mosses – *Fissidens* spp.
Fire moss – *Ceratodon purpureus, Funaria hygrometrica*
Fir moss – *Abietinella abietina*
Fireproof spring moss – *Fontinalis antipyretica*
Fishhook moss – *Campylopus*
Five-pointed leaf little feather moss – *Haplocladium microphyllum*
Flabby thread moss – *Rosulabryum moravicum*
Flat fork moss – *Fissidens dubius*
Flat glaze moss – *Entodon cladorrhizans*
Flat neckera moss – *Alleniella complanata*
Flat-topped bogmoss – *Sphagnum fallax*
Footstool moss – *Dicranum scoparium*
Fork mosses – *Orthodicranium, Dicranum* spp.
Fountain apple moss – *Philonotis fontana*
Fountain feather moss – *Hygroamblystegium tenax*
Fountain lattice moss – *Cinclidotus fontinaloides*
Foxtail feather moss – *Thamnobryum alopecurum*
Fragile fork moss – *Dicranum tauricum*
Fringed bogmoss – *Sphagnum fimbriatum*
Fringed hoarmoss – *Hedwigia ciliata*
Fringe moss – *Niphotrichum canescens*
Fringe mosses – *Racomitrium* spp.
Frizzled crispmoss – *Tortella tortuosa*
Frizzled screwmoss – *Tortella tortuosa*
Furry thuidium – *Thuidiopsis furfurosa*
Giant bryum – *Rhodobryum giganteum*
Giant green moss – *Dicranum majus*
Giant moss – *Dawsonia superba*
Giant rose moss – *Rhodobryum giganteum*
Giant royal moss – *Dawsonia superba*
Glasswort hydnum moss – *Pseudoscleropodium purum*
Glistering feather moss – *Alleniella complanata*
Glistering shrub moss – *Climacium dendroides*
Glittering wood moss – *Hylocomium splendens*
Goblin's gold – *Schistostega pennata*
Golden bulbed moss – *Funaria hygrometrica*
Golden fern moss – *Cratoneuron filicinum*
Golden oreas moss – *Oreas martiana*
Golden thread moss – *Leptobryum pyriforme*
Gold hair moss – *Ditrichum pallidum*
Gold mosses – *Schistostega* spp.
Gold thread moss – *Ditrichum pallidum*
Gooseneck mosses – *Rhytidiadelphus* spp.
Greater forked moss – *Dicranum majus*
Great hairy screwmoss – *Syntrichia ruralis*
Great yew moss – *Fissidens adianthoides*
Green-leaved plant moss – *Calohypnum plumiforme*
Green rose moss – *Rhodobryum* spp.
Green-tufted stubble moss – *Weissia controversa*

Grey cushion moss – *Grimmia pulvinata*
Grimmia mosses – *Schistidium* spp.
Ground mosses – *Hyophila* spp.
Ground pine moss – *Climacium*
Hair grass moss – *Cirriphyllum piliferum*
Hair mosses – *Ditrichum* spp.
Hairy moss – *Trichosteleum* spp.
Hair-pointed feather moss – *Cirriphyllum piliferum*
Haircap moss – *Polytrichum commune*
Hairy cap moss – *Polytrichum commune*
Haldane's moss – *Callicladium haldaneanum*
Handbell moss – *Gemmabryum caespiticium*
Hanging moss – *Antitrichia curtipendula*
Hart's tongue – *Plagiomnium undulatum*
Hedwig's fringe leaf moss – *Hedwigia ciliata*
Hercynian haircap – *Oligotrichum hercynicum*
Hercynian haircap moss – *Oligotrichum hercynicum*
Hidden capsule moss – *Cryphaea* spp.
Hoarmosses – *Hedwigia* spp.
Hoary fringe moss – *Niphotrichum canescens*
Hoary rock moss – *Racomitrium lanuginosum*
Hoary tile moss – *Grimmia pulvinata*
Hokkaido ball moss – *Plagiothecium* spp.
Hook beak tufa moss – *Hymenostylium recurvirostrum*
Hooked moss – *Leucobryum aduncum*
Hookmosses – *Palustriella* spp.
Horn calcareous moss – *Mnium hornum*
Impossible moss – *Takakia sp.*
Incurved hair moss – *Oligotrichum hercynicum*
Irish daltonia – *Daltonia splachnoides*
Isopterygium moss – *Isopterygium* spp.
Joint-toothed moss – *Distichophyllum* spp., *Hydrogonium* spp., *Lembophyllum* spp.
Juicy Lucy – *Pseudoscleropodium purum*
Juniper haircap moss – *Polytrichum juniperinum*
Kidney-leaved liverwort – *Acrobolbus* sp.
Knapwort – *Leptodictyum riparium*
Kneiff's feather moss – *Leptodictyum riparium*
Knight's plume moss – *Ptilium crista-castrensis*
Large-leafed pocket moss – *Fissidens grandifrons*
Large-leafed red peat moss – *Sphagnum magellanicum*
Large-leaf moss – *Pogonatum cirratum*
Large leaf moss – *Rhizomnium glabrescens*
Large mousetail moss – *Isothecium alopecuroides*
Large white moss – *Leucobryum glaucum*
Lateral cryphaea – *Cryphaea* spp.
Lateral daltonia – *Cryphaea* spp.
Lawn moss – *Orthodicranium*
Lesser bird's claw beard moss – *Barbula convulata*
Lesser striated feather moss – *Plasteurhynchium striatulum*
Lipstick thyme moss – *Mnium hornum*
Little shaggy moss – *Rhytidiadelphus loreus*
Log moss – *Hypnum imponens, Thuidium delicatulum*
Long-beaked thyme moss – *Plagiomnium rostratum*
Long-beaked water feather moss – *Rhynchostegium riparioides*
Long-forked moss – *Dicranum elongatum*
Long leaf fork moss – *Paraleucobryum longifolium*
Long-necked bryum – *Leptobryum pyriforme*
Long smooth cap moss – *Atrichum androgynum*
Long tail moss – *Anomodon viticulosus*
Loose-leaved fork moss – *Cynodontium laxifolia*
Luminescent moss – *Schistostega pennata*
Lustrous moss – *Sphagnum subnitens*
Magellanic bogmoss – *Schistostega pennata*
Magellan's peatmoss – *Sphagnum magellanicum*
Magnificent moss – *Plagiomnium ellipticum*
Maidenhair pocket moss – *Fissidens adianthoides*
Many-flowered leskea – *Pylaisia polyantha*
Many-fruited leskea – *Leskea polycarpa*
Many-fruited thread moss – *Plagiomnium ciliare*
Many-fruited thyme moss – *Plagiomnium affine*
Marsh bryum – *Rosulabryum perlimbatum*
Marsh feather moss – *Leskea polycarpa*
Marsh fern moss – *Fissidens adianthoides*
Marsh fork moss – *Dicranum bonjeanii*
Marsh thyme moss – *Plagiomnium ellipticum*

Matted bryum – *Bryum caespiticium*
Medussa moss – *Hedwigia ciliata*
Menzies' tree moss – *Leucolepis acanthoneuron*
Missionary moss – *Octoblepharum albidum*
Montana grimmia – *Grimmia montana*
Mood moss – *Dicranum scoparium*
Mossy rock moss – *Niphotrichum canescens*
Mountain fern moss – *Hylocomium splendens*
Mountain groove moss – *Aulacomnium turgidum*
Mountain haircap moss – *Polytrichum pallidisetum*
Mouse ear cress – *Weymouthia cochlearifolia*
Mousetail mosses – *Isothecium* spp.
Natural sheet moss – *Hypnum imponens*
Neat feather moss – *Pseudoscleropodium purum*
Neckera moss – *Exsertotheca crispa*
Neckera mosses – *Neckera*
Nerved leskea moss – *Pseudoleskeella nervosa*
Net tooth moss – *Cinclidotus*
Nipplewort – *Papillaria crocea*
Noble moss – *Spiridens* spp.
Nodding thread moss – *Pohlia nutans*
Notch leaf moss – *Paraleucobryum longifolium*
Nowell's limestone moss – *Zygodon gracilis*
Nuttall's homalothecium moss – *Homalothecium nuttallii*
Octoblepharum moss – *Octoblepharum albidum*
Odd-sided dalton – *Cryphaea* spp.
Oeder's apple moss – *Plagiopus oederianus*
Ohio archidium moss – *Archidium ohioense*
Ohio haircap moss – *Polytrichum ohioense*
Old rock moss – *Hedwigia ciliata*
Ostrich moss – *Grimmia pulvinata*
Ostrich-plume feather moss – *Ptilium crista-castrensis*
Pale bogmoss – *Sphagnum nemoreum*
Pale-leaved thread moss – *Brachythecium albicans*
Palmer's astrella – *Astrella palmeri*
Palm moss – *Climacium dendroides*
Pastle amarillo – *Dendropogonella rufescens*
Peat mosses – *Sphagnum* spp.
Pendulous barbella moss – *Neodicladiella pendula*
Pendulous wing-moss – *Antitrichia curtipendula*
Petticoat moss – *Splachnum* spp.
Philibert's tamarisk moss – *Thuidium assimile*
Phoenix moss – *Fissidens nobilis*
Pigtail moss – *Weissia controversa*
Pillow moss – *Hypnum cupressiforme*
Pincushion moss – *Leptostomum inclinans, Leucobryum sp.*
Pine-branched moss – *Abietinella abietina*
Pink sphagnum – *Sphagnum divinum*
Pipe-cleaner moss – *Ptychomnion aciculare*
Plume-leaved bogmoss – *Sphagnum subnitens*
Plume moss – *Fissidens adianthoides, F. dubius*
Pocket moss – *Fissidens dubius*
Pocket mosses – *Fissidens* spp.
Pointed spear moss – *Calliergonella cuspidata*
Pointless screwmoss – *Tortula inermis*
Poodle moss – *Pseudanomodon attenuatus*
Pott moss – *Hyophila* spp.
Predictor moss – *Funaria hygrometrica*
Prostate signal moss – *Sematophyllum demissum*
Pulvinate dry rock moss – *Grimmia pulvinata*
Purple fork moss – *Ceratodon purpureus*
Purple horn toothed moss – *Ceratodon purpureus*
Purple rhacocarpus moss – *Rhacocarpus* spp.
Purple-stalked pocket moss – *Fissidens osmundoides*
Puzzling moss – *Takakia* sp.
Queen Catherine's moss – *Atrichum undulatum*
Raincoat moss – *Macromitrium* spp.
Rain moss – *Hyophila* spp.
Rambling tail-moss – *Anomodon viticulosus*
Red beard moss – *Bryoerythrophyllum rubrum*
Red branch moss – *Braunia secunda*
Red parasol – *Splachnum rubrum, S. luteum*
Red penny moss – *Rhizomnium punctatum*
Red roof moss – *Ceratodon purpureus*
Red-shafted hood moss – *Orthotrichum anomalum*
Red shank moss – *Ceratodon purpureus*
Red sphagnum – *Sphagnum magellanicum*
Red-stemmed feather moss – *Pleurozium schreberi*

Red-stem moss – *Pleurozium schreberi*
Red stem moss – *Ptychomnion aciculare*
Ribbed bogmoss – *Aulacomnium palustre*
Rigid bogmoss – *Sphagnum teres*
River mosses – *Philonotis* spp.
Rock bristle moss – *Lewinskya rupestris*
Rock moss – *Niphotrichum canescens*
Rock mosses – *Racomitrium* spp., *Andreaea* spp.
Rolled-leaf wet ground moss – *Hyophila involuta*
Rooftop moss – *Rosulabryum capillare*
Rose moss – *Rhodobryum* sp.
Rose peat moss – *Sphagnum palustre*
Rosy thyme tread moss – *Rhodobryum* sp.
Rough foxtail moss – *Brachythecium rutabulum*
Rough gooseneck moss – *Hylocomiadelphus triquetrus*
Rough moss – *Claopodium crispifolium*
Rough rockmoss – *Andreaea rupestris*
Rough-stalked feather moss – *Brachythecium rutabulum, Brachytheciastrum rutabulum*
Rough-stalked ragged moss – *Brachytheciastrum rutabulum, Brachythecium rutabulum*
Round-stemmed entodon moss – *Entodon seductrix*
Rugose fork moss – *Dicranum polysetum*
Rusty peat moss – *Sphagnum palustre*
Saber-tooth moss – *Plagiomnium ciliare*
Sandhill screwmoss – *Syntrichia ruralis*
Scale leaf moss – *Taxiphyllum taxirameum*
Scarce hedgehog moss – *Grimmia anodon*
Schofield's ctenidium moss – *Ctenidium schofieldii*
Schreber's big red moss – *Pleurozium schreberi*
Screw bryum – *Rosulabryum capillare*
Screw moss – *Cinclidotus* spp.
Screwmosses – *Syntrichia* spp., *Tortula* spp.
Seaside grimmia – *Schistidium maritimum*
Seductive entodon moss – *Entodon seductrix*
Seventy-mile-an-hour moss – *Ceratodon purpureus*
Shaggy mosses – *Rhytidiadelphus* spp.
Shaguma moss – *Cratoneuron* spp.
Sharp-leaved moss – *Plagiomnium acutum*
Sheaf-leaved screwmoss – *Barbula convulata*
Sheet moss – *Thuidium delicatulum*
Shiny sexy moss – *Entodon seductrix*
Showy bristle moss – *Lewinskya speciosum*
Sickle-leaved hook moss – *Sanionia uncinata*
Side-fruited crispmoss –*Tortella squarrosa*
Sidewalk moss – *Bryum caespiticium*
Signal mosses – *Sematophyllum* spp.
Silk moss – *Entodon* spp.
Silk wood moss – *Polytrichum commune*
Silky flatbergium – *Flatbergium* spp.
Silky forklet moss – *Dicranella heteromalla*
Silky wall feather moss – *Camptothecium* sp.
Silver bryum – *Bryum argenteum*
Skull moss – *Tetraplodon mnioides*
Slender comb moss – *Ctenidium fastigiatum*
Slender cruet – *Tetraplodon mnioides*
Slender green feather moss – *Hamatocaulis vernicosus*
Slender tail moss – *Pseudanomodon attenuatus*
Slender yoke moss – *Zygodon gracilis*
Small capsule dung moss – *Splachnum ampullaceum*
Small cord moss – *Funaria microstoma*
Smaller lattice moss – *Cinclidotus fontinaloides*
Smaller white moss – *Leucobryum juniperoideum*
Small-mouth moss – *Pogonatum microstomum*
Small sekra moss – *Cinclidotus fontinaloides*
Small spine moss – *Pogonatum spinulosum*
Small squarrose peat moss – *Sphagnum teres*
Smoky feather moss – *Homalothecium lutescens*
Smooth cap moss – *Atrichum* spp.
Smooth stalk feather moss – *Brachythecium salebrosum*
Spiked white moss – *Leucobryum aduncum*
Spike mosses – *Pogonatum* spp.
Spiky bogmoss – *Sphagnum squarrosum*
Spiral extinguisher moss – *Encalypta streptocarpa*
Spiral web tooth – *Rosulabryum capillare*
Splendid feather moss – *Hylocomium splendens*
Sponge gourd moss – *Pohlia nutans*
Spoon moss – *Bryoandersonia illecebra*

Spreading earthmoss – *Physcomitrium patens*
Spreading-leaved earthmoss – *Physcomitrium patens*
Spring bartram moss – *Philonotis fontana*
Springy turf moss – *Rhytidiadelphus squarrosus*
Spruce tree feather moss – *Abietinella abietina*
Square gooseneck moss – *Rhytidiadelphus squarrosus*
Squirrel-tail moss – *Leucodon sciuroides*
Staircase moss – *Climacium* spp.
Stair-step moss – *Hylocomium splendens*
Starburst moss – *Atrichum undulatum*
Star moss – *Syntrichia ruralis*
Starry thyme moss – *Mnium stellare*
Steel ring moss – *Schistidium maritimum*
Straight-leaved apple moss – *Bartramia ithyphylla*
Stream moss – *Mnium marginatum*
Streamside leptodictyum moss – *Leptodictyum riparium*
Sturm's bristle moss – *Orthotrichum rupestre*
Summer screwmoss – *Tortula muralis*
Surveyor's moss – *Plagiomnium undulatum*
Swamp feather moss – *Hygroamblystegium tenax*
Swamp mosses – *Philonotis* spp.
Swan moss – *Campylopus*
Swan's neck thyme moss – *Mnium hornum*
Swelling thread moss – *Aulacomnium palustre*
Swollen moss – *Aulacomnium turgidum*
Syed's thread moss – *Rosulabryum moravicum*
Tail mosses – *Anomodon* spp., *Dicranum* spp.
Tall clustered thread moss – *Ptychostomum pallescens*
Tamarisk moss – *Thuidium tamariscinum*
Thick point grimmia – *Schistidium crassipilum*
Thin-rib curved tailmoss – *Dicranum bonjeanii*
Thin-teethed moss – *Leptodontium vitculosoides*
Thread cedar moss – *Cryphaea* spp.
Thread moss – *Anomodon* spp., *Aulacomnium palustre, Bryum* spp., *Imbribryum* spp., *Plagiomnium* spp.
Thyme leaf moss – *Rhizomnium punctatum*
Thyme moss – *Plagiomnium undulatum*
Thyme mosses – *Mnion* spp., *Plagiomnium* spp., *Rhizomnium* spp.
Tiger tail moss – *Hedwigia ciliata*
Tiny-leaved haplocladium moss – *Haplocladium microphyllum*
Tongue-leaf copper moss – *Merceyopsis cataractae*
Toothless grimmia moss – *Grimmia anodon*
Toothpick moss – *Entodon seductrix*
Tooth within moss – *Entodon*
Tousled treasure moss – *Callicladium haldaneanum*
Tree beard – *Dendropogonella rufescen*
Tree climacium moss – *Climacium dendroides*
Tree ruffle liverwort – *Porella navicularis*
Tree-shaped feather moss – *Climacium dendroides*
Tree-skirt moss – *Pseudanomodon attenuatus*
Triangular bryum – *Rosulabryum perlimbatum*
Tufa moss – *Cratoneuron* spp.
Tufted bryum moss – *Gemmabryum caespiticium*
Tufted thread moss – *Bryum caespiticium*
Turgid thread moss – *Aulacomnium turgidum*
Twin-stalked fork moss – *Ceratodon purpureus*
Twisted cord moss – *Funaria hygrometrica*
Twisted moss – *Syntrichia ruralis*
Twisted teeth beard moss – *Barbula indica*
Twisting thread moss – *Rosulabryum capillare*
Two-colored beardless moss – *Anoectangium thomsoni*
Two hair moss – *Ditrichum pallidum*
Umbrella moss – *Macromitrium* spp., *Rhodobryum giganteum*
Undulated hair moss – *Atrichum undulatum*
Undulating Catharinea – *Atrichum undulatum*
Urn haircap moss – *Pogonatum urnigerum*
Urn mosses – *Physcomitrium* spp.
Varnished hook moss – *Hamatocaulis vernicosus*
Velvet feather moss – *Brachytheciastrum velutinum*
Velvet tree apron – *Claopodium rostratum*
Vinous comb moss – *Ctenidium robustum*

Water measuring cord moss – *Funaria hygrometrica*
Water moss – *Hyophila* spp.
Wavy dicranum – *Dicranum polysetum*
Wavy-leaf curved-tail moss – *Dicranum polysetum*
Wet ground moss – *Hyophila* spp.
White moss – *Octoblepharum albidum*
White mosses – *Leucobryum* spp., *Octoblepharum* spp.
White-tipped bristle moss – *Orthotrichum diaphanum*
White-tipped moss – *Hedwigia ciliata*
White-toothed peat moss – *Sphagnum girgensohnii*
Whitish feather moss – *Brachythecium albicans*
Whorled tufa moss – *Eucladium verticillatum*
Wood comb moss – *Ctenidium sylvaticum*
Woodsy thyme moss – *Plagiomnium cuspidatum*
Woolly fringe moss – *Racomitrium lanuginosum*
Worm moss – *Bryoandersonia illecebra*
Wrinkle-leaved feather moss – *Rhytidium rugosum*
Yellow curtains – *Dendropogonella rufescen*
Yellow feather moss – *Brachythecium salebrosum*
Yellow moosedung moss – *Splachnum luteum*
Yellow moss – *Dendropogonella rufescen*
Yellow mushroom moss – *Splachnum rubrum, S. luteum*
Yellow starry feather moss – *Campylium stellatum*
Yellow yarn – *Claopodium rostratum*
Yoke mosses – *Zygodon* spp.

Liverworts

Acid frillwort – *Fossombronia wondraczekii*
Alaska liverwort – *Fossombronia alaskana*
Alpine rushwort – *Gymnomitrion alpinum*
Arctic liverwort – *Fossombronia alaskana*
Autumn flapwort – *Syzygiella autumnalis*
Bent round scalewort – *Porella chilensis*
Bent scissorleaf prongwort – *Herbertus aduncus*
Bifid crestwort – *Lophocolea bidentata*
Bitter scalewort – *Porella arboris-vitae*
Brazilian scalewort – *Frullania brasiliensis*
Brown radula – *Dactyloradula brunnea*
Carinthian earwort – *Scapania carinthiaca*
Cheap frillwort – *Fossombronia pusilla*
Chequerwort – *Corsinia coriandrina*
Ciliated fringewort – *Ptilidium ciliare*
Ciliate earwort – *Scapania ciliata*
Cliff waxwort – *Plagiochasma rupestre*
Comb liverwort – *Riccardia multifida*
Common fold-leaf liverwort – *Diplophyllum albicans*
Common kettlewort – *Blasia pusilla*
Common liverwort – *Marchantia polymorpha*
Common mushroom-headed liverwort – *Conocephalum conicum*
Common scissorleaf prongwort – *Herbertus aduncus*
Common snakeskin liverwort – *Conocephalum conicum*
Cordate flapwort – *Jungermannia exsertifolia*
Cowlworts – *Colura* spp.
Craven featherwort – *Pedinophyllum interruptum*
Creeping fingerwort – *Lepidozia reptans*
Crescent cup liverwort – *Lunularia cruciata*
Crestworts – *Heteroscyphus* spp., *Lophocolea* spp.
Crossed-stemmed liverwort – *Chiastocaulon* spp.
Cup liverwort – *Gottschelia* spp.
Cylindrical-leaved liverwort – *Cylindrocolea* spp.
Dangling face liverwort – *Balantiopsis* spp.
Deceptive liverwort – *Gackstroemia* spp.
Dense leaf scalewort – *Porella densifolia*
Dilated scalewort – *Frullania dilatata*
Down liverwort – *Trichocoleopsis* spp.
Dumortier's liverwort – *Dumortiera hirsuta*
Earworts – *Scapania* spp.
Elegant scalewort – *Porella elegantula*
Endive pellia – *Apopellia endiviifolia, Pellia endiviifolia*
Fan liverwort – *Hymenophyton sp.*
Featherworts – *Plagiochila* spp.
Fingerworts – *Lepidozia* spp.
Flapworts – *Nardia* spp.

Flattened radula – *Radula complanata*
Floating crystalwort – *Riccia fluitans*
Flotow's ruffwort – *Moerckia flotoviana*
Flush notchwort – *Saccobasis polita*
Forked veilwort – *Metzgeria furcata*
Fossickwort – *Aneura mirabilis*
Fragrant macewort – *Mannia fragrans*
Frillwort – *Fossombronia pusilla*
Frillworts – *Fossombronia* spp.
Fringed heartwort – *Ricciocarpos natans*
Fringeworts – *Ptilidium* spp.
Ghostwort – *Aneura mirabilis*
Glaucous crystalwort – *Riccia glauca*
Gray hard-scale liverwort – *Mylia taylorii*
Great featherwort – *Plagiochila asplenioides*
Great-scented liverwort – *Conocephalum conicum*
Greater pawwort – *Barbilophozia lycopodioides*
Greater whipwort – *Aneura mirabilis*
Grove earwort – *Scapania nemorea*
Hairy threadwort – *Blepharostoma trichophyllum*
Handsome woollywort – *Trichocolea tomentella*
Hanging millipede liverwort – *Frullania nisquallensis*
Heath earwort – *Scapania irrigua*
Hemispheric liverwort – *Reboulia hemisphaerica*
Hooked frullania – *Frullania hamatiloba*
Inflated notchwort – *Gymnocolea inflata*
Inverted cone scalewort – *Radula obconica*
Irish ruffwort – *Moerckia hibernica*
Jagged germanderwort – *Riccardia chamedryfolia*
Jameson's liverwort – *Syzygiella autumnalis*
Java pennywort – *Jackiella* spp.
Juniper prongwort – *Herbertus aduncus*
Juniper scissorleaf – *Herbertus juniperoideus*
Kidney-leaved liverwort – *Acrobolbus* spp.
Killarney featherwort – *Plagiochila bifaria*
Leafy liverwort – *Frullania ericoides*
Lesser featherwort – *Plagiochila porelloides*
Lesser rough earwort – *Scapania aequiloba*
Lesser whipwort – *Bazzania tricrenata*
Lindenberg's featherwort – *Adelanthus lindenbergianus*
Lindenberg's scalewort – *Radula lindenbergiana*
Little hands liverwort – *Lepidozia reptans*
Long-leaved flapwort – *Liochlaena lanceolata*
Lung liverwort – *Marchantia polymorpha*
Lyon's notchwort – *Tritomaria quinquedentate*
MacKay's pouncewort – *Marchesinia mackaii*
Marsh earwort – *Syzygiella* spp.
Marsh flapwort – *Syzygiella* spp.
Most beautiful fringewort – *Ptilidium pulcherrimum*
Mountain liverwort – *Marchantia polymorpha*
Naked liverwort – *Mylia nuda*
Narrow mushroom-headed liverwort – *Mannia androgyna*
Naugehyde liverworts – *Ptilidium* spp.
New York scalewort – *Frullania squarrosa*
Northern naugehyde liverwort – *Ptilidium ciliare*
Northern prongwort – *Herbertus borealis*
Notched pouchwort – *Calypogeia arguta*
Notched rushwort – *Marsupella emarginata*
Notchworts – *Tritomaria* spp.
One sided pocketwort - *Paraschistochila* spp.
Orkney notchwort – *Anastrepta orcadensis*
Orobus-seed liverwort – *Targionia hypophylla*
Orobus-seed liverwort – *Targionia hypophylla*
Overleaf pellia – *Pellia epiphylla*
Pacific fuzzwort – *Ptilidium californicum*
Pale liverwort – *Chiloscyphus polyanthos*
Pale scalewort – *Frullania monocera*
Palmate germanderwort – *Riccardia palmata*
Peculiar featherwort – *Plagiochila peculiaris*
Pellias – *Pellia* spp.
Plumier's ducks foot – *Marchantia chenopoda*
Pocketwort – *Schistochila* spp.
Pouncewort – *Drepanolejeunea* spp.
Prongworts – *Herbertus* spp.
Questionable veilwort – *Pallavicinia ambigua*
Radula liverworts – *Radula* spp.
Ribbonwort – *Pallavicinia lyellii*

River startip liverwort – *Scapania undulata*
Rock veilwort – *Metzgeria conjugata*
Rose moss – *Notoscyphus lutescens*
Rough earwort – *Scapania aspera*
Ruffworts – *Moerckia* spp.
Rufous scalewort – *Frullania falciloba*
Rushworts – *Marsupella* spp.
Scalewort – *Porella cordaeana*
Scaleworts – *Porella* spp., *Radula* spp.
Shield liverwort – *Cheilolejeunea* spp.
Shiny film liverwort – *Hymenophyton flabellatum*
Small greasewort – *Aneura pinguis*
Small-leaved liverwort – *Leptolejeunea* spp.
Small mushroom-headed liverwort – *Reboulia hemisphaerica*
Snake liverwort – *Conocephalum conicum*
Spoonwort – *Pleurozia* spp.
Square-leaved crestwort – *Chiloscyphus polyanthos*
Squarrose scalewort – *Frullania squarrosula*
St. Winifred's moss liverwort – *Chiloscyphus polyanthos*
Star-headed liverwort – *Marchantia polymorpha*
Starwort – *Asterella wallichiani*
Straggling pouchwort – *Saccogyna viticulosa*
Strapped earwort – *Scapania stephanii*
Tahitian liverwort – *Cyathodium foetidissimum*
Tamarisk scalewort – *Frullania tamarisci*
Taylor's flapwort – *Mylia taylorii*
Taylor's scale sedge – *Lepidolaena taylorii*
Tetragon flapwort – *Solenostoma tetragonum*
Threadworts – *Cephaloziella* spp.
Three-lobed bazzania – *Bazzania trilobata*
Toothed liverwort – *Symphyogyna* spp.
Toothed ribbonwort – *Symphyogyna* spp.
Tourmentine mâle – *Chiloscyphus polyanthos*
Tree fringewort – *Ptilidium pulcherrimum*
Tree ruffle liverwort – *Porella navicularis*
Tri-tip leafy liverwort – *Lophozia ventricosa*
Tumid notchwort – *Lophozia ventricosa*
Two-lobed flapwort – *Nardia insecta*
Umbrella liverwort – *Marchantia polymorpha*
Variable-leaved crestwort – *Lophocolea heterophylla*
Veilwort – *Pallavicinia lyellii*
Veilworts – *Metzgeria* spp.
Viking prongwort – *Herbertus borealis*
Wall scalewort – *Porella platyphylla*
Warty earwort – *Scapania verrucosa*
Water earwort – *Scapania undulata*
Water rushwort – *Marsupella aquatica*
Wax liverwort – *Plagiochasma* spp.
Waxwort – *Plagiochasma* spp.
Wedge flapwort – *Leptoscyphus* spp.
Western naugahyde liverwort – *Ptilidium pulcherrimum*
Whipworts – *Bazzania* spp.
Whip bearing tree liverwort – *Dendromastigophora* spp.
White earwort – *Diplophyllum albicans*
White frostwort – *Gymnomitrion obtusum*
Wood's whipwort – *Mastigophora* spp.
Woolly worm liverwort – *Trichocolea mollissima*
Yellow pouncewort – *Lejeunea flava*

Hornworts

Big hornwort – *Megaceros* spp.
Camphor spurflower – *Plectranthus cylindraceus*
Coon tail – *Ceratophyllum demersum*
Dotted hornwort – *Anthoceros punctatus*
Erect hornwort – *Phaeoceros erectus*
Field hornwort – *Anthoceros agrestis*
Hornwort – *Leiosporoceros*
Hornworts – *Anthoceros* spp.
Rigid hornwort – *Ceratophyllum demersum*
Smooth hornwort – *Phaeoceros laevis*

Resources

ORGANIZATIONS

British Bryological Society new and entertaining finds and stories.

Bryophyte Ecology (five-volume ebook from Michigan Technological University)—excellent resource by Glime; one of the most complete online surveys of mosses with great pictures and citations.

Consortium of Bryophyte Herbaria (Bryophyte Portal website)—thorough and up to date.

Flora of North America—volume 27 is a thorough taxonomic guide.

International Association of Bryologists—professional organization established in 1969.

Mountain Moss (an online resource for moss gardening)—Annie Martin is a recognized moss expert and supplier of moss species.

ESSENCE COMPANIES

Alaskan Essences

First Light Flower Essence of New Zealand

LightBringer Essences

Self Heal Distributing

Yorkshire and Bailey Flower Essences

BOOKS AND FILMS

Bryophytes: The Secret Plants That Surround Us (documentary, 2011)

The Magical World of Moss (documentary available online, 2023)

Mosses Liverworts & Hornworts of the World (book by J. Wilbraham, 2025—a great addition to bryophyte knowledge)

Na Caonaigh, Nowness (video by Orlando FitzGerald, available online, 2020)

Super Moss (video by Bruno Victor-Pujebet, Zadig Productions, available online, 2021)

References

Aasim, M., S. A. Ali, S. Aydin, A. Bakhsh et al. 2023. "Artificial Intelligence-Based Approaches to Evaluate and Optimize Phytoremediation Potential of in vitro Regenerated Aquatic Macrophyte *Ceratophyllum demersum L.*" *Environmental Science and Pollution Research International* 30 (14): 40206–17.

Abay, G., M. Altun, O. C. Karakoc, F. Güll et al. 2013. "Insecticidal Activity of Fatty Acid-rich Turkish Bryophyte Extracts against *Sitophilus granarius* (Coleoptera: Curculionidae)." *Combinatorial Chemistry & High Throughput Screening* 16 (10): 806–16.

Abay, G., M. Altun, S. Koldas, A. R. Tüfekci et al. 2015. "Determination of Antiproliferative Activities of Volatile Contents and HPLC Profiles of *Dicranum scoparium* (Dicranaceae, Bryophyta)." *Combinatorial Chemistry & High Throughput Screening* 18 (5): 453–63.

Abdel-Shafi, S., Y. Hussein, G. A. Sabaa, A. S. Abdel-Monaem. 2017. "An Evaluation of the Antibacterial and Antiviral Activities of Some Bryophytes." *Egyptian Journal of Microbiology* 1 (1): 63–86.

Abdullah, N., Y. Tamimi, S. Dobretsov et al. 2021. "Malformin-A1 (MA1) Sensitizes Chemoresistant Ovarian Cancer Cells to Cisplatin-Induced Apoptosis." *Molecules* 26 (12): 3624.

Adams, C. E., and K. E. Stevens. 2007. "Evidence for a Role of Nicotinic Acetylcholine Receptors in Schizophrenia." *Frontiers in Bioscience* 12: 4755–72.

Adio, A. M., and W. A. König. 2005. "Sesquiterpene Constituents from the Essential Oil of the Liverwort *Plagiochila asplenioides*." *Phytochemistry* 66 (5): 599–609.

Adio, A. M., C. Paul, P. Kloth, W. A. König. 2004. "Sesquiterpenes of the Liverwort *Scapania undulata*." *Phytochemistry* 65 (2): 199–206.

Adio, A. M., C. Paul, W. A. König, H. Muhle. 2003. "Volatile Constituents in the Liverwort *Tritomaria polita*." *Phytochemistry* 64 (2): 637–44.

Adio, A. M., C. Paul, W. A. König, H. Muhle. 2002. "Volatile Components from European Liverworts *Marsupella emarginata, M. aquatica* and *M. alpina*." *Phytochemistry* 61 (1): 79–91.

Adio, A. M., S. H. von Reuss, C. Paul, H. Muhle et al. 2007. "Sesquiterpenoid Constituents of the Liverwort *Marsupella aquatica*." *Tetrahedron: Asymmetry* 18 (10): 1245–53.

Adou, E., R. B. Williams, J. K. Schilling, S. Malone et al. 2005. "Cytoxic Diterpenoids from Two Lianas from the Suriname Rainforest." *Bioorganic and Medicinal Chemistry* 13 (21): 6009–14.

Agelet, A., and J. Valles. 2003. "Studies on Pharmaceutical Ethnobotany in the Region of Pallars (Pyrenees, Catalonia, Iberian Peninsula) Part II. New and Very Rare Uses of Previously Known Medicinal Plants." *Journal of Ethnopharmacology* 84: 211–27.

Ainge, G. D., P. J. Gerard, S. F. R. Hinkley, S. D. Lorimer et al. 2001. "Hodgsonox, a New Class of Sesquiterpene from the Liverwort *Lepidolaena hodgsoniae*. Isolation Directed by Insecticidal Activity." *Journal of Organic Chemistry* 66 (8): 2818–21.

Akatin, M. Y., M. E. Kemal, N. Batan. 2022. "Antimicrobial Activities of Some Bryophytes Collected from Trabzon, Türkiye and Preparation of Herbal Soap and Cream Using *Pellia epiphylla* Extract for the First Time." *Anatolian Bryology* 8 (1): 30–36.

Akiel, M. A., O. Y. Alshehri, S. A. Aljihani, A. Almuaysib et al. 2022. "Viridiflorol Induces Anti-Neoplastic Effects on Breast, Lung and Brain Cancer Cells Through Apoptosis." *Saudi Journal of Biological Sciences* 29 (2): 816–21.

Alam, A., S. C. Sharma, V. Sharma. 2012. "In Vitro Antifungal Efficacies of Aqueous Extract of *Targionia hypophylla* L. against the Growth of Some Pathogenic Fungi." *International Journal of Ayurvedic Medicine* 2: 229–33.

Alam, A., V. Sharma, K. K. Rawat, P. K. Verma. 2015. "Bryophytes—The Ignored Medicinal Plants." *Sikkim Manipal University Medical Journal* 2 (1): 299–316.

Alam, A, V. Sharma, S. Sharma, P. Kumari. 2012. "Antibacterial Activity of the Alcoholic Extracts of *Entodon nepalensis* Mizush. Against Some Pathogenic Bacteria." *Report and Opinion* 4 (10): 44–47.

Alatalo, J. M., A. K. Jägerbrand, M. B. Erfanian, S. Chen et al. 2020. "Bryophyte Cover and Richness Decline after 18 Years of Experimental Warming in Alpine Sweden." *AoB Plants* 12 (6).

Alcorn, J. B. 1984. *Huastec Mayan Ethnobotany*. Austin: University Texas Press.

Aleti, G., S. Lehner, M. Bacher, S. Compant et al. 2016. "Surfactin Variants Medicate Species-Specific Biofilm Formation and Root Colonization in Bacillus." *Environmental Microbiology* 18 (8): 2634–45.

Ali, T., M. Inagaki, H. B. Chai, T. Wieboldt et al. 2017. "Halogenated Compounds from Directed Fermentation of *Penicillium concentricum*, an Endophytic Fungus of the Liverwort *Trichocolea tomentella*." *Journal of Natural Products* 80 (5): 1397–1403.

Alijanpour, S., S. Jafaripour, Z. Ghasemzadeh, F. Khakpai, M. R. Zarrindast. 2021. "Harmaline Potentiates Morphine-Induced Antinociception via Affecting the Ventral Hippocampal GABA-A Receptors In Mice." *European Journal of Pharmacology* 893: 173806.

Allen, D. E. and G. Hatfield. 2004. *Medicinal Plants in Folk Tradition. An Ethnobotany of Britain & Ireland*. Portland, OR: Timber Press.

Althoff, F., L. Wegner, K. Ehlers, H. Buschmann et al. 2022. "Developmental Plasticity of the Amphibious Liverwort *Riccia fluitans*." *Frontiers in Plant Science* 13: 909327.

Altuner, E. M. 2008. "Bazi karayosunu türlerinin antimikrobiyal aktivitesinin belirlenmesi" Doctoral dissertation, Ankara Üniversitesi Fen Bilimleri Enstitüsü Biyoloji Anabilim Dalı.

Altuner, E. M., and B. Cetin. 2009. "Antimicrobial Activity of *Thuidium delicatulum* (Bryopsida) Extracts." *Kafkas Üniversitesi Fen Bilimleri Enstitüsü Dergisl* 2 (2): 85–92.

Altuner, E. M., K. Canli, A. Ilgaz. 2014. "Antimicrobial Screening of *Calliergonella cuspidate, Dicranum polysetum* and *Hypnum cupressiforme.*" *Journal of Pure and Applied Microbiology* 8 (1): 539–45.

Altuner, E. M., and B. Cetin. 2018. "Antimicrobial Activity of *Isothecium alopecuroides* and Potential Effect of Some Climate Elements on the Activity of This Bryophyte Sample." *Kastamonu University Journal of Forestry Faculty* 18 (2): 126–37.

Alves, R. J. M., T. G. Miranda, R. O. Pinheiro, W. B. de Souza Pinheiro et al. 2022. "Volatile Chemical Composition of *Octoblepharum albidum* Hedw. (Bryophyta) from the Brazilian Amazon." *BMC Chemistry* 16: 76.

Amina, M., P. Alam, M. K. Parvez, N. M. Al-Musayeib et al. 2018. "Isolation and Validated HPTLC Analysis of Four Cytotoxic Compounds, Including a New Sesquiterpene from Aerial Parts of *Plectranthus cylindraceus.*" *Natural Product Research* 32 (7): 804–9.

Anaya-Eugenio, G. D., T. Ali, L. H. Rakotondraibe, E. C. de Blanco. 2019. "Cytotoxic Constituents from *Penicillium concentricum*, an Endophytic Fungus from *Trichocolea tomentella.*" *Anticancer Drugs* 30 (4): 323–29.

Andersson, M. A., R. Mikkola, R. M. Kroppenstedt, F. A. Rainey et al. 1998. "The Mitochondrial Toxin Produced by *Streptomyces griseus* Strains Isolated from an Indoor Environment Is Valinomycin." *Applied and Environmental Microbiology* 64 (12): 4767–73.

Ando, H., and A Matsuo. 1984. *Applied Bryology. Advances in Bryology.* Hiroshima: Botanical Institute, Hiroshima University. Available online.

Anh, L. H., V. Q. Lam, A. Takami, T. D. Khanh et al. 2022. "Cytotoxic Mechanism of Momilactones A and B Against Acute Promyelocytic Leukemia and Multiple Myeloma Cell Lines." *Cancers* (Basel) 14 (19): 4848.

Antinori, S., M. Corbellino, L. Meroni, F. Resta et al. 2012. "*Aspergillus* meningitis: A Rare Clinical Manifestation of Central Nervous System Aspergillosis. Case Report And Review of 92 Cases." *Journal of Infection* 66 (3): 218–38.

Aponte, J. C., H. Yang, A. J. Vaisberg, D. Castillo et al. 2010. "Cytotoxic and Anti-Infective Sesquiterpenes Present in *Plagiochila disticha* (Plagiochilaceae) and *Ambrosia peruviana* (Asteraceae)." *Planta Medica* 76 (7): 705–7.

Araque, I., J. Ramírez, R. Vergara, J. Mella et al. 2023. "Cytotoxic Activity, Topoisomerase I Inhibition and In Silico Studies of New Sesquiterpene-aryl Ester Derivatives of (-) Drimenol." *Molecules* 28 (9): 3959.

Arias, H. R., D. Feuerbach, B. Schmidt, M. Heydenreich et al. 2018. "Drimane Sesquiterpenoids Noncompetitively Inhibit Human *a3ß4* Nicotinic Acetylcholine Receptors with Higher Potency Compared to Human *a*3ß4 and *a*7 Subtypes." *Journal of Natural Products* 81 (4): 811–17.

Aris, P., Y. L. Wei, M. Mohamadzadeh, X. H. Xia. 2022. "Griseofulvin: An Updated Overview of Old and Current Knowledge." *Molecules* 27 (20): 7034.

Ariyo, O. A., O. Shonubi, O. O. Oyesiku, A. O. Akande. 2011. "Antimicrobial Activity of the Indigenous Liverwort, *Ricca nigerica* Jones, from Southwestern Nigeria." *Evansia* 28: 43–48.

Aruna, K. B., and M. Krishnappa. 2018. "Phytochemistry and Antimicrobial Activities of *Pogonatum microstomum* (R. Br. Ex Schwagr.) Brid. (Bryophyta; Musci: Polytrichaceae)." *Phytochemistry* 3 (1): 120–25.

Asai, H., K. Kato, M. Suzuki, M. Takahashi et al. 2022. "Potential Anti-Allergic Effects of Bibenzyl Derivatives from Liverworts, *Radula perrottetii*." *Planta Medica* 88 (12): 1069–77.

Asakawa, Y. 1981. "Biologically Active Substances Obtained from Bryophytes." *The Journal of the Hattori Botanical Laboratory* 50: 123–42.

Asakawa, Y. 1982. "Chemical Constituents of the Hepaticae." In *Fortschritte der Chemie organischer Naturstoffe. Progress in the Chemistry of Organic Natural Products*, vol. 42, edited by W. Herz, H. Grisebach, and G. W. Kirby. Vienna: Springer.

Asakawa, Y. 1990. "Terpenoids and Aromatic Compounds with Pharmacological Activity from Bryophytes." In *Bryophtes: Their Chemistry and Chemical Taxonomy*, edited by H. D. Zinsmeister and R. Mues. New York: Oxford University Press.

Asakawa, Y. 1995a. "Chemical Constituents of the Bryophytes." In *Progress in the Chemistry of Organic Natural Products*, vol. 65, edited by W. Herz, W. B. Kirby, R. E. Moore, W. Steglich et al. Vienna: Springer.

Asakawa, Y. 1995b. "Polyphenols in Bryophytes: Structures, Biological Activities, and Bio- and Total Syntheses." *Recent Advances in Research on Polyphenols* 5: 36–66.

Askawa, Y. 1999. "Phytochemistry of Bryophytes: Biologically Active Terpenoids and Aromatic Compounds from Liverworts," in *Phytochemicals in Human Health Protections, Nutrition, and Plant Defense, Edition 33* edited by J. Romeo. New York: Kluwer Academic/Plenum Publishers.

Asakawa, Y. 2007. "Biological Active Compounds from Bryophytes." *Pure Applied Chemistry* 79 (4): 557–80.

Asakawa, Y. 2008. "Liverworts Potential Source of Medicinal Compounds." *Current Pharmaceutical Design* 14 (29): 3067–88.

Asakawa, Y. 2015. "Search for New Liverwort Constituents of Biological Interest." In *Natural Produces: Recent Advances*, edited by A. K. Chauhan, P. Pushpangadan, and V. George. New Delhi: Write and Print Publications, Educationist Press.

Asakawa, Y., and A. Ludwiczuk. 2013. "Bryophytes: Liverworts, Mosses and Hornworts: Extraction and Isolation Procedures." *Methods in Molecular Biology* 1055: 1–20.

Asakawa, Y., A. Ludwiczuk, F. Nagashima. 2013. "Chemical Constituents of Bryophytes: Bio- and Chemical Diversity, Biological Activity, and Chemosystemics."

Asakawa, Y., A. Ludwiczuk, M. Novakovic, D. Bukvicki et al. 2022. "Bis-bibenzyls, Bibenzyls and Terpenoids in 33 Genera of the Marchantiophyta (Liverworts): Structures, Synthesis, and Bioactivity." *Journal of Natural Products* 85 (3): 729–62.

Asakawa, Y., A. Ludwiczuk, T. Hashimoto. 2013. "Cytotoxic and Antiviral Compounds from Bryophytes and Inedible Fungi." *Journal of Pre-Clinical and Clinical Research* 7 (2): 73–85.

Asakawa, Y., and E. O. Campbell. 1982. "Terpenoids and Bibenzyls from Some New Zealand Liverworts." *Phytochemistry* 21: 2663–67.

Asakawa, Y., F. Nagashima, A. Ludwiczuk. 2022. "Distribution of Bibenzyls, Prenyl Bibenzyls, and Terpenoids in the Liverwort Genus *Radula*." *Journal of Natural Products* 83 (3): 756–69.

Asakawa, Y., K. Kondo, and M. Tori. 1991a. "Cyclopropanochroman Derivatives from the Liverwort *Radula javanica*." *Phytochemistry* 30 (1): 325–28.

Asakawa, Y., K. Nil, M. Higuchi. 2015. "Identification of Sesquiterpene Lactones in the Bryophyta (Mosses) *Takakia*: *Takakia* Species Are Closely Related Chemically to the Marchantiophyta (Liverworts)." *Natural Product Communications* 10 (1): 5–8.

Asakawa, Y., M. Tori, K. Takikawa, H.G. Krishnamurty et al. 1987. "Cyclic Bis (Bibenzyls) and Related Compounds from the Liverworts *Marchantia polymorpha* and *Marchantia palmata*." *Phytochemistry* 26 (6): 1811–16.

Asakawa, Y., M. Toyota, A. Ueda, M. Tori, Y. Fukazawa. 1991. "Sesquiterpenoids from the Liverwort *Bazzania japonica*." *Phytochemistry* 30 (9): 3037–40.

Asakawa, Y., M. Toyota, F. Nagashima, T. Hashimoto. 2007. "Chemical Constituents of Selected Japanese and New Zealand Liverworts." *Natural Product Communications* 3 (2): 289–300.

Asakawa, Y., M. Toyota, F. Nagashima, T. Hashimoto. 2008a. "Chemical Constituents of Selected Japanese and New Zealand Liverworts." *Natural Product Communications* 3 (2): 289–300.

Asakawa, Y., M. Toyota, M. von Konrat, J. E. Braggins. 2003. "Volatile Components of Selected Species of the Liverwort Genera *Frullania* and *Schusterella* (Frullaniaceae) from New Zealand, Australia and South America: A chemosystematic approach." *Phytochemistry* 62 (3): 439–52.

Asakawa, Y., T. Takemoto, M. Toyota, and T. Aratani. 1977. "Sacculatal and Isosacculatal, Two New Exceptional Diterpenedials from the Liverwort, *Trichocoleopsis sacculata*." *Tetrahedron Letters* 18 (16): 1407–10.

Asakawa, Y., Y. Tada, T. Hashimoto. 1994. "Naphthalene Derivatives from the New Zealand Liverwort, *Wettsteinia schusterana*." *Phytochemistry* 35 (6): 1555–57.

Asakura, K., T. Kanemasa, K. Minagawa, K. Kagawa et al. 2000. "Alpha-eudesmol, a P/Q-type $Ca(2^+)$ Channel Blocker, Inhibits Neurogenic Vasodilation and Extravasation Following Electrical Stimulation of Trigeminal Ganglion." *Brain Research* 873 (1): 94–101.

Asif, A., S. Ishtiaq, S. H. Kamran, R. Waseem et al. 2023. "UHPLC-MS and GC-MS Phytochemical Profiling, Amelioration of Pain and Inflammation with Chloroform Extract of *Funaria hygrometrica* Hedw. via Modulation of Inflammatory Biomarkers." *Inflammopharmacology* 31 (4): 1879–92.

Ayinke, A. B., M. A. Morakinyo, I. M. Olalekan, T. O. Philip et al. 2015. "In vitro Evaluation of Membrane Stabilizing Potential of Selected Bryophyte Species." *European Journal of Medicinal Plants* 6 (3): 181–90.

Azevedo, M. M. B., C. A. Almeida, F. C. M. Chaves, I. A. Rodrigues et al. 2016. "7-hydroxycalamenene Effects on Secreted Aspartic Proteases Activity and Biofilm Formation of *Candida* spp." *Pharmacognosy Magazine* 12 (45): 36–40.

Azimi, H., M. Fallah-Tafti, M. Karimi-Darmiyan, M. Abdollahi. 2011. "A Comprehensive Review of Vaginitis Phytotherapy. *Pakistan Journal of Biological Sciences* 14 (21): 960–66.

Azuelo, A. G., L. G. Sariana, M. P. Pabualan. 2011. "Some Medicinal Bryophytes: Their Ethnobotanical Uses and Morphology." *Asian Journal of Biodiversity* 2 (1): 50–80.

Baek, S. H., N. Perry, S. D. Lorimer. 2003. "Ent-Costunolide from the Liverwort *Hepatostolonophora paucistipula.*" *Journal of Chemical Research* (1): 14–15.

Baek, S. H., R. K. Phipps, N. B. Perry. 2004. "Antimicrobial Chlorinated Bibenzyls from the Liverwort *Riccardia marginata.*" *Journal of Natural Products* 67 (4): 718–20.

Bailey, A. 1996. *The Handbook of Bailey Flower Essences.* West Yorkshire, England: Bailey Flower Essences Ltd.

Bailly, C. 2023. "Discovery and Anticancer Activity of the Plagiochilins from the Liverwort Genus *Plagiochila.*" *Life* 13 (3): 758.

Bakar, M. F. A., F. A. Karim, M. Suleiman, A. Isha et al. 2015. "Phytochemical Constituents, Antioxidant and Antiproliferative Properties of a Liverwort, *Lepidozia borneensis* Stephani from Mount Kinabalu, Sabah, Malaysia." *Evidence Based Complementary and Alternative Medicine* 2015: 936215.

Baldry, M., A. Nielsen, M. S. Bojer, Y. Zhao et al. 2016. "Norlichexanthone Reduces Virulence Gene Expression and Biofilm Formation in *Staphyloccus aureus.*" *PLoS One* 11 (12): e0168305.

Bardón, A., G. B. Mitre, N. Kamiya, M. Toyota et al. 2002. "Eremophilanolides and Other Constituents from the Argentine Liverwort *Frullania brasiliensis.*" *Phytochemistry* 59 (2): 205–13.

Bargagli, R., F. Monaci, F. Borghini, F. Bravi et al. 2002. "Mosses and Lichens as Biomonitors of Trace Metals. A Comparison Study on *Hypnum cupressiforme* and *Parmelia caperata* in a Former Mining District in Italy." *Environmental Pollution* 116 (2): 279–87.

Barot, N. S., and H. K. Bagla. 2009. "Extraction of Humic Acid from Biological Matrix—Dry Cow Dung Powder." *Green Chemistry Letters & Review* 2 (4): 217–21.

Basile, A., S. Giordano, J. A. López-Sáez, R. C. Cobianchi. 1999. "Antibacterial Activity of Pure Flavonoids Isolated from Mosses." *Phytochemistry* 52 (8): 1479–82.

Basile, A., S. Giordano, S. Sorbo, M. L. Vuotto et al. 1998. "Antibiotic Effects of *Lunularia cruciata* (Bryophyta) Extract." *Pharmaceutical Biology* 36 (1): 25–28.

Basile, A., S. Sorbo, B. Conte, B. Golia et al. 2011. "Antioxidant Activity in Extracts from *Leptodictyum riparium* (Bryophyte), Stressed by Heavy Metals, Heat Shock, and Salinity." *Plant Biosystems* 145 (1): 77–80.

Basile, A., S. Sorbo, S. Giordano, A. Lavitola et al. 1998. "Antibacterial Activity in *Pleurochaete squarrosa* Extract (Bryophyta)." *International Journal of Antimicrobial Agents* 10 (2): 169–72.

Basile, A., W. L. Vuotto, M. T. L. Ielpo, V. Moscatiello et al. 1998. "Antibacterial Activity in *Rhynchostegium riparioides* (Hedw.) Card. Extract (Bryophyta)." *Phytotherapy Research* 12 (1): S146–48.

Bay, G., N. Nahar, M. Oubre, M. J. Whitehouse et al. 2013. "Boreal Feather Mosses Secrete Chemical Signals to Gain Nitrogen." *New Phytologist* 200 (1): 54–60.

Beerling, D. 2019. *Making Eden: How Plants Transformed a Barren Planet*. Oxford, U.K.: Oxford University Press.

Beever, J. E., and J. E. Greeson. 1995. "*Polytrichum commune* Hedw. and *Polytrichadelphus magellanicus* (Hedw.) Mitt. Used as Decorative Material on New Zealand Maori Cloaks." *Journal of Bryology* 18 (4): 819–23.

Beike, A. K., V. Spagnuolo, V. Lüth, F. Steinhart et al. 2015. "Clonal In vitro Propagation of Peat Mosses (*Sphagnum* L.) as Novel Green Resources for Basic and Applied Research." *Plant Cell Tissue Organ Cultivation* 120 (3): 1037–49.

Belcher, H., and E. Swale. 1998. "Moss That Grows on Skulls: A Curious Old Remedy Run to Earth in Cambridge." *Nature in Cambridgeshire* 40: 74–75.

Belcik, F. P., and N. Weigner. 1980. "Antimicrobial Activities or Antibiosis of Certain Eastern U.S. Liverwort, Lichen and Moss Extracts." *Journal of Elisha Mitchell Science Society* 96: 94.

Belkin, M., D. B. Fitzgerald, M. D. Felix. 1952. "Tumor-Damaging Capacity of Plant Materials. II. Plants Used as Diuretics." *Journal of the National Cancer Institute* 13 (3): 741–44.

Benek, A., K. Canli, E. M. Altuner. 2022. "Traditional Medicinal Uses of Mosses." *Anatolian Bryology* 8 (1): 57–65.

Benesova, V., Z. Samek, V. Herout, F. Sorm. 1969. "On Terpenes. Isolation and Structure of Pinguisone from *Aneura pinguis* (L.) Dum." *Collection of Czechoslovak and Chemical Communications* 34 (2): 582–92.

Benke, D., A. Barberis, S. Kopp, K. H. Altmann et al. 2009. "GABA A Receptors as In Vivo Substrate for the Anxiolytic Action of Valerenic Acid, a Major Constituent of Valerian Root Extracts." *Neuropharmacology* 56 (1): 174–81.

Benny, A. T., P. Rathinam, S. Dev, B. Mathew et al. 2022. "Perillaldehyde Mitigates Virulence Factors and Biofilm Formation of *Pseudomonas aeruginosa* Clinical Isolates, by Acting on the Quorum Sensing Mechanism In Vitro." *Journal of Applied Microbiology* 133 (2): 385–99.

Bhattarai, H. D., B. Paudel, H. S. Lee, Y. K. Lee et al. 2008. "Antioxidant Activity of *Sanionia uncinate*, a Polar Moss Species from King George Island, Antarctica." *Phytotherapy Research* 22 (12): 1635–39.

Bhattarai, H. D., B. Paudel, H. K. Lee, H. Oh et al. 2008. "In Vitro Antioxidant Capacities of Two Benzonaphthoxanthenones: Ohioensins F and G, Isolated from the Antarctic Moss *Polytrichastrum alpinum*." *Zeitschrift für Naturforschung C* 64 (3–4): 197–200.

Bing, H. J., Y. H. Wu, J. Zhou, H. Y. Sun. 2016. "Biomonitoring Trace Metal Contamination by Seven Sympatric Alpine Species in Eastern Tibetan Plateau." *Chemosphere* 165: 388–98.

Birladeanu, L. 2003. "The stories of Santonin and Santonic Acid." *Angewandte Chemin* 42 (11): 1202–8.

Bishnoi, A., A. Alam, V. Sharma. 2015. "Comparative Assessment of Antifungal Efficacy of *Anoectangium clarum* Mitt. and *Hyophila spathulata* (Harv.) A. Jaeger." *Mycopath* 13 (2): 89–92.

Bishnoi, A., V. Singh, V. Sharma, A. Alam. 2016. "Antibacterial Activity of *Anoectangium clarum* Mitt. (Bryophyta: Pottiaceae) against Some Pathogenic Bacteria." *Sikkim Manipal University Medical Journal* 3 (1): 650.

Bland, J. 1971. *Forests of Lilliput: The Realms of Mosses and Lichens*. Englewood Cliffs, N.J.: Prentice-Hall.

Bläs, B., J. Zapp, H. Becker. 2004. "Ent-clerodane Diterpenes and Other Constituents from the Liverwort *Adelanthus lindenbergianus* (Lehm.) Mitt." *Phytochemistry* 65 (1): 127–37.

Blatt-Janmaat, K. L., S. Neumann, J. Zeigler, K. Peters. 2023. "Host Tree and Geography Induce Metabolic Shifts in the Epiphytic Liverwort *Radula complanata*." *Plants* (Basel) 12 (3): 571.

Boas, F. 1966. *Ethnography of the Kwakiutl*, edited by H. Codere. Chicago: University of Chicago Press.

Bodade, R. G., P. S. Borkar, S. Arfeen, C. N. Khobragade. 2008. "In Vitro Screening of Bryophytes for Antimicrobial Activity." *Journal of Medicinal Plants* 7 (S4): 23–28.

Bomfim, D. S., R. P. C. Ferraz, N. C. Carvalho, M. B. P. Soares et al. 2013. "Eudesmol Isomers Induce Caspase-Mediated Apoptosis in Human Hepatocellular Carcinoma HepG2 Cells." *Basic and Clinical Pharmacology and Toxicology* 113 (5): 300–306.

Boom, B. M. 1996. *Ethnobotany of the Chácobo Indians, Beni, Bolivia*. Advances in Economic Botany, vol. 4. New York: New York Botanical Garden.

Borel, C., D. H. Welti, I. Fernandez, M. Colmenares. 1993. "Dicranin, an Antimicrobial and 15-Lipoxygenase Inhibitor from the Moss *Dicranum scoparium*." *Journal of Natural Products* 56 (7): 1071–77.

Bowman, J. L. 2016. "A Brief History of Marchantia from Greece to Genomics." *Plant and Cell Physiology* 57 (2): 210–29.

Brown, R. 2011. "Some Observations on the Parts of Fructification In Mosses; with Characters and Descriptions of Two New Genera Of That Order," in *The Transactions of the Linnean Society of London Vol. X*, 312–24.

Brunshwig, H. 1500. *Liber de arte distillandi*. Strasbourg.

Bucar, M., V. Segota, A. Rimac, N. Koletic et al. 2022. "Green Christmas: Bryophytes as Ornamentals in Croatian Traditional Nativity Scenes." *Journal of Ethnobiology and Ethnomedicine* 18 (1): 15.

Buchanan, M. S., T. Hashimoto, Y. Asakawa. 1996. "Phytl Esters and Phaeophytins from the Hornwort *Megacros flagellaris*." *Phytochemistry* 41 (5): 1373–76.

Bukvicki, D., A. K. Tyagi, D. G. Gottardi, M. M. Veljic et al. 2013. "Assessment of the Chemical Composition and in Vitro Antimicrobial Potential of Extracts of the Liverwort *Scapania aspera*." *Natural Product Communications* 8 (9): 1313–16.

Bukvicki, D., D. Gottardi, L. Vannini, A. Dzamic et al. 2015. "Chemical Composition and Antimicrobial Assessment of Liverwort *Lopozia ventricosa* Extracts." *Revista Brasileira de Botanica* 38: 25–30.

Bukvicki, D., D. Gottardi, M. Veljic, P. D. Marin et al. 2012. "Identification of Volatile Components of Liverwort (*Porella cordaeana*) Extracts Using GC/MS-SPME and Their Antimicrobial Activity." *Molecules* 17 (6): 6982–95.

Bukvicki, D., M. Novakovic, I. Tomic, J. Nikodinovic-Runic et al. 2021. "Biotransformation of Perrottetin F by *Aspergillus niger*: New Bioactive Secondary Metabolites." *Records of Natural Products* 15 (4): 281–92.

Bukvicki, D., M. Veljic, M. Sokovic, S. Grujic et al. 2012. "Antimicrobial Activity of Methanol Extracts of *Abietinella abietina, Neckera crispa, Platyhypnidium riparoides, Cratoneuron filicinum* and *Campylium protensum* Mosses." *Archives of Biological Sciences* 64 (3): 911–16.

Burgess, E. J., L. Larsen, N. B. Perry. 2000. "A Cytotoxic Sesquiterpene Caffeate from the Liverwort *Bazzania novae-zelandiae*." *Journal of Natural Products* 63 (4): 537–39.

Burgos, V., C. Paz, K. Saavedra, M. Saavedra et al. 2020. "Drimenol, Isodrimeninol and Polygodial Isolated from *Drimys winteri* Reduce Monocyte Adhesion to Stimulated Human Endothelial Cells." *Food and Chemical Toxicology* 145: 111775.

Byeon, H. E., S. H. Um, J. H. Yim, H. K. Lee et al. 2012. "Ohioensin F Suppresses TNF-*a*-Induced Adhesion Molecule Expression by Inactivation of the MAPK, Akt and NF-$_k$B Pathways in Vascular Smooth Muscle Cells." *Life Sciences* 90 (11–12): 396–406.

Cagno, V., M. Donalisio, A. Civra, C. Cagliero et al. 2015. "In Vitro Evaluation of the Antiviral Properties of Shilajit and Investigation of Its Mechanisms of Action." *Journal of Ethnopharmacology* 166: 129–34.

Cai, H., and H. Hu. 2021. "Costunolide Induces Apoptosis of K562/ADR Cells through PI3K/AKT Pathway." *Zhongguo Shi Yan Xue Ye Xue Za Zhi* 29 (1): 68–71.

Calder, V. L., A. L. J. Cole, J. R. L. Walker. 1986. "Antibiotic Compounds from New Zealand Plants. III: A Survey of Some New Zealand Plant for Antibiotic Substances." *Journal of the Royal Society of New Zealand* 16 (2): 169–81.

Canli, K., E. M. Altuner, I. Akata. 2015. "Antimicrobial Screening of *Mnium stellare*." *Bangladesh Journal of Pharmacology* 10 (2): 321–25.

Cannone, N., T. Corinti, F. Malfasi, P. Gerola et al. 2017. "Moss Survival Through in Situ Cryptobiosis after Six Centuries of Glacier Burial." *Scientific Reports* 7 (1): 4438.

Cansu, T. B., B. Yayli, T. Özdemir, N. Batan et al. 2013. "Antimicrobial Activity and Chemical Composition of the Essential Oils of Mosses (*Hylocomium splendens* (Hedw.) Schimp. and *Leucodon sciuroides* (Hedw.) Schwägr.) Growing in Turkey." *Turkish Journal of Chemistry* 37 (2): 213–19.

Cao, H., J. B. Xiao, M. Xu. 2007. "Comparison of Volatile Components of *Marchantia convoluta* Obtained by Supercritical Carbon Dioxide Extraction and Petrol Ether Extraction." *Journal of Food Composition and Analysis* 20 (1): 45–51.

Caputo, L., F. Capozzolo, G. Amato, V. de Feo et al. 2022. "Chemical Composition, Antibiofilm, Cytotoxic, and Anti-Acetylcholinesterase Activities of *Myrtus communis* L. Leaves Essential Oil." *BMC Complementary Medicine and Therapies* 22 (1): 142.

Carroll, J. F., G. Paluch, J. Coats, M. Kramer. 2010. "Elemol and Amyris Oil Repel the Ticks *Ixodes scapularis* and *Amblyomma americanum* (Acari: Ixodidae) in Laboratory Bioassays." *Experimental and Applied Acarology* 51 (4): 383–92.

Castaldo-Cobianchi, R., S. Giordano, A. Basile, U. Violante. 1988. "Occurrence of Antibiotic Activity in *Conocephalum conicum, Mnium undulatum* and *Leptodictyum riparium* (Bryophytes)." *Plant Biosystems* 122 (5–6): 303–11.

Catanzaro, E., E. Turrini, T. Kerre, S. Sioen et al. 2022. "Perillaldehyde Is a New Ferroptosis Inducer with a Relevant Clinical Potential for Acute Myeloid Leukemia Therapy." *Biomedicine and Pharmacotherapy* 154: 113662.

Celik, G. 2020. "Antimicrobial Properties and Chemical Composition of the Essential Oil of *Leucobryum glaucum* (Leucobryaceae)." *Anatolian Bryology* 6 (2): 112–18.

Celik, G., H. Sahin, N. Baltas, N. Batan et al. 2023. "Chemical Analysis of Biological Activity of the Essential Oils and Extracts of Two Liverwort Species Growing in Turkey." *Botanica Serbica* 47 (1): 31–40.

Chandra, S., D. Chandra, A. Barh, Pankaj, R. K. Pandey et al. 2016. "Bryophytes: Hoard of Remedies, an Ethno-Medicinal Review." *Journal of Traditional and Complementary Medicine* 7 (1): 94–98.

Chang, A. X., L. M. Sun, X. Z. Wu, H. X. Lou. 2009. "The Inhibitory Effect of a Macrocyclic Bisbibenzyl Riccardin D on the Biofilms of *Candida albicans*." *Biological and Pharmaceutical Bulletin* 32 (8): 1417–21.

Chaudhary, A., B. S. Yadav, S. Singh, P. K. Maurya et al. 2017. "Docking-Based Screening of *Ficus religiosa* Phytochemicals as Inhibitors of Human Histamine H2 Receptor." *Pharmacognosy Magazine* 13 (suppl 3): S706–S714.

Chen, F., A. Ludwiczuk, G. Wei, X. Chen et al. 2018. "Terpenoid Secondary Metabolites in Bryophytes: Chemical Diversity, Biosynthesis and Biological Functions." *Critical Reviews in Plant Sciences* 37 (2–3): 210–31.

Chen, X., C. Wang, H. Qiu, Y. Yuan et al. 2019. "Asperpyrone A Attenuates RANKL-Induced Osteoclast Formation through Inhibiting NFATc1, Ca^{2+} Signalling and Oxidative Stress." *Journal of Cellular and Molecular Medicine* 23 (12): 8269–79.

Cheng, X. X., Y. P. Xiao, P. Wang, X. B. Wang et al. 2013. "The Ethyl Acetate Fraction of *Polytrichum commune* L. ex Hedw Induced Cell Apoptosis via Reactive Oxygen Species in L1210 Cells." *Journal of Ethnopharmacology* 148 (3): 926–33.

Chicca, A., M. A. Schafroth, I. Reynoso-Moreno et al. 2018. "Uncovering the Psychoactivity of a Cannabinoid from Liverworts Associated with a Legal High." *Science Advances* 4 (10): eaat2166.

Chimplee, S., P. Graidist, T. Srisawat, S. Sukrong et al. 2019. "Anti-Breast Cancer Potential of Frullanolide from *Grangea maderaspatana* Plant by Inducing Apoptosis." *Oncology Letters* 17 (6): 5283–91.

Chobot, V., L. Kubicová, S. Nabbout, L. Jahodar et al. 2008. "Evaluation of Antioxidant Activity of Some Common Mosses." *Zeitschrift für Naturforschung C Journal of Biosciences* 63 (7–8): 476–82.

Choi, W. S., J. W. Jeong, S. O. Kim, G. Y. Kim et al. 2014. "Anti-Inflammatory Potential of Peat Moss Extracts in Lipopolysaccharide-Stimulated RAW 264.7 Macrophages." *International Journal of Molecular Medicine* 34 (4): 1101–9.

Chou, A., R. Sucgang, R. J. Hamill, L. Zechiedrich et al. 2023. "Mortality Difference from *Klebsiella aerogenes* vs *Enterobacter cloacae* Bloodstream Infections." *Access Microbiology* 5 (2): acmi000421.

Chowdhuri, S. R., A. B. Raha, S. Mitra, J. Datta. et al. 2018. "'Dicranin' in the Membrane Phospholipids of a Dicranaceae and Pottiaceae Moss Member of the Eastern Himalayan Biodiversity Hotspot." *Lipids* 53 (5): 539–45.

Cianciullo, P., F. Cimmino, V. Maresca, S. Sorbo et al. 2022. "Anti-Tumor Activities from Secondary Metabolites and Their Derivatives in Bryophytes: A Brief Review." *Applied Biosciences* 1 (1): 73–94.

Classen, B, A. Baumann, J. Utermoehlen. 2019. "Arabinogalactan-Proteins in Spore-Producing Land Plants." *Carbohydrate Polymers* 210: 215–24.

Colak, E., R. Kara, T. Ezer, G. Y. Celik et al. 2011. "Investigation of Antimicrobial Activity of Some Turkish Pleurocarpic Mosses." *African Journal of Biotechnology* 10 (60): 12905–8.

Colonna, F. 1616. *Minus cognitarum rariorumque nostro coelo orientium stirpium εκφρασις, qua non pauacae ab antiquioribus Theophrasto, Dioscoride, Plinio, Galeno, aliisque descriptae . . . Item de aqualilibus aliisque nonnullis anibalibus.* Rome: Apud Iacobum Mascardum.

Compton, B. D. 1993. "Upper North Wakashan and Southern Tsimshian Ethnobotany: The Knowledge and Usage of Plants and Fungi among the Oweekeno, Hanaksiala (Kitlope and Kemano), Haisla (Kitamaat) and Kitasoo Peoples of the Central and North Coasts of British Columbia." Doctoral dissertation, University of British Columbia.

Conart, C., and H. T. Simonsen. 2025. "Tamariscol Biosynthesis in *Frullania tamarisci*." *Phytochemistry* 229: 114301.

Connolly, J. D. 1982. "New Diterpenoids from the Hepaticae." *Revista Latinoamericana de Quimica* 12: 121–26.

Cornejo, A., J. M. Jimenez, L. Caballero, F. Mello et al. 2011. "Fulvic Acid Inhibits Aggregation and Promotes Disassembly of Tau Fibrils Associated with Alzheimer's Disease." *Journal of Alzheimer's Disease* 27 (1): 143–53.

Corrigan, D., C. Kloos, C. S. O'Connor, R. F. Timoney. 1976. "Lipid Components of Sphagnum Mosses." *Planta Medica* 29 (3): 261–67.

Coulerie, P., M. Nour, L. Thouvenot, Y. Asakawa. 2014. "Sesquiterpene Hydrocarbons from the Liverwort *Treubia isignensis* var. *isignensis* with Chemotaxonomic Significance." *Natural Product Communications* 9 (8): 1059–60.

Crusco, A., R. Baptista, S. Bhowmick, M. Beckmann et al. 2019. "The Anti-Mycobacterial Activity of a Diterpenoid-Like Molecule Operates Through Nitrogen and Amino Acid Starvation." *Frontiers in Microbiology* 10: 1444.

Csicsor, A., and E. Tombacz. 2022. "Screening of Humic Substances Extracted from Leonardite for Free Radical Scavenging Activity Using DPPH Method." *Molecules* 27 (19): 6334.

Csupor, D., T. Kurtán, M. Vollár, N. Kúsz et al. 2020. "Pigments of the Moss *Paraleucobryum longifolium*: Isolation and Structure Elucidation of Prenyl-Substituted 8,8'-Linked 9,10-Phenanthrenequinone Dimers." *Journal of Natural Products* 83 (2): 268–76.

Cullmann, F., and H. Becker. 1999. "Lignans from the Liverwort *Lepicolea ochroleuca*." *Phytochemistry* 52 (8): 1651–56.

Culpeper, N. 1653. *The English Physitian*. Reprinted in 2009 as *Culpeper's Complete Herbal* London: Arcturus Publishing.

Dague, A. L., L. R. Valeeva, N. M. McCann, M. R. Sharipova et al. 2023. "Identification and Analysis of Antimicrobial Activities from a Model Moss *Ceratodon purpureus*." *Metabolites* 13 (3): 350.

Dang, X., S. Chalkias, I. J. Koralnik. 2015. "JC Virus-iLOV Fluorescent Strains Enable the Detection of Early and Late Viral Protein Expression." *Journal of Virological Methods* 223: 25–29.

de Faria Garcia, E., M. A. de Oliveira, A. M. Godin et al. 2010. "Antiedematogenic Activity and Phytochemical Composition of Preparations from *Echinodorus grandifloras* Leaves." *Phytomedicine* 18 (1): 80–86.

dei Cas, L., F. Pugni, G. Fico. 2015. "Tradition of Use on Medicinal Species in Valfurva (Sondrio, Italy)." *Journal of Ethnopharmacology* 163: 113–34.

de la Cruz, M., and J. Badiano. 1939. *Libellus de Medicinalibus Indorum Herbis*. Translated by W. Gates as *The De la Cruz-Badiano Aztec Herbal of 1552*. London: Maya Society.

de la Maza, M. G. 1889. *Ensayo de farmacofitologia Cubana. Resumen de las propiodades medicinales, especialidad las recientemente estudiadas, de muchas plantas indígenas ó de cultivo, nuevos productos*. Havana, Cuba: La Propaganda Literaria.

de Oliveira, D. P., T. do Valle Moreira, N. V. Batista, J. D de Souza Filho et al. 2018. "Esterification of Trans-aconitic Acid Improves Its Anti-Inflammatory Activity in LPS-Induced Acute Arthritis." *Biomedicine and Pharmacotherapy* 99: 87–95.

de Oliveira, D. P., G. G. Augusto, N. V. Batista et al. 2018. "Encapsulation of Trans-aconitic Acid in Mucoadhesive Microspheres Prolongs the Anti-Inflammatory Effect in LPS-Induced Acute Arthritis." *European Journal of Pharmaceutical Sciences* 119: 112–20.

de Oliveira, P. F., C. C. Munari, H. D. Nicolella, R. C. S. Veneziani et al. 2016. "Manool, a *Salvia officinalis* Diterpene, Induces Selective Cytotoxicity in Cancer Cells." *Cytotechnology* 68 (5): 2139–43.

de Sousa, D. P., E. Raphael, U. Brocksom, T .J. Brocksom. 2007. "Sedative Effect of Monoterpene Alcohols in Mice: A Preliminary Screening." *Zeitschrift für Naturforschung C Journal of Biosciences* 62 (7–8): 563–66.

Deora, G. S. and N. Guhil. 2016. "Studies on Antifungal Potential of *Bryum cellulare* (a Moss) Crude Extracts against Spore Germination of Fungus *Curvularia lunata*." *International Journal of Pharmaceutical Sciences and Research* 44: 353–57.

Dey, A., and J. de Nath. 2011. "Antifungal Bryophyte: A Possible Role against Human Pathogens and in Plant Protection." *Research Journal of Botany* 6: 129–40.

Dey, A., and A. Mukherjee. 2015 "Therapeutic Potential of Bryophytes and Derived Compounds against Cancer." *Journal of Acute Disease* 4 (3): 236–48.

Dhondiyal, P. B., B. Pande, K. Bargali. 2013. "Antibiotic Potential of *Lunularia cruciata* (L.) Dum ex Lindb (bryophyta) of Kumaon Himalaya." *African Journal of Microbiology Research* 7 (34): 4350–54.

Dickson, J. H., K. D. Oeggi, W. Kofler, W. K. Hofbauer et al. 2019. "Seventy-Five Mosses and Liverworts Found Frozen with the late Neolithic Tyrolean Iceman: Origins, Taphonomy and the Iceman's Last Journey." *PLoS One* 14 (10): e0223752.

Ding, H. 1982. *Medicinal Spore-Bearing Plants of China*. Shanghai: Science and Technology Press.

Ditta, L. A., E. Rao, F. Provenzano, J. L. Sanchez et al. 2020. "Agarose/$_{\kappa}$-carragenan-Based Hydrogel Film Enriched with Natural Plant Extracts for the Treatment of Cutaneous Wounds." *International Journal of Biological Macromolecules* 164: 2818–30.

Dixon, H. N. 1896. *The Student's Handbook of British Mosses*. Reprinted 1954, 3rd Ed. London: Sumfield and Day.

Dodoens, R. 1557. *La premiere parties de l'historie des plantes, contenant les especes, differences, forme, noms, vertus & operations de herbs*. Paris: de l'Imprimerie de Iean Loë.

Dogan, M., M. Karatas, M. Aasim. 2018. "Cadmium and Lead Bioaccumulation Potentials of an Aquatic Macrophyte *Ceratophyllum demersum* L.: A Laboratory Study." *Ecotoxicology and Environmental Safety* 148: 431–40.

Doskotch, R. W., and F. S. el-Feraly. 1969. "Antitumor Agents. II. Tulipinolide, a New Germacranolide Sesquiterpene, and Constunolide (*sic*). Two Cyctotoxic Substances from *Liriodendron tulipifera* L." *Journal of Pharmaceutical Sciences* 58 (7): 877–80.

Doskotch, R. W., and F. S. el-Feraly. 1970. "Antitumor Agents. IV. Structure of Tulipinolide and Epitulipinolide. Cytotoxic Sesquiterpenes from *Liriodendron tulipifera* L." *Journal of Organic Chemistry* 35 (6): 1928–36.

Drieshen, C. 2024. "A Cure from the Crypt: Weapon Salve in the Library of John Dee." Cambridge University Library Special Collections.

Drobnik, J., and A. Stebel. 2020. "Central European Ethnomedical and Officinal Uses of Peat, with Special Emphasis on the Tolpa Peat Preparation (TPP): An Historical Review." *Journal of Ethnopharmacology* 246: 112248.

Drobnik, J., and A. Stebel. 2021. "Four Centuries of Medicinal Mosses and Liverworts in European Ethnopharmacy and Scientific Pharmacy: A Review." *Plants* (Basel) 10 (7): 1296.

Du, Z. X. 1997. "A Study of Medicinal Bryophytes Used in Guangxi Province, S China." *Chenia* 3: 123–24.

Duan, W. B., A. T. Peng, S. N. Yuan, S. N. Wang et al. 2023. "Two New Benzophenones from the Moss *Pogonatum spinulosum*." *Natural Products Research* 38 (13): 2201–6.

Duarté, X., C. T. Anderson, M. Grimson, R. D. Barabote et al. 2000. "*Erwinia chrysanthemi* Strains Cause Death of Human Gastrointestinal Cells in Culture and Express an Initimin-like Protein." *FEMS Microbiology Letters* 190 (1): 81–86.

Duffin, C. J. 2022. "The Periwig of a Dead Cranium: Medical Skull Moss." *Pharmaceutical Historian* 52 (3): 75–85.

Duong, T. H., T. Aree, T. K. D. Le, V. S. Dang, N. H. Nguyen et al. 2025. "Chemical Constituents with Their Alpha-Glucosidase Inhibitory Activity from the Whole Plant of *Ceratophyllum demersum*." *Phytochemistry* 229: 114290.

Durán-Peña, M. J., J. M. Botubol Ares, J. R. Hanson, I. G. Collado, et al. 2015. "Biological Activity of Natural Sesquiterpenoids Containing a Gem-Dimethylcyclopropane Unit." *Natural Product Reports* 32: 1236–48.

Eastman, J. and A. Hansen. 1995. *The Book of Swamp and Bog: Trees, Shrubs and Wildflowers of the Eastern Freshwater Wetlands*. Mechanicsburg, PA: Stackpole Books.

Edwards, S. R. 2012. *English Names for British Bryophytes*. Special vol. 5. Wootton, Northampton, U.K.: British Bryological Society.

Ehsani, M., S. Bartsch, S. M. M. Rasa, J. Dittmann et al. 2022. "The Natural Compound Atraric Acid Suppresses Androgen-Regulated Neo-angiogenesis of Castration-Resistant Prostate Cancer Through Angiopoietin 2." *Oncogene* 41 (23): 3263–77.

Ekwealor, J. T. B., and K. M. Fisher. 2020. "Life under Quartz: Hypolithic Mosses in the Mojave Desert." *PLoS One* 15 (7): e0235928.

Elbert, W., B. Weber, S. Burrows, J. Steinkamp et al. 2012. "Contribution of Cryptogamic Covers to the Global Cycles of Carbon and Nitrogen." *Nature Geoscience* 5: 459–62.

Eldridge, D. J., E. Guirado, P. B. Reich, R. Ochoa-Hueso et al. 2023. "The Global Contribution of Soil Mosses to Ecosystem Services." *Nature Geoscience* 16: 430–38.

Elibol, B., T. Ezer, R. Kara, G. Y. Celik et al. 2011. "Antifungal and Antibacterial Effects of Some Acrocarpic Mosses." *African Journal of Biotechnology* 10 (6): 986–89.

Ellingwood, F. 1915. *The American Materia Medica. Therapeutics and Pharmacognosy*. Evanston, IL: Ellingwood's Therapeutist.

El-Shiekh, R. A., M. A. Elhemely, I. A. Naguib, S. I. Bukhari, R. Elshimy. 2023. "Luteolin 4'-Neohesperidoside Inhibits Clinically Isolated Resistant Bacteria in Vitro and in Vivo." *Molecules* 28 (6): 2609.

Emadi, A., J. Y. Law, E. T. Strovel, R. G. Lapidus et al. 2018. "Asparaginase *Erwinia chrysanthemi* Effectively Depletes Plasma Glutamine in Adult Patients with Relapsed/Refractory Acute Myeloid Leukemia." *Cancer Chemotherapy and Pharmacology* 81 (1): 217–22.

Endo, A., K. Hirano, R. Ose, S. Maeno et al. 2020. "Impact of Kestose Supplementation on the Healthy Adult Microbiota in In Vitro Fecal Batch Cultures." *Anaerobe* 61: 102076.

Erturk, O., H. Sahin, E. Y, Erturk, H. E. Hotaman et al. 2015. "The Antimicrobial and Antioxidant Activities of Extracts Obtained from Some Moss Species in Turkey." *Herba Polonica* 61 (4): 52–65.

Fabure, J., H. Plaisance, F. Cazier, A. Delbende. 2010. "Potential Use of *Syntrichia ruralis* Form Monitoring Atmospheric BTEX." *International Journal of Environment and Health* 4 (2–3): 201–5.

Faleva, A. V., N. V. Ul'yanovskii, D. I. Falev, A. A. Onuchina et al. 2022. "New Oligomeric Dihydrochalcones in the Moss *Polytrichum commune*: Identification, Isolation and Antioxidant Activity." *Metabolites* 12 (10): 974.

Fan, H. H., G. Wei, X. L. Chen, H. Guo et al. 2021. "Sesquiterpene Biosynthesis in a Leafy Liverwort *Radula lindenbergiana* Gottsche ex C. Hartm." *Phytochemistry* 190: 112847.

Fan, J. H., S. Sun, C. Y. Lv, Z. Z. Li et al. 2022. "Discovery of Myctotoxin Alternariol as a Potential Lead Compound Targeting Xanthine Oxidase." *Chemico-Biological Interactions* 360: 109948.

Fan, S., R. Zhu, Y. Li, Y. Qiao et al. 2019. "Prenyl Bibenzyls Isolated from Chinese Liverwort *Radula amoena* and Their Cytotoxic Activities." *Phytochemistry Letters* 31: 53–57.

Fang, J. M., R. Li, Y. Zhang, P. K. Oduro et al. 2022. "Aristolone in *Nardostachys jatamansi* DC. Induces Mesenteric Vasodilation and Ameliorates Hypertension via Activation of the K_{atp} Channel and PDK1-Akt-eNOS Pathway." *Phytomedicine* 104: 154257.

Fang, X., L. Kang, Y. F. Qiu, Z. S. Li et al. 2023. "*Yersinia enterocolitica* in Crohn's Disease." *Frontiers in Cellular and Infection Microbiology* 13: 1129996.

Fareed, M. F., A. M. Haroon, S. A. Rabeh. 2008. "Antimicrobial Activity of Some Macrophytes from Lake Manzalah (Egypt)." *Pakistan Journal of Biological Sciences* 11 (21): 2454–63.

Fatima, R., A. Naim, S. Naeem. 2019. "Ligand Based Screening of Chemical Constituents from African Medicinal Plants for the Identification of MAOB Inhibitors." *Pakistan Journal of Pharmaceutical Sciences* 32 (3 suppl.): 1207–13.

Feld, H., D. S. Rycroft, J. Zapp. 2014. "Chromenes and Prenylated Benzoic Acid Derivatives from the Liverwort *Pedinophyllum interruptum*." *Zeitschrift für Naturforschung B* 59 (7): 825–28.

Feld, H. J., J. Zapp, H. Becker. 2003. "Secondary Metabolites from the Liverwort *Tylimanthus renifolius*." *Phytochemistry* 64 (8): 1335–40.

Fernandes, A. da Silva., L. B. Brito, G. A. R. Oliveira, E. R. A. Ferraz et al. 2019. "Evaluation of the Acute Toxicity, Phototoxicity and Embryotoxicity of a Residual Aqueous Fraction from Extract of the Antarctic moss *Sanionia uncinata*." *BMC Pharmacology & Toxicology* 20 (suppl 1): 77.

Fesenko, I., R. Azarkina, I. Kirov, A. Kniazev et al. 2019. "Phytohormone Treatment Induces Generation of Cryptic Peptides with Antimicrobial Activity in the Moss *Physcomitrella patens*." *BMC Plant Biology* 19 (1): 9.

Figueiredo, A. C., M. Sim-Sim, J. G. Barroso, L.G. Pedro et al. 2002. "Composition of the Essential Oil from the Liver *Marchesinia mackaii* (Hook.) S. F. Gray Grown in Portugal." *Journal of Essential Oil Research* 14 (6): 439–42.

Flowers, S. 1957. "Ethnobryology of the Gosiute Indians of Utah." *The Bryologist* 60: 11–14.

Frahm, J. P. 2004. "New Frontiers in Bryology and Lichenology: Recent Developments of Commercial Products from Bryophytes." *Bryologist* 107 (3): 277–83.

Frangedakis, E., M. Shimamura, J. C. Villarreal, F. W. Li et al. 2022. "The Hornworts: Morphology, Evolution and Development." *New Phytologist* 229 (2): 735–54.

Franquemont, C. 1990. "The Ethnobotany of Chinchero, an Andean Community in Southern Peru." *Fieldiana Botany* 24: 1–126.

Frediansyah, A., F. Sofyantoro, S. Alhumaid, A. A. Mutair et al. 2022. "Microbial Natural Products with Antiviral Activities, Including Anti-SARS-CoV-2: A Review." *Molecules* 27 (13): 4305.

Fu, P., S. Lin, L. Shan, M. Lu et al. 2009. "Constituents of the Moss *Polytrichum commune*." *Journal of Natural Products* 72 (7): 1335–37.

Fuchs, L. 1549. *De Historia Stirpium Commentarii Insignes*. Lugduni, France: Balthazarus Arnollet.

Fujii, K., D. Morita, K. J. Onoda, T. Kuroda et al. 2016. "Minimum Structural Requirements for Cell Membrane Leakage-Mediated Anti-MRSA Activity of Macrocyclic Bis(bibenzyl)s." *Bioorganic and Medicinal Chemistry Letters* 26 (9): 2324–27.

Fukada, R., J. Kawano, T. Tsuruta, T. Nonaka et al. 2023. "Two New Eremophilane-Type Sesquiterpenoids from Japanese Liverwort *Bazzania japonica*." *Chemistry and Biodiversity* 20 (4): e202300131.

Fukuyama, Y., and Y. Asakawa. 1991a. "Novel Neurotrophic Isocuparane-Type Sesquiterpene Dimers, Mastigophorenes A, B, C and D, Isolated from the Liverwort *Mastigophora diclados*." *Journal of the Chemical Society, Perkin Transactions* 1 (11): 2737–41.

Fukuyama, Y., and Y. Asakawa. 1991b. "Neurotrophic Secoaromadendrane-Type Sesquiterpenes from the Liverwort *Plagiochila fruticosa*." *Phytochemistry* 30: 4061–65.

Fukuyama, Y., M. Kubo, K. Harada. 2020. "The Search for, and Chemistry and Mechanism of, Neurotrophic Natural Products." *Journal of Natural Medicine* 74 (4): 648–71.

Fukuyama, Y., M. Tori, M. Wakamatsu, Y. Asakawa. 1988. "Norpinguisone Methyl Ester and Norpinguisanolide, Pinguisane-Type Norsesquiterpenoids from *Porella elegantula*." *Phytochemistry* 27 (11): 3557–61.

Furusawa, M., T. Hashimoto, Y. Noma, Y. Asakawa. 2006. "Isolation and Structures of New Cyclomyltaylane and ent-chamigrane-type Sesquiterpenoids from the Liverwort *Reboulia hemishaerica* and Their Biotransformation by the Fungus *Aspergillus niger*." *Chemical and Pharmaceutical Bulletin* (Tokyo) 54 (7): 996–1003.

Furuyama, Y., T. Motoyama, T. Nogawa, T. Kamakura et al. 2021. "Dihydropyriculol Produced by *Pyricularia oryzae* Inhibits the Growth of *Streptomyces griseus*." *Bioscience Biotechnology and Biochemistry* 85 (5): 1290–93.

Gahtori, D., and P. Chaturvedi. 2011. "Antifungal and Antibacterial Potential of Methanol and Chloroform Extracts of *Marchantia polymorpha* L." *Archives of Phytopathology and Plant Protection* 44: 726–31.

Gao, C. Y., X. Y. Ma, Z. Zhang, Q. S. Lu et al. 2022. "Asparaginase *Erwinia chrysanthemi* for Acute Lymphoblastic Leukemia and Lymphoblastic Lymphoma." *Drugs Today* (Barcelona) 58 (6): 261–71.

Gao, G. Q., G. W. Wang, H. K. Zhang. 2004. "Investigation of the Effect, Mechanism and Activity of *Rhodobryum roseum* on Curing Lack of Blood and Cardiovascular Disease." *Chinese Journal of Integrated Traditional and Western Medicine* 24: 929.

Gao, P., X. P. Huang, T. T. Liao, G. S. Li et al. 2019. "Daucosterol Induces Autophagic-Dependent Apoptosis in Prostate Cancer via JNK Activation." *BioScience Trends* 13 (2): 160–67.

Gaok, Y. X., X. J. Xu, S. Chang, Y. J. Wang et al. 2015. "Totarol Prevents Neuronal Injury In Vitro and Ameliorates Brain Ischemic Stroke: Potential Roles of Akt Activation and HO-1 Induction." *Toxicology and Applied Pharmacology* 289 (2): 142–54.

Garcia, D. G., C. F. G de Albuquerque, C. I. da Silva, R. Kiss et al. 2018. "Effect of Polygodial and Its Direct Derivatives on the Mammalian Na^+/K^+-ATPase Activity." *European Journal of Pharmacology* 831: 1–8.

Garrido, A., J. G. Ledezma, A. A. Durant-Archibold, N. S. Allen et al. 2019. "Chemical Profiling of Volatile Components of the Gametophyte and Sporophyte Stages of the Hornwort *Leiosporoceros dussi* (Leiosporocerotaceae) from Panama by HS-SPME-GC-MS." *Natural Product Communications* 14 (8): 1–4.

Gauvin-Bialecki, A., C. Ah-Peng, J. Smadja, D. Strasberg. 2010. "Fragrant Volatile Compounds in the Liverwort *Drepanolejeuna madagascariensis* (Steph.) Grolle: Approach by the HS-SPME Technique." *Chemistry and Biodiversity* 7 (3): 639–48.

Gawel-Beben, K., P. Osika, Y. Asakawa, B. Antosiewicz et al. 2019. "Evaluation of Anti-Melanoma and Tyrosinase Inhibitory Properties of Marchantin A, a Natural Macrocyclic Bisbibenzyl Isolated from Marchantia Species." *Phytochemistry Letters* 31: 192–95.

Geiger, H., and T. Seeger. 2000. "Triflavones and a Biflavone from the Moss *Rhizogonium distichum*." *Zeitschrift für Naturforschung Section C Journal of Biosciences* 55 (11–12): 870–73.

Geis, W., and H. Becker. 2000. "Sesqui- and Diterpenes from the Liverwort *Gackstroemia decipiens*." *Phytochemistry* 53 (2): 247–52.

Geis, W., and H. Becker. 2001. "Odoriferous Sesquiterpenoids from the Liverwort *Gackstroemia decipiens*." *Flavour and Fragrance Journal* 16 (6): 422–24.

Gellerman, J. L., W. H. Anderson, D. G. Richardson, H. Schlenk. 1975. "Distribution of Arachidonic and Eixosapentaenoic Acids in the Lipids of Mosses." *Biochimica et Biophysica Acta* 388 (2): 277–90.

Gerard, J. 1597. *The Herball or Generall Historie of Plants*. London: J. Norton.

Gilabert, M., K. Marcinkevicius, S. Andujar, M. Schiavone et al. 2015. "Sesqui- and Triterpenoids from the Liverwort *Lepidozia chordulifera* Inhibitors of Bacterial Biofilm and Elastase Activity of Human Pathogenic Bacteria." *Phytomedicine* 22 (1): 77–85.

Gilabert, M., A. N. Ramos, M. M. Schiavone, M. E. Arena et al. 2011. "Bioactive Sesqui- and Diterpenoids from the Argentine Liverwort *Porella chilensis*." *Journal of Natural Products* 74 (4): 574–79.

Giuliani, C., G. Pieraccini, C. Santilli, C. Tani et al. 2020. "Anatomical Investigation and GC/MC Analysis of 'Coco de Mer,' *Lodoicea maldivica* (Arecaceae)." *Chemistry and Biodiversity* 17 (11): e2000707.

Glime, J. M. 2007. "Economic and Ethnic Uses of Bryophytes." In *Bryophytes: Mosses*. Vol. 27 of *Flora of North America*, edited by Flora of North America Editorial Committee. United Kingdom: Oxford University Press.

Glime, J. M. 2013. "Household and Personal Uses." Chapter 1-1 in *q*, vol. 5. ebook: Michigan Technological University and the International Association of Bryologists.

Glime, J. M. 2017. "Medical Uses: Medical Conditions." Chap. 2. in *Bryophyte Ecology*, vol. 5. ebook: Michigan Technological University and the International Association of Bryologists.

Glime, J. M. 2022. "Bryophyte Defenses Against Bacteria." Chap. 19-3 in *Bryophyte Ecology*, vol. 2. ebook: Michigan Technological University and the International Association of Bryologists.

Gomes, M. P., J. C. M de Brito, E. M. Bicalho, J. G. Silva et al. 2018. "Ciprofloxacin vs. Temperature: Antibiotic Toxicity in the Free-Floating Liverwort *Ricciocarpus natans* from a Climate Change Perspective." *Chemosphere* 202: 410–19.

Grecco, S. D, E. G. A. Martins, N. Girola, C. R. de Figueiredo et al. 2015. "Chemical Composition and In Vitro Cytotoxic Effects of the Essential Oil from *Nectandra leucantha* Leaves." *Pharmaceutical Biology* 53 (1): 133–37.

Greeshma, G., K. Dineshbabu, K. Murugan. 2016. "Chromatographic Analysis (RP-HPLC) of Phenolic Acids and FTIR Spectra in *Brachythecium buchananii* (Hook.) A. Jaeger." *Journal of Phytochemistry Photon* 117: 410–16.

Greeshma, G., and K. Murugan. 2018. "Comparison of Antimicrobial Potentiality of the Purified Terpenoids from Two Moss Species *Thuidium tamariscellum* (C. Muell.) Bosch. & Sande-Lac and *Brachythecium buchananii* (Hook.) A. Jaeger." *Journal of Analytical and Pharmaceutical Research* 7 (5): 530–38.

Grohmann, G. 1989. *The Plant, Vol. 1.* The Biodynamic Farming and Gardening Association.

Guichardant, M., M. Michel, C. Borel, L. Fay et al. 1992. "Effects of 9, 12, 15-Octadecatrien-6-Ynoic Acid on Metabolism of Arachidonic Acid in Platelets and on Platelet Aggregation." *Thrombosis Research* 65 (6): 687–98.

Gulabani, A. 1974. "Bryophytes as Economic Plants." *Botanica* 14: 73–75.

Guo, C. Q., D. Edwards, P. C. Wu, J. G. Duckett et al. 2012. "*Riccardiothallus devonicus* gen. et sp. nov., the Earliest Simple Thalloid Liverwort from the Lower Devonian of Yunnan, China." *Review of Palaeobotany and Palynology* 176–177: 35–40.

Guo, D. X., Y. Du, Y. Y. Wang, L. M. Sun et al. 2009. "Secondary Metabolites from the Liverwort *Ptilidium pulcherrimum*." *Natural Product Communications* 4 (10): 1319–22.

Guo, D. X., F. Xiang, X. N. Wang et al. 2010. "Labdane Diterpenoids and Highly Methoxylated Bibenzyls from the Liverwort Frullania Inouei." *Phytochemistry* 71: 1573–78.

Guo, L., J. Z. Wu, T. Han, T. Cao et al. 2008. "Chemical Composition, Antifungal and Antitumor Properties of Ether Extracts of *Scapania verrucosa* Heeg. and Its Endophytic Fungus *Chaetomium fusiforme*." *Molecules* 13 (9): 2114–25.

Guo, M., G. B. Ding, S. J. Guo, Z. Y. Li et al. 2015. "Isolation and Antitumor Efficacy Evaluation of a Polysaccharide from *Nostoc commune* Vauch." *Food and Function* 6 (9): 3035–44.

Guo, M., G. B. Ding, P. Yang, L. C. Zhang et al. 2016. "Migration Suppression of Small Cell Lung Cancer by Polysaccharides from *Nostoc commune* Vaucher." *Journal of Agricultural and Food Chemistry* 64 (32): 6277–85.

Guo, M., and Z. Y. Li. 2019. "Polysaccharides Isolated from *Nostoc commune* Vaucher Inhibit Colitis-Associated Colon Tumorigenesis in Mice and Modulate Gut Microbiota." *Food and Function* 10 (10): 6873–81.

Guo, M., Z. Y. Li, Y. X. Huang, M. G. Shi. 2019. "Polysaccharides from *Nostoc commune* Vaucher Activate Macrophages via NF-kB and AKT/$JNK_{1/2}$ Pathways to Suppress Colorectal Cancer Growth In Vivo." *Food and Function* 10 (7): 4269–79.

Guo, X. L., P. Leng, Y. Yang, L. G. Yu et al. 2008. "Plagiochin E, a Botanic-Derived Phenolic Compound, Reverses Fungal Resistance to Fluconazole Relating to the Efflux Pump." *Journal of Applied Microbiology* 104 (3): 831–38.

Guo, Y. X., Z. M. Lin, M. J. Wang, Y. W. Dong et al. 2016. "Jungermannenone A and B Induce ROS- and Cell Cycle-Dependent Apoptosis in Prostate Cancer Cell in Vitro." *Acta Physiologica Sinica* 37 (6): 814–24.

Guo, Z. F., G. M. Bi, Y. H. Zhang, J. H. Li et al. 2020. "Rare Benzonaphthoxanthenones from Chinese Folk Herbal Remedy *Polytrichum commune* and Their Anti-Neuroinflammatory Activities In Vitro." *Bioorganic Chemistry* 102: 104087.

Gupta, A., S. S. Thakur, P. L. Uniyal, R. Gupta. 2001. "A Survey of Bryophytes for Presence of Cholinesterase." *American Journal of Botany* 88 (12): 2133–35.

Gupta, K.G., and B. Singh. 1971. "Occurrence of Antibacterial Activity in Moss Extracts." *Research Bulletin*, Punjab University, 22: 237–39.

Gupta, K. K., K. K. Sharma, H. Chandra. 2022. "*Micrococcus luteus* Strain CGK112 Isolated from Cow Dung Demonstrated Efficient Biofilm-Forming Ability and Degradation Potential Toward High-Density Polyethylene (HDPE)." *Archives of Microbiology* 204 (7): 402.

Hackl, T., W. A. König, H. Muhle. 2004. "Isogermacrene A, a Proposed Intermediate in Sesquiterpene Biosynthesis." *Phytochemistry* 65 (15): 2261–75.

Hackl, T., W. A. König, H. Muhle. 2006. "Three Ent-eudesmenones from the Liverwort *Plagiochila bifaria*." *Phytochemistry* 67 (8): 778–83.

Halsor, M. J., A. Liamer S. Pandur, I. L. U. Ræder et al. 2019. "Draft Genome Sequence of the Symbiotically Competent Cyanobacterium *Nostoc* sp. Strain KVJ20." *Microbiology Resource Announcements* 8 (45): e01190-19.

Ham, J. Y., W. Lim, K. W. Kim, Y. M. Heo et al. 2019. "Gentisyl Alcohol Inhibits Proliferation and Induces Apoptosis via Mitochondrial Dysfunction and Regulation of MAPK and PI3K/AKT Pathways in Epithelial Ovarian Cancer Cells." *Marine Drugs* 17 (6): 331.

Han, B., P. Jiang, W. Y. Liu, H. S. Xu et al. 2018. "Role of Daucosterol Linoleate on Breast Cancer: Studies on Apoptosis and Metastasis." *Journal of Agricultural and Food Chemistry* 66 (24): 6031–41.

Han, H. Y., A. M. M. Alsayed, Y. Wang, Q. Yan et al. 2023. "Discovery of ß-cyclocitral-Derived Mono-carbonyl Curcumin Analogs as Anti-Hepatocellular Carcinoma Agents via Suppression of MAPK Signaling Pathway." *Bioorganic Chemistry* 132: 106358.

Han, J. J., Y. Li, J. C. Zhou, X. Y. Qi et al. 2021. "Dolabrane Diterpenoids from the Chinese Liverwort *Notoscyphus lutescens*." *Journal of Natural Products* 84 (11): 2929–36.

Han, J. J., Y. Li, J. C. Zhou, J. Z. Zhang et al. 2021. "Terpenoids from Chinese Liverworts *Scapania* spp." *Journal of Natural Products* 84 (4): 1210–15.

Han J. J., J. Z. Zhang, R. X. Zhu, Y. Li et al. 2018. "Plagiochianins A and B, Two Ent-2,3-seco-Aromadendrane Derivatives from the Liverwort *Plagiochila duthiana*." *Organic Letters* 20 (20): 6550–53.

Haq, I., and A. Kilaru. 2020. "An Endocannabinoid Catabolic Enzyme FAAH and Its Paralogs in an Early Land Plant Reveal Evolutionary and Functional Relationship with Eukaryotic Orthologs." *Scientific Reports* 10 (1): 3115.

Harinantenaina, L., and Y. Asakawa. 2007. "Chemical Constituents of Malagasy Liverworts. 6. A Myltaylane Caffeate with Nitric Oxide Inhibitory Activity from *Bazzania nitida*." *Journal of Natural Products* 70 (5): 856–58.

Harinantenaina, L., R. Kurata, S. Takaoka, Y. Asakawa. 2006. "Chemical Constituents of Malagasy Liverworts: Cyclomyltaylanoids from *Bazzania madagassa*." *Phytochemistry* 67 (24): 2616–22.

Harinantenaina, L., D. N. Quang, T. Nishizawa, T. Hashimoto et al. 2005. "Bis(bibenzyls) from Liverworts Inhibit Lipopolysaccharide-Inducible NOS in RAW 264.7 Cells: A Study of Structure-Activity Relationships and Molecular Mechanism." *Journal of Natural Products* 68: 1779–81.

Harinantenaina, L., R. Kurata, Y. Asakawa. 2005. "Chemical Constituents of Malagasy Liverworts, Part III: Sesquiterpenoids from *Bazzania decrescens* and *Bazzania madagassa*." *Chemical and Pharmaceutical Bulletin* (Tokyo) 53 (5); 515–18.

Harinantenaina, L., Y. Takahara, T. Nishizawa, C. Kohchi et al. 2006. "Chemical Constituents of Malagasy Liverworts, Part V: Prenyl Bibenzyls and Clerodane Diterpenoids with Nitric Oxide Inhibitory Activity from *Radula appressa* and *Thysananthus spathulistipus*." *Chemical and Pharmaceutical Bulletin* 54 (7): 1046–49.

Harrigan, G. G., A. Ahmad, N. Baj, T. E. Glass et al. 1993. "Bioactive and Other Sesquiterpenoids from *Porella cordaeana*." *Journal of Natural Products* 56 (6): 921–25.

Harris, E. S. J. 2008. "Traditional Uses and Folk Classification of Bryophytes." *Bryologist* 111 (2): 169–217.

Hart, J. A. 1981. "The Ethnobotany of the Northern Cheyenne Indians of Montana." *Journal of Ethnopharmacology* 4: 1–55.

Hayashi, S., A. Matsuo. 1970. "Bazzanenol, a New Sesquiterpene Alcohol Having a Skeleton of Bicyclo (5.3.1) Undecane System from Hepaticae, *Bazzania pompeana* (Lac.) Mitt." *Experientia* 26 (4): 347–48.

Hashimoto, T., H. Tanaka, Y. Asakawa. 1994. "Stereostructure of Plagiochiline A and Conversion of Plagiochiline A and Stearoylvelutinal into Hot-tasting Compounds by Human Saliva." *Chemical and Pharmaceutical Bulletin* 42 (7): 1542–44.

Hegazy, M. E. F., A. M. Gamal-Eldeen, A. el Halawany, B. H. Mohamed. 2012. "Steroidal Metabolites Transformed by *Marchantia polymorpha* Cultures Block Breast Cancer Estrogen Biosynthesis." *Cell Biochemistry and Biophysics* 63 (1): 85–96.

Hegde, P., B. R. Sindhura, S. Ballal, B. M. Swamy et al. 2021. "*Rhizoctonia bataticola* Lectin Induces Apoptosis and Inhibits Metastasis in Ovarian Cancer Cells by Interacting with CA 125 Antigen Differentially Expressed on Ovarian Cells." *Glycoconjugate Journal* 38 (6): 669–88.

Heinrichs, J., A. Scheben, G. E. Lee, J. Vana et al. 2015. "Molecular and Morphological Evidence Challenges the Records of the Extant Liverwort *Ptilidium pulcherrimum* in Eocene Baltic Amber." *PLoS One* 10 (11): e0140977.

Hennessey, W. M., ed. and trans. (1871) 2012. *The Annals of Loch Cé: A Chronicle of Irish Affairs from AD 1014 to AD 1590*, vol. 2. Cambridge University Press.

Hernández-Rodríguez, E., C. Delgadillo-Moya. 2020. "The Ethnobotany of Bryophytes in Mexico." *Botanical Sciences* 99: 13–27.

Hernández-Rodriguez, E., and J. López-Santiago. 2021. "Uses and Traditional Knowledge of *Dendropogonella rufescens* (Bryophyta: Cryphaeaceae) in a Zapotec Community of Southeastern Mexico." *Botanical Sciences* 100: 153–68.

Hernick, L. V., E. Landing, K. E. Bartowski. 2008. "Earth's Oldest Liverworts *Metzgeriothallus sharonae* sp. nov. from the Middle Devonian (Givetian) of Eastern New York, USA." *Review of Palaeobotany and Palynology* 148: 154–62.

Herrick, J. W. 1995. *Iroquois Medical Botany*. Syracuse, NY: Syracuse University Press.

Hertewich, U., J. Zapp, H. Becker, K. P. Adam. 2001. "Biosynthesis of a Hopane Triterpene and Three Diterpenes in the Liverwort *Fossombronia alaskana*." *Phytochemistry* 58 (7): 1049–54.

Hertewich, U. M., J. Zapp, H. Becker. 2003. "Secondary Metabolites from the Liverwort *Jamesoniella colorata*." *Phytochemistry* 63 (2): 227–33.

Hieu, H. V., V. B. Tatipamula, K. N. Killari, S. T. Koneru. 2022. "HPTLC Analysis, Antioxidant and Antidiabetic Activities of Ethanol Extract of Moss *Fissidens grandiflora*." *Indian Journal of Pharmaceutical Sciences* 82: 449–55.

Hijaz, M., S. Das, I. Mert, A. Gupta et al. 2016. "Folic Acid Tagged Nanoceria as a Novel Therapeutic Agent in Ovarian Cancer." *BMC Cancer* 16 (1): 220.

Hoffman, A., and F. Shahidi. 2009. "Paclitaxel and Other Taxanes in Hazelnut." *Journal of Functional Foods* 1 (1): 33–37.

Hoof, L. van, D. A. Berghe, P. E. Vanden, A. J. Vlietnick. "Antimicrobial and Antiviral Screening of Bryophyta." *Fitoterapia* 52: 223–29.

Hong, M. J., T. H. Kim, K. Sowndhararajan, S. M. Kim. 2021. "Chemical Composition of Common Liverwort (*Marchantia polymorpha* L.) and Racomitrium Moss (*Racomitrium canescens* (Hedw.) Brid) in Korea." *Weed and Turfgrass Science* 10 (4): 365–74.

Hong, W. S. 1980. "A Study of the Distribution of *Diplophyllum* in Western North America." *Bryologist* 83: 497–504.

Hook, V., L. Funkestein, J. Wegrzyn, S. Bark et al. 2012. "Cysteine Cathepsins in the Secretory Vesicle Produce Active Peptides: Cathepsin L Generates Peptide Neurotransmitters and Cathepsin B Produces Beta-amyloid of Alzheimer's Disease." *Biochimica et Biophysica Acta* 2824 (1): 89–104.

Hossen, S. M. M., M. J. Islam, R. Hossain, A. Barua et al. 2021. "CNS Anti-Depressant, Anxiolytic and Analgesic Effects of *Ganoderma applanatum* (Mushroom) along with Ligand-Receptor Binding Screening Provide New Insights: Multi-Disciplinary Approaches." *Biochemical and Biophysics Reports* 27: 101062.

Hou, T., Y. Z. Wang, W. C. Dan, Y. Wei et al. 2023. "β-Ionone Represses Renal Cell Carcinoma Progression through Activating LKB1/AMPK-Triggered Autophagy." *Journal of Biochemical and Molecular Toxicology* 37 (6): e23331.

Hsieh, T. C., X. H. Lu, Z. R. Wang, J. M. Wu. 2006. "Induction of Quinone Reductase NQ01 by Resveratrol in Human K562 Cells Involves the Antioxidant Response Element ARE and Is Accompanied by Nuclear Translocation of Transcription Factor Nrf2." *Medicinal Chemistry* 2 (3): 275–85.

Hu, H. T., X. Y. Liu, P. L. Zhang, H. M. Gao et al. 2020. "Novel Secondary Metabolites from the Endobryophytic Fungus *Botrysphaeria laricina* and Their Biological Activity." *Fitoterapia* 143: 104599.

Hu, Y., D. H. Guo, P. Liu, K. Rahman et al. 2009. "Antioxidant Effects of a *Rhodobryum roseum* Extract and Its Active Components in Isoproterenol-Induced Myocardial Injury in Rats and Cardiac Myocytes against Oxidative Stress-Triggered Damage." *Pharmazie* 64 (1): 53–57.

Hu, Z. Y, D. L. Zhang, D. Wang, B. Sun et al. 2016. "Bisbibenzyls, Novel Proteasome Inhibitors, Suppress Androgen Receptor Transcriptional Activity and Expression Accompanied by Activation of Autophagy in Prostate Cancer LNCaP Cells." *Pharmaceutical Biology* 54 (2): 364–74.

Hu, T., H. Feng, Y.P. Zhao, W. Yang et al. 2021. "Biochemical and Functional Characterization of Two Microbial Type Terpene Synthases from Moss *Stereodon submimpoens*." *Plant Physiology and Biochemistry* 166: 750–60.

Huang, F. Y., Y. N. Li, W. L. Mei, H. F. Dai et al. 2012. "Cytochalasin D, a Tropical Fungal Metabolite, Inhibits CT26 Tumor Growth and Angiogenesis." *Asian Pacific Journal of Tropical Medicine* 5 (3): 169–74.

Huang, W. J., C. L. Wu, C. W. Lin, L. L. Chi et al. 2010. "Marchantin A, a Cyclic Bis(bibenzyl Ether), Isolated from the Liverwort *Marchantia emarginata* subsp. Tosana Induces Apoptosis in Human MCF-7 Breast Cancer Cells." *Cancer Letters* 291: 108–19.

Huang, W. S., J. T. Yang, C. C. Lu, S. F. Chang et al. 2015. "Fulvic Acid Attenuates Resistin-Induced Adhesion of HCT-116 Colorectal Cancer Cells to Endothelial Cells." *International Journal of Molecular Sciences* 16 (12): 29370–82.

Hueber, F. 1961. "Hepaticites devonicus: A New Fossil Liverwort from the Devonian of New York." Annals of the Missouri Botanical Garden 48 (2): 125–31.

Huneck, S. 1983. "Chemistry and Biochemistry of Bryophytes." In *New Manual of Bryology*, edited by R. M. Shuster. Nichinan, Japan: Hattori Botanical Laboratory.

Huneck, S, Y. Asakawa, Z. Taira, A. F. Cameron et al. 1983. "Gymnocolin, a New Cis-clerodane Diterpenoid from the Liverwort *Gymnocolea inflata*. Crystal Structure Analysis." *Tetrahedron Letters* 24: 115–16.

Hussain, S., F. Al-Nsour, A. B. Rice, J. Marshburn et al. 2012. "Cerium Dioxide Nanoparticles Induce Apoptosis and Autophagy in Human Peripheral Blood Monocytes." *ACS Nano* 6 (7): 5820–29.

Hutschenreuther, A., C. Birkemeyer, K. Grötzinger, R. K. Straubinger et al. 2010. "Growth Inhibiting Activity of Volatile Oil from *Cistus creticus* L. against *Borrelia burgdorferi* s.s. in Vitro." *Pharmazie* 65 (4): 290–95.

Iglesias-Aguirre, C. E., F. Vallejo, D. Beltrán, E. Aguilar-Aguilar et al. 2022. "Lunularin Producers Versus Non-Producers: Novel Human Metabotypes Associated with the

Metabolism of Resveratrol by the Gut Microbiota." *Journal of Agricultural and Food Chemistry* 70 (34): 10521–31.

Ikeda, M., Y. Kurotobi, A. Namikawa, S. Kuranuki et al. 2011. "Norlichexanthone Isolated from Fungus P16 Promotes the Secretion and Expression of Adiponectin in Cultured ST-13 Adipocytes." *Medicinal Chemistry* 7 (4): 250–56.

Ikegami, S., M. Nakamura, T. Honda, T. Yamamura et al. 2023. "Efficacy of 1-kestose Supplementation in Patients with Mild to Moderate Ulcerative Colitis: A Randomised, Double-Blind, Placebo-Controlled Pilot Study." *Alimentary Pharmacology and Therapeutics* 57 (11): 1249–57.

Ikram, N. K. B. K., A. B. Kashkooli, A. V. Peramuna, A. R. van der Krol et al. 2017. "Stable Production of the Antimalarial Drug Artemisinin in the Moss *Physcomitrella patens*." *Frontiers in Bioengineering and Biotechnology* 5: 47.

Ilhan, S., F. Saveroglu, F. Colak, C. F. Iscen et al. 2006. "Antimicrobial Activity of *Palustriella commutata* (Hedw.) Ochyra Extracts (Bryophyta)." *Turkish Journal of Biology* 30: 149–52.

Ingólfsdóttir, K., G. F. Gudmundsdóttir, H. M. Ogmundsdóttir, K. Paulus et al. 2002. "Effects of Tenuiorin and Methyl Orsellinate from the Lichen *Peltigera leucophlebia* on 5-/15-lipogenases and Proliferation of Malignant Cell Lines In Vitro." *Phytomedicine* 9 (7): 654–58.

Irita, H., T. Hashimoto, Y. Fukuyama, Y. Asakawa. 2000. "Herbertane-Type Sesquiterpenoids from the Liverwort *Herbertus sakuraii*." *Phytochemistry* 55 (3): 247–53.

Islam, M. T., M. Martorell, C. González-Contreras, M. Villagran et al. 2023. "An Updated Overview of Anticancer Effects of Alternariol and Its Derivatives: Underlying Molecular Mechanisms." *Frontiers in Pharmacology* 14: 1099380.

Isoe, S. 1983. "Terpenedials. Biological Activity and Synthetic Study." In *Proceedings Papers II*, 849–50. 48th Annual Meeting of the Chemical Society of Japan.

Itoh, D., R. P. Karunagoda, T. Fushie, K. Katoh, K. Nabeta. 2000. "Nonequivalent Labeling of the Phytyl Side Chain of Chlorophyll A in Callus of the Hornwort *Anthoceros punctatus*." *Journal of Natural Products* 53 (8): 1090–93.

Ivanova, V., M. Kolarova, K. Aleksieva, K.J. Dornberger et al. 2007. "Sanionins: Anti-Inflammatory and Antibacterial Agents with Weak Cytotoxicity from the Antarctic Moss *Sanionia georgico-uncinata*." *Preparative Biochemistry and Biotechnology* 37 (4): 343–52.

Ivkovic, I., M. Novakovic, M. Veljjic, M. Mojsin et al. 2021. "Bis-Bibenzyls from the Liverwort *Pellia Endiviifolia* and Their Biological Activity." *Plants* 10 (6): 1063.

Iwai, Y., K. Murakami, Y. Gomi, T. Hashimoto et al. 2011. "Anti-Influenza Activity of Marchantins, Macrocyclic Bisbibenzyls Contained in Liverworts." *PLoS One* 6 (5): e19825.

Jaikhan, P., C. Boonyarat, K. Arunrungvichian, P. Taylor. 2016. "Design and Synthesis of Nicotinic Acetylcholine Receptor Antagonists and the Effect on Cognitive Impairment." *Chemical Biology and Drug Design* 87 (1): 39–56.

Jaiswal, R., T. K. Bleuria, R. Mohan, S. K. Mahajan et al. 2007. "Totarol Inhibits Bacterial Cytokinesis by Perturbing the Assembly Dynamics of FtsZ." *Biochemistry* 46 (14): 4211–20.

Jambi, E. J., and F. A. Alshubaily. 2022. "Shilajit Potentiates the Effect of Chemotherapeutic Drugs and Mitigates Metastasis Induced Liver and Kidney Damages in Osteosarcoma Rats." *Saudi Journal of Biological Sciences* 29 (9): 103393.

Jang, J., S. M. Kim, S. M. Yee, E. M. Kim et al. 2019. "Daucosterol Suppresses Dextran Sulfate Sodium (DDS)-Induced Colitis in Mice." *International Immunopharmacology* 72: 124–30.

Janovec, L., J. Janocková, M. Matejová, E. Konkol'ová et al. 2019. "Proliferation Inhibition of Novel Diphenylamine Derivatives." *Bioorganic Chemistry* 83: 487–99.

Jarukas, L., L. Ivanauskas, G. Kasparaviciene, J. Baranauskaite et al. 2021. "Determination of Organic Compounds, Fulvic Acid, Humic Acid, and Humin in Peat and Sapropel Alkaline Extracts." *Molecules* 26 (10): 2995.

Jensen, J. S., R. E. Omarsdottir, J. B. Thorsteinsdottir, H. M. Ogmundsdottir et al. 2012. "Synergistic Cytotoxic Effect of the Microtubule Inhibitor from Marchantia Polymorpha and the Aurora Kinase Inhibitor MLN8237 on Breast Cancer Cells in Vitro." *Planta Medica* 78: 448–54.

Ji, M., Y. Shi, H. Lou. 2011. "Overcoming the P-Glycoprotein-Mediated Multidrug Resistance in K562/A02 Cells Using Riccardin F and Pakyonol, Bisbibenzyl Derivatives from Liverworts." *Bioscience Trends* 5: 192–97.

Jian-Bo, X., R. Feng-Lian, M. Xu. 2005. "Anti-Hepatitis B Virus Activity of Flavonoids from *Marchantia convoluta. Iran Journal of Pharmacology and Therapeutics* 42 (2): 128–31.

Jiang, H., J. Sun, Q. Xu, S. Liu et al. 2013. "Marchantin M: A Novel Inhibitor of Proteasome Induces Autophagic Cell Death in Prostate Cancer Cells." *Cell Death Discovery* 3: e761.

Jiang, L. H., X. L. Yuan, N. Y. Yang, L. Ren et al. 2015. "Daucosterol Protects Neurons against Oxygen-Glucose Deprivation/Reperfusion-Mediated Injury by Activating IGF1 Signaling Pathway." *Journal of Steroid Biochemistry and Molecular Biology* 152: 45–52.

Jimenez-Aleman, G. H., V. Castro, A. Londaitsbehere, et al. 2021. "SARS-CoV-2 Fears Green: The Chlorophyll Catabolite Pheophorbide A Is a Potent Antiviral." *Pharmaceuticals* (Basel) 14 (10): 1048.

Jin, X. M., C. C. Wang, L. Wang. 2020. "Costunolide Inhibits Osteosarcoma Growth and Metastasis via Suppressing STAT3 Signal Pathway." *Biomedicine and Pharmacotherapy* 121: 109659.

Jin, Y., M. A. Tomeh, P. Zhang, M. Z. Su et al. 2023. "Microfluidic Fabrication of Photo-Responsive Ansamitocin P-3 Loaded Liposomes for the Treatment of Breast Cancer." *Nanoscale* 15 (8): 3780–95.

Jockovic, N., P. B. Andrade, P. Valentao, M. Sabovljevic. 2008. "HPLC-DAD of Phenolics in Bryophtyes *Lunularia cruciata, Brachytheciastrum velutinum* and *Kindbergia praelonga*." *Journal of the Serbian Chemical Society* 73 (12): 1161–67.

Joshi, B. P., V. V. Bhandare, M. Vankawaia, P. Patel et al. 2022. "Friedelin, a Novel Inhibitor of CYP17A1 in Prostate Cancer from *Cassia tora*." *Journal of Biomolecular Structure and Dynamics* 14: 1–26.

Joshi, S., S. Singh, R. Sharma, S. Vats et al. 2023. "Gas Chromatography-Mass Spectrometry (GC-MS) Profiling of Aqueous Ethanol Fraction of *Plagiochasma appendiculatum* Lehm. & Lindenb. and *Sphagnum fimbriatum* Wilson for Probable Antiviral Potential." *Vegetos* 36: 87–92.

Joshi, S., S. Singh, R. Sharma, S. Vats et al. 2022. "Phyochemical Screening and Antioxidant Potential of *Plagiochasma appendiculatum* Lehm. & Lindenb. and *Sphagnum fimbriatum* Wilson." *Plant Science Today* 9 (4): 986–90.

Joung, Y. H., E. J. Lim, M. S. Kim, S. D. Lim et al. 2008. "Enhancement of Hypoxia-Induced Apoptosis of Human Breast Cancer Cells via STAT5b by Momilactone B." *International Journal of Oncology* 33 (3): 477–84.

Jung, H., H. J. Kim, E. S. Choi, J. Y. Lee et al. 2021. "Effectiveness of Oral Phloroglucinol as a Premedication for Unsedated Esophagogastroduodenoscopy: A Prospective, Double-Blinded, Placebo-Controlled, Randomized Trial." *PLoS One* 16 (8): e0255016.

Kahriman, N., T. Ozdemir, T. B. Cansu, C. Volga. 2009. "Essential Oils in Mosses (*Brachythecium salebrosum*, *Eurhynchium pulchellum* and *Plagiomnium undulatum*) Grown in Turkey." *Asian Journal of Chemistry* 21 (7): 5505–09.

Kamada, T., M. L. Johanis, S. Y. Ng, C. S. Phan et al. 2020. "A New Epi-Neovarrucosane-Type Diterpenoid from the Liverwort *Pleurozia subinflata* in Borneo." *Natural Products and Bioprospecting* 10 (1): 51–56.

Kamory, E., G. M. Keseru, B. Papp. 1995. "Isolation and Antibacterial Activity of Marchantin A, A Cyclic Bis(bibenzyl) Constituent of Hungarian *Marchantia polymorpha*." *Planta Medica* 61 (4): 387–88.

Kandpal, V., P. Chaturvedi, K. Negi, S. Gupta et al. 2016. "Evaluation of Antibiotic and Biochemical Potential of Bryophytes from Kumaun Hills and Tarai Belt of Himalayas." *International Journal of Pharmacy and Pharmaceutical Sciences* 8: 65–68.

Kang, D. Y., S. P. Nipin, P. Darvin, Y. H. Joung et al. 2017. "Momilactone B Inhibits Ketosis In Vitro by Regulating the ANGPTL3-LPL Pathway and Inhibiting HMGCS2." *Animal Biotechnology* 28 (3): 189–97.

Kang, S. J., S. H. Kim, P. Liu, E. Jovel et al. 2007. "Antibacterial Activities of Some Mosses Including *Hylocomium splendens* from South Western British Columbia." *Fitoterapia* 78 (5): 373–76.

Kang, Y. H., and J. M. Pezzuto. 2004. "Induction of Quinone Reductase as a Primary Screen for Natural Product Anticarcinogens." *Methods in Enzymology* 382: 380k–414.

Kang, Y. Q., J. C. Zhou, P. H. Fan, S. Q. Wang et al. 2015. "Scapaundulin C, a Novel Labdane Diterpenoid Isolated from Chinese Liverwort *Scapania undulata*, Inhibits Acetylcholinesterase Activity." *Chinese Journal of Natural Medicine* 13: 933–36.

Kara, R., C. Aydin, S. B. Diler. 2020. "Cytotoxic and Genotoxic Activity of Turkish Pale Liverwort (*Chiloscyphus polyantos* (L.) Corda) Against Human Periferal (*sic*) Blood Lymphocytes." *Anatolian Bryology* 6 (1): 1–7.

Karaoglu, S. A., S. Biyik, C. Nisbet, R. Akpinar et al. 2023. "Use of *Dicranum polysetum* Extract Against Paenibacillus Larvae Causing American Foulbrood under In Vivo and In Vitro Conditions." *International Microbiology* 26 (4): 1087–1101.

Karim, F. A., M. Suleiman, A. Rahmat, M. F. A. Bakar. 2014. "Phytochemicals, Antioxidant and Antiproliferative Properties of Five Moss Species from Sabah, Malaysia." *International Journal of Pharmacy and Pharmaceutical Sciences* 6: 292–97.

Karpinski, T. M., and A. Adamczak. 2017. "Antibacterial Activity of Ethanolic Extracts of Some Moss Species." *Herba Polonica* 63: 3.

Katariya, L., P. B. Ramesh, T. Gopalappa, S. Desireddy et al. 2017. "Fungus-Farming Termites Selectively Bury Weedy Fungi That Smell Different from Crop Fungi." *Journal of Chemical Ecology* 43 (10): 986–95.

Kaur, S., P. Kumar, D. Kumar, M. D. Kharya et al. 2013. "Parasympathomimetic Effect of Shilajit Accounts for Relaxation of Rat Corpus Cavernosum." *American Journal of Men's Health* 7 (2): 119–27.

Kenmoku, H., H. Tada, M. Oogushi, T. Esumi et al. 2014. "Seed Dormancy Breaking Diterpenoids from the Liverwort *Plagiochila sciophila* and Their Differentiation Inducing Activity in Human Promyelocytic Leukemia HL-60 Cells." *Natural Product Communications* 9 (7): 915–20.

Khan, M. M., Q. A. Bhatti, M. Akhlaq, M. Ishaq et al. 2022. "Assessment of Antimicrobial Potential of *Plagiochasma rupestre* Coupled with Healing Clay Bentonite and AGNPS." *BioMed Research International* 2022: 4264466.

Khatami, Z., S. Herdlinger, P. Sarkhail, M. Zehi et al. 2020. "Isolation and Characterization of Aceytylcholinesterase Inhibitors from *Piper longum* and Binding Mode Predictions." *Planta Medica* 86 (15): 1118–24.

Kim, D. Y., and B. Y. Choi. 2019. "Costunolide—A Bioactive Sesquiterpene Lactone with Diverse Therapeutic Potential." *International Journal of Molecular Sciences* 20 (12): 2926.

Kim, S. J., H. R. Park, E. Park, S. C. Lee. 2007. "Cytotoxic and Antitumor Activity of Momilactone B from Rice Hulls." *Journal of Agricultural and Food Chemistry* 55: 1702–6.

Kim, S. Y., M. J. Hong, T. H. Kim, K. Y. Lee et al. 2021. "Anti-Inflammatory Effect of Liverwort (*Marchantia polymorpha* L.) and Racomitrium Moss (*Racomitrium canescens* (Hedw.) Brid.) Growing in Korea." *Plants* (Basel) 10 (10): 2075.

Kim, Y. C., V. da S. Bolzani, N. Baj, A. A. Gunatilaka et al. 1996. "A DNA-Damaging Sesquiterpene and Other Constituents from *Frullania nisquallensis*." *Planta Medica* 62 (1): 61–63.

Kimb, S. H. et al. 2007. "Antibacterial Activities of Some Mosses including *Hylocomium splendens* from South Western British Columbia." Institute for Aboriginal Health 78 (5): 373–76.

Kimmerer, R. W. 2003. *Gathering Moss: A Natural and Cultural History of Mosses.* Corvallis: Oregon State University Press.

Kirisanth, A., M. N. M. Nafras, R. K. Dissanayake, J. Wjayabandara. 2020. "Antimicrobial and Alpha-Amylase Inhibitory Activities of Organic Extracts of Selected Sri Lankan Bryophytes." *Evidence Based Complementary Alternative Medicine* 2020: 3479851.

Klavina, L., G. Springe, V. Nikolajeva, I. Martsinkevich et al. 2015. "Chemical Composition Analysis, Antimicrobial Activity and Cytotoxicity Screening of Moss Extracts (Moss Phytochemistry)." *Molecules* 20 (9): 17221–43.

Klegin, C., N. F. de Moura, M. H. O de Sousa, R. Frassini et al. 2021. "Chemical Composition and Cytotoxic Evaluation of the Essential Oil of *Phyllogonium viride* (Phyllogoniaceae, Bryophyta)." *Chemistry and Biodiversity* 18 (3): e2000794.

Klein, O. I., N. A. Kulikova, A. I. Konstantinov, M. V. Zykova et al. 2021. "A Systemtic Study of the Antioxidant Capacity of Humic Substances Against Peroxyl Radicals: Relation to Structure." *Polymers* (Basel) 13 (19): 3262.

Klöcking, R., K. D. Thiel, M. Sprössig. 1976. "Antiviral Activity of Humic Acids from Peat Water." In *Proceedings of the 5th International Peat Congress*, vol. 1, 446–55. Pozabn, Poland.

Ko, F. N., C. H. Liso, C. L. Wu. 1995. "Marchantinquinone, Isolated from *Reboulia hemisphaerica*, as Inhibitor of Lipid Peroxidation and as Free Radical Scavenger." *Chemico-Biologica Interactions* 98 (2): 131–43.

Kohn, E. O. 1992. "Some Observations on the Use of Medicinal Plants from Primary and Secondary Growth by the Runa of Eastern Lowland Ecuador." *Journal of Ethnobiology* 12 (1): 141–52.

Koid, C. W., N. F. M. Shaipulah, G. E. Lee, S. R. Gradstein et al. 2022. "Volatile Organic Compounds of Bryophytes from Peninsular Malaysia and Their Roles in Bryophytes." *Plants* 11 (19): 2575.

Komala, I., T. Ito, F. Nagashima, Y. Yagi et al. 2010. "Cytotoxic, Radical Scavenging and Antimicrobial Activities of Sesquiterpenoids from the Tahitian Liverwort *Mastigophora diclados* (Brid.) Nees (Mastigophoraceae)." *Journal of Natural Medicines* 64 (4): 417–22.

Komala, I., T. Ito, F. Nagashima, Y. Yagi et al. 2011. "Cytotoxic Bibenzyls, and Germacrene- and Pinguisane-Type Sesquiterpenoids from the Indonesian, Tahitian and Japanese Liverwort *Chandonanthus hirtellus*." *Natural Products Communication* 6 (3): 303–9.

Komala, I., T. Ito, F. Nagashima, Y. Yagi, et al. 2010. "Zierane Sesquiterpene Lactone, Cembrane and Fusicoccane Diterpenoids, from the Tahitian Liverwort *Chandonanthus Hirtellus*." *Phytochemistry* 71 (11–12): 1387–94.

Komala, I., T. Ito, Y. Yagi, Y. Asakawa. 2010. "Volatile Components of Selected Liverworts, and Cytotoxic, Radical Scavenging and Antimicrobial Activities of Their Crude Extracts." *Natural Products Communication* 5 (9): 1375–80.

Kondoh, M., F. Nagashima, K. Suzuki, M. Harada et al. 2005. "Induction of Apoptosis by New Ent-kaurene-Type Diterpenoids Isolated from the New Zealand Liverwort *Jungermannia* Species." *Planta Medica* 71 (11): 1005–9.

Kraut, L., and R. Mues. 1998. "The First Biflavone Found in Liverworts and Other Phenolics and Terpenoids from *Chandonanthus hirtellus* ssp. *giganteus* and *Plagiochila asplenioides*." *Zeitschrift für Naturforschung* 54C: 6–10.

Krzaczkowski, L., M. Wright, D. Rebérioux, G. Massiot et al. 2009. "Pharmacological Screening of Bryophyte Extracts that Inhibit Growth and Induce Abnormal Phenotypes in Human HeLa Cancer Cells." *Fundamental and Clinical Pharmacology* 23 (4): 473–82.

Kubo, I., and M. Himejima. 1991. "Anethole, a Synergist of Polygodial Against Filamentous Microorganisms." *Journal of Agricultural and Food Chemistry* 39 (12): 2290–92.

Kumar, A., M. Premoli, F. Aria, S. A. Bonini et al. 2019. "Cannabimimetic Plants: Are They New Cannabinodergic Modulators?" *Planta* 249 (6): 1681–94.

Kumar, P., and B. L. Chaudhary. 2010. "Antibacterial Activity of Moss *Entodon myurus* (Hook) Hamp. Against Some Pathogenic Bacteria." *Bioscan* 5 (4): 605–8.

Kumar, K., V. Nath, A. K. Asthana. 2007. "Concept of Bryophytes in Classical Text of Indian Ethnobotanical Prospective." In *Current Trends in Bryology*, edited by V. Nath and A. K. Asthana. Dehra Dun, India: Bishen Singh Mahendra Pal Singh.

Kumar, K., K. K. Singh, A. K. Asthana, V. Nath. 2000. "Ethnotherapeutics of Bryophyte *Plagiochasma appendiculatum* among the Gaddi Tribes of Kangra Valley, H.P., India." *Pharmaceutical Biology* 38 (5): 353–56.

Kuroda, W., and W. Ogawa. 2017. "Search for Novel Antibacterial Compounds and Targets." *Yakugaku Zasshi* 137 (4): 383–88.

Labbé, C., F. Faini, C Villigrán, J. Coll et al. 2005. "Antifungal and Insect Antifeedant 2-Phenylethanol Esters from the Liverwort *Balantiopsis cancellata* from Chile." *Journal of Agricultural and Food Chemistry* 53 (2): 247–49.

Labbé, C., F. Faini, C. Villagran, J. Coll et al. 2007. "Bioactive Polychlorinated Bibenzyls from the Liverwort *Riccardia polyclada*." *Journal of Natural Products* 70 (12): 2019–21.

Lahlou, E. H., T. Hashimoto, Y. Asakawa. 2000. "Chemical Constituents of the Liverworts *Plagiochasma japonica* and *Marchantia tosana*." *Journal of the Hattori Botanical Laboratory* 88: 271–75.

Lashin, G. M. A, S. Abdel-Shafi, Y. Hussein, A. Osman et al. 2015. "Efficient Inhibition of Pathogenic Bacteria and Potential Toxicity by Secondary Metabolites of Some Bryophyte." *Egyptian Journal of Botany and Microbiology* 3: 475–97.

Latif, E. S., N. F. Kamaludin, R. Rajasegaran. 2019. "Cytotoxicity of *Pogonatum cirratum* Extracts Against CCL-119, a Human T-Cell Acute Lymphoblastic Leukaemia Cell Line." Frontiers Pharmacology Conference abstract in *International Conference on Drug Discovery and Translational Medicine 2018:* "Seizing Opportunities and Addressing Challenges of Precision Medicine." Putrajaya, Malaysia.

Law, D. M., D. V. Basile, M. R. Basile. 1985. "Determination of Endogenous Indole-3-Acetic Acid in *Plagiochila arctica* (Hepaticae)." *Plant Physiology* 77 (4): 926–29.

Lee, J. Y., J. W. Park, J. S. Choi, S. H. Yun, B. H. Rhee et al. 2024. "Aromadendrin Inhibits Lipopolysaccaride-Induced Inflammation in BEAS-2B Cells and Lungs of Mice." *Biomolecules and Therapeutics* 32 (5): 546–55.

Lee, M. K., H. Y. Yang, J. S. Yoon, E. J. Jeong et al. 2008. "Antifibrotic Activity of Diterpenes from *Biota orientalis* Leaves on Hepatic Stellate Cells." *Archives of Pharmacal Research* 31 (7): 866–71.

Lee, S. C., I. M. Chung, Y. J. Jin, Y. S. Song et al. 2008. "Momilactone B, an Allelochemical of Rice Hulls, Induces Apoptosis on Human Lymphoma Cells (Jurkat) in a Micromolar Concentration." *Nutrition and Cancer* 60 (40): 542–51.

Lee, S. H., Y. C. Cho, J. S. Lim. 2021. "Costunolide, a Sesquiterpene Lactone, Suppresses Skin Cancer via Induction of Apoptosis and Blockage of Cell Proliferation." *International Journal of Molecular Sciences* 22 (4): 2075.

Lee, Y. S., M. H. Kang, S. Y. Cho, C. S. Jeong. 2007. "Effects of Constituents of *Amomum xanthioides* on Gastritis in Rats and on Growth of Gastric Cancer Cells." *Archives of Pharmacal Research* 30 (4): 436–43.

Leguy, E., C. Meyer, D. Vienneau, C. Berr et al. 2022. "Modeling Exposure to Airborne Metals Using Moss Biomonitoring in Cemeteries in Two Urban Areas Around Paris and Lyon in France." *Environmental Pollution* 303: 119097.

Lewington, A. 1990. *Plants for People*. Oxford University Press.

Li, F., Y. H. Han, X. Wu, X. Q Cao et al. 2022. "Gut Microbiota-Derived Resveratrol Metabolites, Dihydroresveratrol and Lunularin, Significantly Contribute to the Biological Activities of Resveratrol." *Frontiers in Nutrition* 9: 912591.

Li, F. W., T. Nishiyama, M. Waller, E. Frangedakis et al. 2020. "Anthoceros Genomes Illuminate the Origin of Land Plants and the Unique Biology of Hornworts." *Nature Plants* 6 (3): 259–72.

Li, F. W., J. C. Villarreal, P. Szövényi. 2017. "Hornworts: An Overlooked Window into Carbon-Concentrating Mechanisms." *Trends in Plant Science* 22 (4): 275–77.

Li, J., S. P. Jiang, C. Y. Huang, X. L. Yang. 2022. "Atraric Acid Ameliorates Hyperpigmentation Through the Downregulation of the PKA/CREB/MITF Signaling Pathway." *International Journal of Molecular Science* 23 (24): 15952.

Li, J. L., L. L. Wie, C. Chen, D. Liu et al. 2020. "Bioactive Constituents from the Bryophyta *Hypnum plumaeforme*." *Chemistry and Biodiversity* 17 (12): e2000552.

Li, M. Y., L. Y. Wang, S. Q. Li, C. L. Hua et al. 2022. "Chemical Composition, Antitumor Properties, and Mechanism of the Essential Oil from *Plagiomnium acutum* T. Kop." *International Journal of Molecular Science* 23 (23): 14790.

Li, M. Z., R. Wang, P. Wang. 2023. "Galaxolide and Irgacure 369 Are Novel Environmental Androgens." *Chemosphere* 324: 138329.

Li, R. J., Z. M. Lin, Y. Q. Kang, Y. X. Guo et al. 2014. "Cembrane-Type Diterpenoids from the Chinese Liverworts *Chandonanthus hirtellus* and *C. birmensis*." *Journal of Natural Products* 77 (2): 339–45.

Li, R. J., Y. Sun, B. Sun, X. N. Wang et al. 2014. "Phytotoxic Cis-clerodane Diterpenoids from the Chinese Liverwort *Scapania stephanii*." *Phytochemistry* 105: 85–91.

Li, R. J., S. Wang, G. Li, J. C. Zhou et al. 2016. "Four New Kaurane Diterpenoids from the Chinese Liverwort *Jungermannia comata* Nees." *Chemistry and Biodiversity* 13 (12): 1685–90.

Li, R. J., R. X. Zhu, Y. Y. Li, J. C. Zhou et al. 2013. "Secondary Metabolites from the Chinese Liverwort *Cephaloziella kiaeri*." *Journal of Natural Products* 76 (9): 1700–1708.

Li, R. J., R. Z. Zhu, Y. Zhao, S. L. Morris-Natschke et al. 2014. "Two New Cadinene-Type Sesquiterpenes from the Chinese Liverwort *Frullania serrata*." *Natural Products Research* 28 (19): 1519–24.

Li, S., H. Niu, Y. Qiao, R. Zhu et al. 2018. "Terpenoids Isolated from Chinese Liverworts *Lepidozia reptans* and Their Anti-Inflammatory Activity." *Bioorganic and Medicinal Chemistry* 26 (9): 2392–400.

Li, S. W., H. Z. Shi, W. Q. Chang, Y. M. Zhang et al. 2017. "Eudesmane Sesquiterpenes from Chinese Liverwort Are Substrates of Cdrs and Display Antifungal Activity by Targeting Erg6 and Erg11 of *Candida albicans*." *Bioorganic and Medicinal Chemistry* 25 (20): 5764–71.

Li, W., Z. H. Xu, Y. Z. Wei, Y. Y. Liu et al. 2022. "Trilobatin Induces Apoptosis and Attenuates Stemness Phenotype of Acquired Gefitinib Resistant Lung Cancer Cells via Suppression of NF-kB Pathway." *Nutrition and Cancer* 74 (2): 735–46.

Li, X., Q. Q. Liu, J. Y. Yu, R. T. Zhang et al. 2021. "Costunolide Ameliorates Intestinal Dysfunction and Depressive Behaviour in Mice with Stress-Induced Irritable Bowel Syndrome via Colonic Mast Cell Activation and Central 5-hydroxytryptamine Metabolism." *Food and Function* 12 (9): 4142–51.

Li, X., B. Sun, C. J. Zhu, H. Q. Yuan et al. 2009. "Reversal of P-Glycoprotein-Mediated Multidrug Resistance by Macrocyclic Bisbibenzyl Derivatives in Adriamycin-Resistant Human Myelogenous Leukemia (K562/A02) Cells." *Toxicology in Vitro* 23: 29–36.

Li, X., W. K. K. Wu, B. Sun, M. Cui et al. 2011. "Dihydroptychantol A, a Macrocyclic Bisbibenzyl Derivative, Induces Autophagy and Following Apoptosis Associated with p53 Pathway in Human Osteosarcoma U2OS Cells." *Toxicology and Applied Pharmacology* 251 (2): 146–54.

Li, X. B., F. Xie, S. S. Liu, Y. Li et al. 2013. "Naphtho-y-pyrones from Endophyte *Aspergillus niger* Occurring in the Liverwort *Heteroscyphus tener* (Steph.) Schiffn." *Chemistry and Biodiversity* 10 (7): 1193–201.

Li, Y., X. B. Li, J. C. Zhou, Z. J. Xu et al. 2023. "Pallamins A-C, Ent-labdane and Pallavicinin Based Dimers from the Chinese Liverwort *Pallavicinia ambigua* (mitt.) stephani." *Phytochemistry* 212: 113702.

Li, Y., Y. K. Ma, L. Zhang, F. Guo et al. 2012. "In Vivo Inhibitory Effect on the Biofilm Formation of *Candida albicans* by Liverwort Derived Riccardin D." *PLoS One* 7 (4): e35543.

Li, Y., Y. Sun, M. Z. Zhu, R. X. Zhu et al. 2019. "Sacculatane Diterpenoids from the Chinese Liverwort *Pellia epiphylla* with Protection Against H2O2-Induced Apoptosis of PC12 Cells." *Phytochemistry* 162: 173–82.

Li, Y., R. X. Zhu, J. Z. Zhang, X. Y. Wu et al. 2018. "Clerodane Diterpenoids from the Chinese Liverwort *Jamesoniella autumnalis* and Their Anti-Inflammatory Activity." *Phytochemistry* 154: 85–93.

Li, Z., Z. C. Tu, H. Wang, L. Zhang. 2020. "Ultrasound-Assisted Extraction Optimization of *a*-glucosidase Inhibitors from *Ceratophyllum demersum* L. and Identification of Phytochemical Profiling by HPLC-QTOF-MS/MS." *Molecules* 25 (19): 4507.

Li, Z. Y., and M. Guo. 2017. "Healthy Efficacy of *Nostoc commune* Vaucher." *Oncotarget* 9 (18): 14669–79.

Li, L., X. R. Wu, J. L. Gong, Z. Q. Wang, W. B. Dai et al. 2024. "Activation of GABA Type A Receptor is Involved in the Anti-insomnia Effect of Huanglian Wendan Decoction." *Frontiers in Pharmacology* 15: 1389768.

Liao, C. H., F. N. Ko, C. L. Wu, C. M. Teng. 2000. "Antiplatelet Effect of Marchantinquinone, Isolated from *Reboulia hemisphaerica*, in Rabbit Washed Platelets." *Journal of Pharmacy and Pharmacology* 52 (3): 353–59.

Lightfoot, J. 1777. *Flora Scotica: Or, a Systematitic Arrangement, in the Linnaean Method, of the Native Plants of Scotland and the Hebrides.* London: B. White at Horace's Head.

Lin, H. R. 2105. "Lepidozenolide from the Liverwort *Lepidoza fauriana* Acts as a Farnesoid X Receptor Agonist." *Journal of Asian Natural Products Research* 17 (2): 149–58.

Lin, P., J. F. Zhang, G. N. Xie, J. C. Li et al. 2023. "Innate Immune Responses to *Sporothrix schenckii*: Recognition and Elimination." *Mycopathologia* 188 (1–2): 71–86.

Lin, W., Y. W. Huang, X. D. Zhou, Y. Ma. 2006. "Toxicity of Cerium Oxide Nanoparticles in Human Lung Cancer Cells." *International Journal of Toxicology* 25 (6): 451–57.

Lin, Z. M., Y. X. Guo, S. Q. Wang et al. 2014. "Diterpenoids from the Chinese Liverwort *Heteroscyphus tener* and Their Antiproliferative Effects." *Journal of Natural Products* 77: 1336–44.

Lin, Z. Y., S. Huang, X. T. LingHu, Y. X. Wang et al. 2022. "Perillaldehyde Inhibits Bone Metastasis and Receptor Activator of Nuclear Factor-$_k$B Ligand (RANKL) Signaling-Induced Osteoclastogenesis in Prostate Cancer Cell Lines." *Bioengineered* 13 (2): 2710–19.

Linde, J., S. Combrinck, S. Van Vuuren, J. Van Rooy et al. 2016. "Volatile Constituents and Antimicrobial Activities of Nine South African Liverwort Species." *Phytochemistry Letters* 16: 61–69.

Liu, C. M., R. L. Zhu, R. H. Liu, H. L. Li et al. 2009. "Cis-Clerodane Diterpenoids from the Liverwort *Gottschelia schizopleura* and Their Cytotoxic Activity." *Planta Medica* 75 (15): 1597–601.

Liu, H., G. Li, B. Zhang, D. Sun et al. 2018. "Suppression of the NF-kB Signaling Pathway in Colon Cancer Cells by the Natural Compound Riccardin D from *Dumortiera hirsuta*." *Molecular Medicine Reports* 17: 5837–43.

Liu, H. J., C. L. Wu, H. Becker, J. Zapp. 2000. "Sesquiterpenoids and Diterpenoids from the Chilean Liverwort *Lepicolea ochroleuca*." *Phytochemistry* 53 (8): 845–49.

Liu, H. J., C. L. Wu, T. Hashimoto, Y. Asakawa. 1996. "Nudenoic Acid: A Novel Tricyclic Sesquiterpenoid from the Taiwanese Liverwort *Mylia nuda*." *Tetrahedron Letters* 37 (52): 9307–9.

Liu, H. P., Z. H. Gao, S. X. Cui, D. F. Sun et al. 2012. "Inhibition of Intestinal Adenoma Formation in APCMin/+ Mice by Riccardin D, a Natural Product Derived Liverwort Plant *Dumortiera Hirsuta*." *PLoS One* 7:e33243.

Liu, N., D. X. Guo, S. Q. Wang, Y. Y. Wang et al. 2012. "Bioactive Sesquiterpenoids and Diterpenoids from the Liverwort *Bazzania albifolia*." *Chemistry and Biodiversity* 9: 2254–61.

Liu, N., D. X. Guo, Y. Y. Wang, L. N. Wang et al. 2011. "Aromatic Compounds from the Liverwort *Conocephalum japonicum*." *Natural Product Communications* 6 (1): 49–52.

Liu, N., R. J. Li, X. N. Wang, R. X. Zhu et al. 2013. "Highly Oxygenated Ent-pimarane-Type Diterpenoids from the Chinese Liverwort *Pedinophyllum interruptum* and Their Alleopathic Activities." *Journal of Natural Products* 76 (9): 1647–53.

Liu, N., L. Zhang, S. Wang, X. N Wang et al. 2012. "Eudesmane-Type Sesquiterpenes from the Liverwort *Apomarsupella revolte*." *Phytochemistry Letters* 5 (2): 346–50.

Liu, N., R. X. Zhu, S. Wang, J. Z. Zhang et al. 2013. "Cis-clerodane Diterpenes from the Liverwort *Scapania ciliata*." *Chemistry and Biodiversity* 10 (9): 1606–12.

Liu, S. G., C. Y. Zhang, J. C. Zhou, J. J. Han et al. 2022. "Diels-Alder Adducts of a labdane Diterpenoid from the Chinese Liverwort *Pallavicinia subciliata*." *Organic Chemistry Frontiers* 9: 1790–96.

Liu, X. L., S. L. Liu, M. Liu, B. H. Kong et al. 2014. "A Primary Assessment of the Endophytic Bacterial Community in a Xerophilous Moss (*Grimmia montana*) Using Molecular Method and Cultivated Isolates." *Brazilian Journal of Microbiology* 45 (1): 163–73.

Liu, Y. Q., M. Wang, D. Wang, X. B. Li et al. 2016. "Malformin A1 Promotes Cell Death Through Induction of Apoptosis, Necrosis and Autophagy in Prostate Cancer Cells." *Cancer Chemotherapy and Pharmacology* 77 (1): 63–75.

Liu, Z. W., Z. H. Luo, Q. Q. Meng, P. C. Zhong et al. 2020. "Network Pharmacology-Based Investigation on the Mechanisms of Action of *Morinda officinalis* How. in the Treatment of Osteoporosis." *Computers in Biology and Medicine* 127: 104074.

Lopez, A., J. B. Hudson, G. H. Towers. "Antiviral and Antimicrobial Activities of Columbian Medicinal Plants." *Journal of Ethnopharmacology* 77 (2–3): 189–96.

López-Sáez, J. A., M. J. Pérez-Alonso, A. Velasco-Negueruela. 1995. "The Bioflavonoid Pattern of the Moss *Bartramia ithyphylla* (Bartramiaceae, Musci)." *Zeitschrift für Naturforschung C Journal of Bioscience* 50 (3): 311–12.

Lorimer, S. D., E. J. Burgess, N. B. Perry. 1997. "Diplophyllolide: A Cytotoxic Sesquiterpene Lactone from the Liverworts *Clasmatocolea vermicularis* and *Chiloscyphus subporosa*." *Phytomedicine* 4: 261–63.

Lorimer, S. D., and N. B. Perry. 1994. "Antifungal Hydroxy-acetophenones from the New Zealand Liverwort *Plagiochila fasciculata*." *Planta Medica* 60: 386–87.

Lorimer, S. D., N. B. Perry, E. J. Burgess, L. M. Foster. 1997. "1-Hydroxyditerpenes from Two New Zealand Liverworts, *Paraschistochila pinnatifolia* and *Trichocolea mollissima*." *Journal of Natural Products* 6 (4): 421–24.

Lorimer, S. D., N. B. Perry, R. S. Tangney. 1993. "An Antifungal Bibenzyl from the New Zealand Liverwort, *Plagiochila stephensoniana*. Bioactivity-Directed Isolation, Synthesis, and Analysis." *Journal of Natural Products* 56: 1444–50.

Lou, H. X., G. Y. Li, F. Q. Wang. 2002. "A Cytotoxic Diterpenoid and Antifungal Phenolic Compounds from *Frullania muscicola* Steph." *Journal of Asian Natural Products Research* 4 (2): 87–94.

Lu, Q. L., Y. Ding, Y. Li, Q. L. Lu. 2020. "5-HT Receptor Agonist Valerenic Acid Enhances the Innate Immunity Signal and Suppresses Glioblastoma Cell Growth and Invasion." *International Journal of Biological Sciences* 16 (12): 2104–15.

Lu, R. H., C. Paul, S. Basar, W. A. König et al. 2003. "Sesquiterpene constituents from the liverwort *Bazzania japonica*." *Phytochemistry* 63 (5): 581–87.

Lu, Y., F. F. Eriksson, M. Thorsteinsdóttir, N. Cronberg et al. 2023. "Lipidomes of Icelandic Bryophytes and Screening of High Contents of Polyunsaturated Fatty Acids by Using Lipidomics Approach." *Phytochemistry* 206: 113560.

Lu, Z. Q., P. H. Fan, M. Ji, H. X. Lou. 2006. "Terpenoids and Bisbibenzyls from Chinese Liverworts *Conocephalum conicum* and *Dumortiera hirsuta*." *Journal of Asian Natural Product Research* 8: 187–92.

Lubaina, A. S., D. Pradeep, J. M. Aswathy, Remya Krishnan et al. 2014. "Traditional Knowledge of Medicinal Bryophytes by the Kani Tribes of Agasthiyarmalai Biosphere Reserve, Southern Western Ghats." *Indo American Journal of Pharmaceutical Research* 4: 2116–21.

Ludwiczuk, A., and Y. Asakawa. 2017. "GC/MS Fingerprinting of Solvent Extracts and Essential Oils Obtained from Liverwort Species." *Natural Product Communications* 12 (8): 1301–5.

Ludwiczuk, A., and Y. Asakawa. 2021. "Chemical Diversity of Liverworts from *Frullania Genus*." *Natural Product Communications* 16 (2): 1–15.

Lunic, T. M., M. R. Mandic, M. M. O. Paviovic, A. D. Sabovljevic et al. 2022. "The Influence of Seasonality on Secondary Metabolite Profiles and Neuroprotective Activities of Moss *Hynum cupressiforme* Extracts: In Vitro and In Silico Study." *Plants* (Basel) 11 (1): 123.

Lunic, T. M., M. M. Oalde, M. R. Mandic, A. D. Sabovljevic et al. 2020. "Extracts Characterization and In Vitro Evaluation of Potential Immunomodulatory Activities of the Moss *Hypnum cupressiforme* Hedw. *Molecules* 25 (5): 3343.

Luo, X. R. 2000. *Handbook Series of Useful Medicinal Herbs with Color Illustrations.* Vol. 5. Guangzhon: Guangdong Science & Technological Press.

Luthfiah, L., D. Setyati, S. Arimurti. 2021. "Antibacterial Activity of Liverworts of *Dumortiera hirsuta* (Sw.) Nees Ethyl Acetate Extract Against Pathogenic Bacteria." *Berkala Sainstek* 9: 75–80.

Luu, M., S. Pautz, V. Kohl, R. Singh et al. 2019. "The Short-Chain Fatty Acid Pentanoate Suppresses Autoimmunity by Modulating the Metabolic-Epigenetic Crosstalk in Lymphocytes." *Nature Communications* 10 (1): 760.

Lv, Q., Y. Xing, D. Dong, Y. Hu et al. 2021. "Costunolide Ameliorates Colitis via Specific Inhibition of HIF1*a*/glycolysis-Mediated Th17 Differentiation." *International Immunopharmacology* 97: 107688.

Lv, Y., Q. Song, Q. Shao, W. Gao et al. 2012. "Comparison of the Effects of Marchantin C and Fucoidan on SFlt-1 and Angiogenesis in Glioma Microenvironment." *Journal of Pharmacy and Pharmacology* 64: 604–9.

Ma, S., H. Xu, W. Huang, Y. Gao et al. 2021. "Chrysophanol Relieves Cisplatin-Induced Nephrotoxicity via Concomitant Inhibition of Oxidative Stress, Apoptosis, and Inflammation." *Frontiers in Physiology* 12: 794302.

Ma, Z. G., Y. P. Yuan, X. Zhang, S. C. Xu et al. 2017. "Piperine Attenuates Pathological Cardiac Fibrosis via PPAR-y/AKT Pathways." *EBioMedicine* 18: 179–87.

Maccarrone, M. 2006. "Fatty Acid Amide Hydrolase: A Potential Target for Next Generation Therapeutics." *Current Pharmaceutical Design* 12 (6): 759–72.

Madsen, G. C. and A. Pates. 1952. "Occurrence of Antimicrobial Substances in Chlorophyllose Plants Growing in Floria." *Environmental Science, Biology, Agricultural and Food Sciences* 113 (3): 293–300.

Magnone, M., L. Sturla, L. Guida, S. Spinelli et al. 2020. "Abscisic Acid: A Conserved Hormone in Plants and Humans and a Promising Aid to Combat Prediabetes and the Metabolic Syndrome." *Nutrients* 12 (6): 1724.

Makajanma, M. M., I. Taufik, A. Faizal. 2020. "Antioxidant and Antibacterial Activity of Extract from Two Species of Mosses: *Leucobryum aduncum* and *Campylopus schmidii*." *Biodiversitas* 21 (6): 2751–58.

Makar, S., T. Saha, S. K. Singh. 2019. "Naphthalene, a Versatile Platform in Medicinal Chemistry: Sky-High Perspective." *European Journal of Medicinal Chemistry* 161: 252–76.

Makinde, A. M., E. A. Fajuyigbe, M. O. Isa. 2015. "Secondary Metabolites and Bioactivity of *Hyophila involuta* (Hook) Jaeg." *Notulae Scientia Biologicae* 7 (4): 456–59.

Mandic, M. R., M. M. Olade, T. M. Lunic, A. D. Sabovljevic et al. 2021. "Chemical Characterization and In Vitro Immunomodulatory Effects of Different Extracts of Moss *Hedwigia ciliata* (Hedw.) P. Beauv. from the Vrsacke Planine Mts., Serbia." *PloS One* 16 (2): e0246810.

Manoharan, R. K., J. H. Lee, Y. G. Kim, S. I. Kim et al. 2017. "Inhibitory Effects of the Essential Oils a-longipinene and Linalool on Biofilm Formation and Hyphal Growth of *Candida albicans*." *Biofouling* 33 (2): 143–55.

Manoj, G. S., J. M. Aswathy, K. Murugan. 2016. "Bactericidal Potential of Selected Bryophytes *Plagochila beddomei*, *Leucobryum bowringii* and *Octoblepharum albidum*." *International Journal of Advanced Research* 4 (4): 370–82.

Manoj, G. S., T. R. S. Kumar, S. Varghese, K. Murugan. 2012. "Effect of Methanolic and Water Extract of *Leucobryum bowringii* Mitt. on Growth, Migration and Invasion of MCF 7 Human Breast Cancer Cells In Vitro." *Indian Journal of Experimental Biology* 50 (9): 602–11.

Manoj, G. S., and K. Murugan. 2012a. "Phenolic Profiles, Antimicrobial and Antioxidant Potentiality of Methanolic Extract of a Liverwort, *Plagiochila beddomei* Steph." *Indian Journal of Natural Product and Resources* 3: 173–83.

Manoj, G. S., and K. Murugan. 2012b. "Wound Healing Activity of Methanolic and Aqueous Extracts of *Plagiochila beddomei* Steph. Thallus in Rat Model." *Indian Journal of Experimental Biology* 50 (8): 551–58.

Marles, R. J., C. Clavelle, L. Monteleone, N. Tays et al. 2000. *Aboriginal Plant Use in Canada's Northwest Boreal Forest*. Vancouver: University of British Columbia Press.

Marques, R. V., A. Guillaumin, A. B. Abdelwahab, A. Salwinski et al. 2021. "Collagenase and Tyrosinase Inhibitory Effect of Isolated Constituents from the Moss *Polytrichum formosum*." *Plants* (Basel) 10 (7): 1271.

Marques, R. V., S. E. Sestito, F. Bourgaud, S. Miguel et al. 2022. "Anti-Inflammatory Activity of Bryophytes Extracts in LPS-Stimulated RAW264.7 Murine Macrophages." *Molecules* 27 (6): 1940.

Martin, A. 2015. *The Magical World of Moss Gardening*. Portland, OR: Timber Press.

Maslyk, M., T. Lenard, M. Olech, A. Martyna, M. Poniewozik et al. 2024. "*Ceratophyllum demersum* the Submerged Macrophyte from the Mining Subsidence Reservoir Nadrybie Poland as a Source of Anticancer Agents." *Scientific Reports* 14 (1): 6661.

Mathieu, V., A. Chantôme, F. Lefranc, A. Cimmino et al. 2015. "Sphaeropsidin A Shows Promising Activity Against Drug-Resistant Cancer Cells by Targeting Regulatory Volume Increase." *Cellular and Molecular Life Sciences* 72 (19): 3731–46.

Matsuo, A., H. Nozaki, M. Nakayama, D. Takaoka et al. 1980. "Structure of (-)-Neoverrucosan-5 β-Ol, a Diterpenoid from *Mylia verrucosa* (Liverwort) containing a Novel Carbon Skeleton: X-Ray Crystal and Molecular Structure of the Benzoate." *Journal of the Chemical Society, Chemical Communications* 17: 822–23.

Matsuo, A., N. Kubota, M. Nakayama, S. Hayashi. 1981. "(-)-Lepidozenal, a Sesquiterpenoid with a Novel Trans-fused Bicyclo Undecane System from the Liverwort *Lepidozia vitrea*." *Chemistry Letters* 10 (8): 1097–100.

Matsuo, A., S. Yuki, M. Nakayama, S. Hayashi. 1982. "Three New Sesquiterpene Phenols of the Ent-herbertane Class from the Liverwort *Herberta adunca*." *Chemical Letters* 11 (4): 463–66.

Mayaba, N., F. Minibayeva, R. P. Beckett. 2002. "An Oxidative Burst of Hydrogen Peroxide During Rehydration Following Dessication in the Moss *Atrichum androgynum*." *New Phytologist* 155: 275–83.

McCleary, J. A., P. S. Sypherd, D. L. Walkington. 1960. "Mosses as Possible Sources of Antibiotics." *Science* 131: 108.

McCleary, J. A., and D. L. Walkington. 1966. "Mosses and Antibiotics." *Revue Bryologique et Lichenologique* 34: 309–14.

McCuaig, B., S. C. Dufour, R. A. Raguso, A. P. Bhatt et al. 2015. "Structural Changes in Plastids of Developing *Splachnum ampullaceum* Sporophytes and Relationship to Odour Production." *Plant Biology* (Stuttgard) 17 (2): 466–73.

McCutcheon, A. R., T. E. Roberts, E. Gibbons, S. M. Ellis et al. 1995. "Antiviral Screening of British Columbia Medicinal Plants." *Journal of Ethnopharmacology* 49 (20): 101–10.

Meka, M., N. Panatula, S. K. Nemal, S. Nallapaty et al. 2022. "Impact of Antioxidant Rich Fractions Isolated from Moss *Fissidens grandiflora* on Alcohol-Induced Oxidative Stress." *Research Journal of Pharmacy and Technology* 15 (11): 5289–94.

Mekuria, T., U. Steiner, H. Hindorf, J.P. Frahm et al. 2005. "Bioactivity of Bryophyte Extracts Against *Botrytis cinerea*, *Alternaria solani* and *Phytophthora infestans*." *Journal of Applied Botany and Food Quality* 70 (2): 89–93.

Melo, I. S., S. N. Santos, L. H. Rosa, M. M. Parma et al. 2014. "Isolation and Biological Activities of an Endophytic *Mortierella alpina* Strain from the Antarctic Moss *Schistidium antarctici*." *Extremophiles* 18 (1): 15–23.

Métoyer, B., A. Benatrehina, L. H. Rakotondriabe, L. Thouvenot et al. 2020. "Dimeric and Esterified Sesquiterpenes from the Liverwort *Chiastocaulon caledonicum*." *Phytochemistry* 179: 112495.

Métoyer, B., N. Lebouvier, E. Hnawia, G. Herbette, et al. 2018. "Chemotypes and Biomarkers of Seven Species of New Caledonian Liverworts from the Bazzanioideae Subfamily." *Molecules* 23 (6): 1353.

Métoyer, B., N. Lebouvier, E. Hnawia, L. Thouvenot et al. 2021. "Chemotaxonomy and Cytotoxicity of the Liverwort *Porella viridissima*." *Natural Products Research* 35: 2099–102.

Mewari, N., and P. Kumar. 2008. "Antimicrobial Activity of Extracts of *Marchantia polymorpha*." *Pharmaceutical Biology* 46: 819–22.

Michelfelder, S., J. Parsons, L. L. Bohlender, S. N. W. Hoernstein et al. 2017. "Moss-Produced, Glycosylation-Optimized Human Factor H for Therapeutic Application in Complement Disorders." *Journal of the American Society for Nephrology* 28 (5): 1462–74.

Micheli, P. A. 1729. *Nova plantarum genera iuxta Tournefortii methodum disposita quibus plantae 1900 recensentur, sciliceet fere 1400 nondum obervatae*. Florentiae, Italy: Typis Bernardi Paperinii, Typographi r. c. Magnae Principis Viduae ab Etruri;.

Millar, K. D. L., B. J. Crandall-Stotler, J. F. S. Ferreira, K. V. Wood. 2007. "Antimicrobial Properties of Three Liverworts in Axenic Culture: *Blassia pusilla, Pallavicinia lyellii* and *Radula obconica*." *Cryptogamie, Bryologie* 28 (3): 197–210.

Minibayeva, F., and R. P. Beckett. 2001. "High Rates of Extracellular Superoxide Production in Bryophytes and Lichens, and an Oxidative Burst in Response to Rehydration Following Desiccation." *New Phytologist* 152: 333–41.

Miranda, T. G., R. J. M. Alves, R. F. de Souza, J. G. S. Mala et al. 2021. "Volatile Concentrate from the Neotropical Moss *Neckeropsis undulata* (Hedw.) Reichart, Existing in the Brazilian Amazon." *BMC Chemistry* 15 (7): 7.

Misra, S., T. Sanyal, D. Sarkar, P. K. Bhattacharya et al. 1989. "Evaluation of Antileishmanial Activity of Trans-aconitic Acid." *Biochemical Medicine and Metabolic Biology* 42 (3): 171–78.

Mitchell, J. C. 1981. "Industrial Aspects of 112 Cases of Allergic Contact Dermatitis from *Frullania* in British Columbia During a 10-Year Period." *Contact Dermatitis* 7 (5): 268–69.

Mitra, S. 2017. "High Content of Dicranin in *Anisothecium spirale* (Mitt.) Broth., a Moss from Eastern Himalayas and Its Chemotaxonomic Significance." *Lipids* 52 (2): 173–78.

Mitre, G. B., N. Kamiya, A. Bardon, Y. Asakawa. 2004. "Africane-Type Sesquiterpenoids from the Argentine Liverwort *Porella swartziana* and Their Antibacterial Activity." *Journal of Natural Products* 67 (1): 31–36.

Miyagawa, T., S. Hamagami, N. Tanigawa. 2000. "Cryptococcus Albidus-Induced Summer-Type Hypersensitivity Pneumonitis." *American Journal of Respiratory and Critical Care Medicine* 161 (3 Pt1): 961–66.

Modolo, L.V., A. X. de Souza, L .P. Horta, D. P. Araujo et al. 2015. "An Overview on the Potential of Natural Products as Ureases Inhibitors: A Review." *Journal of Advanced Research* 6 (1): 35–44.

Moerman, D. E. 1998. *Native American Ethnobotany*. Portland OR: Timber Press.

Mohammad, N., N. Ali, N. Uddin, S. F. Wadood et al. 2018. "Evaluation of Informants' Consensus Factor of Medicinal Uses of Bryophytes in Swegalai Valley KPK, Pakistan." *JBES* 12 (5): 57–63.

Mohandas, G. G., and M. Kumaraswamy. 2018. "Antioxidant Activities of Terpenoids from *Thuidium tamariscellum* (C. Muell.) Bosch. and Sande-Lac. A Moss." *Pharmacognosy Journal* 10 (4): 645–49.

Monaci, F., S. Ancora, N. Bianchi, I. Bonini et al. 2021. "Combined Use of Native and Transplanted Moss for Post-Mining Characterizations of Metal (Loid) River Contamination." *Science of The Total Environment* 750: 141669.

Monteiro, A. S. E. N., D. R. Campos, A. A. S. Albuquerque et al. 2020. "Effect of Diterpene Manool on the Arterial Blood Pressure and Vascular Reactivity in Normotensive and Hypertensive Rats." *Arquivos brasileiros de Cardiologia* 115 (4): 669–77.

Montenegro, G., M. C. Portaluppi, F. A. Salas, M. F. Diaz. 2009. "Biological Properties of the Chilean Native Moss *Sphagnum magellanicum*." *Biological Research* 42 (2): 233–37.

Moo-Puc, R. E., G. J. Mena-Rejon, L. Quijano, R. Cedillo-Rivera. 2007. "Antiprotozoal Activity of *Senna racemosa*." *Journal of Ethnopharmacology* 112 (2): 415–16.

Morita, H., Y. Tomizawa, T. Tsuchiya, Y. Hirasawa et al. 2009. "Antimiotic Activity of Two Macrocyclic Bis(Bibenzyls), Isoplagiochins A and B from the Liverwort *Plagiochila fruticosa*." *Bioorganic and Medicinal Chemistry Letters* 19: 493–96.

Mort, J. S., and D. J. Buttle. 1997. "Cathepsin B." *International Journal of Biochemistry and Cell Biology* 29 (5): 715–20.

Motti, R., A. Di Palma, B. de Falco. 2023. "Bryophytes Used in Folk Medicine: An Ethnobotanical Overview." *Horticulturae* 9: 137.

Mukhia, S., P. Mandal, D. K. Singh, D. Singh. 2019. "Comparison of Pharmacological Properties and Phytochemical Constituents of in Vitro, Propagated and Naturally Occurring Liverwort *Lunularia cruciata*." *BMC Complementary and Alternative Medicine* 19: 1–6.

Müller, C. A., V. Perz, C. Provasnek, F. Quartinello et al. 2017. "Discovery of Polyesterases from Moss-Associated Microorganisms." *Applied and Environmental Microbiology* 83 (4): e02641–16.

Mulyaningsih, S., F. Sporer, S. Zimmermann, J. Reichling et al. 2010. "Synergistic Properties of the Terpenoids Aromadendrene and 1,8-cineole from the Essential Oil of *Eucalyptus globulus* against Antibiotic-Susceptible and Antibiotic-Resistant Pathogens." *Phytomedicine* 17 (13): 1061–66.

Munoz, C., K. Schröder, B. Henes, J. Hubert et al. 2024. "Phytochemical Exploration of Ceruchinol in Moss: A Multidisciplinary Study on Biotechnological Cultivation of *Physcomitrium patens* (Hedw.) Mitt." *Applied Sciences* 14: 1274.

Nagashima, F., and Y. Asakawa. 2001. "Sesqui- and Diterpenoids from Two Japanese and Three European Liverworts." *Phytochemistry* 56 (4): 347–52.

Nagashima, F., M. Kondoh, M. Kawase, S. Simizu et al. 2003. "Apoptosis-Inducing Properties of Ent-Kaurene-Type Diterpenoids from the Liverwort *Jungermannia truncata*." *Planta Medica* 69: 377–79.

Nagashima, F., M. Kondoh, T. Uematsu, A. Nishiyama et al. 2002. "Cytotoxic and Apoptosis-Inducing Ent-Kaurane-Type Diterpenoids from the Japanese Liverwort *Jungermannia truncata* NEES." *Chemical and Pharmaceutical Bulletin* 50 808–13.

Nagashima, F., S. Momosaki, Y. Watanabe, M. Toyota et al. 1996. "Terpenoids and Aromatic Compounds from Six Liverworts." *Phytochemistry* 41 (1): 207–11.

Nagashima, F., M. Murakami, S. Takaoka, Y. Asakawa. 2004. "New Sesquiterpenoids from the New Zealand Liverwort *Chiloscyphus subporosus*." *Chemical and Pharmaceutical Bulletin* 52 (8): 949–52.

Nagashima, F., Y. Ohi, T. Nagai, M. Tori et al. 1993. "Terpenoids from Some German and Russian Liverworts." *Phytochemistry* 33: 1444–48.

Nagashima, F., T. Sekiguchi, Y. Asakawa. 2005. "New Sesquiterpenoid from the New Zealand Liverwort *Lepidozia spinosissima*." *Natural Products Research* 19 (7): 679–83.

Nagashima, F., M. Suzuki, S. Takaoka, Y. Asakawa. 2001. "Sesqui- and Diterpenoids from the Japanese Liverwort *Jungermannia infusca*." *Journal of Natural Products* 64 (10): 1309–17.

Nagashima, F., M. Toyota, Y. Asakawa. 2006. "Bazzanane Sesquiterpenoids from the New Zealand Liverwort *Frullania falciloba*." *Chemical and Pharmaceutical Bulletin* (Tokyo) 54 (9): 1347–49.

Nagashima, F., Y. Kuba, Y. Asakawa. 2006. "Diterpenoids and aromatic compounds from the three New Zealand liverworts *Jamesoniella kirkii*, *Balantiopsis rosea*, and *Radula* species." *Chemical and Pharmaceutical Bulletin* 54 (6): 902–6.

Naidu, K. K., S. Satya, A. Priya, B. T Vinay. 2020. "In-Vitro Anti-Inflammatory and Anticancer Activities of *Octoblepharum albidum* Hedw." *American Journal of Medical and Natural Sciences* 1 (1): 19–24.

Nedeljko, L., M. S. Sabovijevic, M. Vujicic, J. Latinovic et al. 2019. "Bryophyte Extracts Suppress Growth of the Plant Pathogenic Fungus *Botrytis cinerea*." *Botanica Serbica* 43 (1): 9–12.

Negi, K., and P. Chaturvedi. 2016. "In Vitro Antimicrobial Efficacy of *Rhynchostegium vagans* A. Jaeger (Moss) Against Commonly Occurring Pathogenic Microbes of Indian Sub-Tropics." *Asian Pacific Journal of Tropical Disease* 6 (1): 10–14.

Negi, K., S. D. Tewarib, P. Chaturvedic. 2018. "Antibacterial Activity of *Marchantia papillata* Raddi subsp. *grossibarba* (Steph.) Bischl. Against *Staphylococcus aureus.*" *Indian Journal of Traditional Knowledge* 17 (4): 763–69.

Neltner, T. J., P. K. Sahoo, R. W. Smith, J. P. V Anders et al. 2022. "Effects of 8 Weeks of Shilajit Supplementation on Serum Pro-c1*a*1, a Biomarker of Type 1 Collagen Synthesis: A Randomized Control Trial." *Journal of Dietary Supplements* 21 (1): 1–12.

Nerlo, H., and A. Kosior. 1977. "Identification of Sterols in the Moss *Climacium dendroides.*" *Acta Poloniae Pharmaceutica* 34 (1): 89–92.

Neves, M., R. Morais, S. Gafner, K. Hostettmann. 1998. "Three Triterpenoids and One flavonoid From the Liverwort *Astrella blumeana* Grown In Vitro." *Phytotherapy Research* 12: 21–24.

Ng, S. Y., L. P. Ang, V. L. Hau, M. Suleiman et al. 2021. "Structural Diversity, Antifungal Activity and Chemosystematics of Borean Liverwort *Bazzania harpago* (De. Not.) Schiffner." *Sains Malaysiana* 50 (1): 101–7.

Ng, S. Y., T. Kamada, M. Suleiman, C. S. Vairappan. 2016a. "A New Cembrane-Type Diterpenoid from Bornean liverwort *Chandonanthus hirtellus.*" *Journal of Asian Natural Products Research* 18 (7): 690–96.

Ng, S. Y., T. Kamada, M. Suleiman, C. S. Vairappan. 2016b. "A New Seco-Clerodane-Type Diterpenoid from Bornean Liverwort *Schistochila acuminata.*" *Natural Product Communications* 11 (8): 1071–72.

Ng, S. Y., T. Kamada, M. Suleiman, C. S. Vairappan. 2018. "Two New Clerodane-Type Diterpenoids from Bornean Liverwort *Gottschelia schizopleura* and Their Cytotoxic Activity." *Natural Product Research* 32 (15): 1832–37.

Ng, S. Y., T. Kamada, C. S. Vairappan. 2017. "New Pimarane-Type Diterpenoid and Ent-Eudesmane-Type Sesquiterpenoid from Bornean Liverwort *Mastigophora diclados.*" *Records of Natural Products* 11 (6): 508–13.

Nicholson, W. A., ed. 1914. *A Flora of Norfolk*. London: West, Newman.

Nicolella, H. D., A. B. Ribeiro, M. R. S de Melo et al. 2022. "Antitumor Effect of Manool in a Murine Melanoma Model." *Journal of Natural Products* 85 (2): 426–32.

Nicolella, H. D., A. B. Ribeiro, C. C. Munari, M. R. Melo et al. 2023. "Antimelanoma Effect of Manool in 2D Cell Cultures and Reconstructed Human Skin Models." *Journal of Biochemical and Molecular Toxicology* 37 (3): e23282.

Niewes, D., M. Huculak-Maczka, M. Braun-Giwerska, K. Marecka et al. 2022. "Ultrasound-Assisted Extraction of Humic Substances from Peat: Assessment of Process Efficiency and Products' Quality." *Molecules* 27 (11): 3413.

Nikolajeva, V., L. Liepina, Z. Petrina, M. Grube et al. 2012. "Antibacterial Activity of Extracts from Some Bryophytes." *Journal of Advances in Microbiology* 2: 345–53.

Niu, C., J. B. Qu, H. X. Lou. 2006. "Antifungal Bis[bibenzyls] from the Chinese Liverwort *Marchantia polymorpha* L." *Chemistry and Biodiversity* 3 (1): 34–40.

Niu, H. M., L. L. Qian, B. Sun, W. J. Liu et al. 2019. "Inactivation of TFEB and NF-kB by Marchantin M Alleviates the Chemotherapy-Driven Pro-Tumorigenic Senescent Secretion." *Acta Pharmaceutica Sinica* 9 (5): 923–36.

Niu, L. L., J. T. Deng, F. H. Zhu, N. Zhou et al. 2014. "Anti-Inflammatory Effect of Marchantin M Contributes to Sensitization of Prostate Cancer Cells to Docetaxel." *Cancer Letters* 348 (1–2): 126–34.

Nordström, U. 2019. *Moss: From Forest to Garden, a Guide to the Hidden World of Moss.* New York: W. W. Norton.

Norred, W. P. 1993. "Fumonisins—Mycotoxins Produced by *Fusarium moniliforme.*" *Journal of Toxicology and Environmental Health* 38 (3): 309–28.

Novakovic, M., D. Bukvicki, B. Andjelkovic, T. Ilic-Tomic et al. 2019. "Cytotoxic Activity of Riccardin and Perrottetin Derivatives from the Liverwort *Lunularia cruciata.*" *Journal of Natural Products* 82 (4): 694–701.

Novakovic, M., A. Ludwiczuk, D. Bukvicki, Y. Asakawa. 2021. "Phytochemicals from Bryophytes: Structures and Biological Activity." *Journal of the Serbian Chemical Society* 86: 1139–75.

Nowaczynski, F., R. Nicoletti, B. Zimowska, A. Ludwiczuk. 2025. "*Marchantia polymorpha* as a Source of Biologically Active Compounds." *Molecules* 30 (3): 558.

Ohta, Y., N. H. Andersen, C. B. Liu. 1977. "Sesquiterpene Constituents of Two Liverworts of Genus Diplophyllum: Novel Eudesmanolides and Cytotoxicity Studies for Enantiomeric Methylene Lactones." *Tetrahedron* 33 (6): 617–28.

Okamoto, H., D. Yoshida, Y. Saito, S. Mizusaki. 1983. "Inhibition of 12-O-Tetradecanolyphorbol-13-Acetate-Induced Ornithine Decarboxylase Activity in Mouse Epidermis by Sweetening Agents and Related Compounds." *Cancer Letters* 21 (1): 29–35.

Onbasli, D., and G. Yuvali. 2021. "In Vitro Medicinal Potentials of *Bryum capillare*, a Moss Sample, from Turkey." *Saudi Journal of Biological Sciences* 28 (1): 478–83.

Önder, A., and H. Özenoglu. 2019. "Evaluation of Cytotoxic Effects of Ethereal Extracts of Some Selected Liverworts." *FABAD Journal of Pharmaceutical Sciences* 44 (2): 119–25.

Önder, A., A. Yildiz, A. S. Cinar, G. Zengin et al. 2022. "The Comparison of the Phytochemical Composition, Antioxidant and Enzyme Inhibition Activity of Two Moss Species: *Plagiomnium ellipticum* (Brid) T. Kop. and *Antitrichia californica* Sull., from Southwest Ecological Region in Turkey." *Natural Product Research* 36 (10): 2660–65.

Ong, K. L., L. H. Gould, D. L. Chen, T. F. Jones et al. 2012. "Changing Epidemiology of *Yersinia enterocolitia* Infections: Markedly Decreased Rates in Young Black Children, Foodborne Diseases Active Surveillance Network (FoodNet), 1996–2009." *Clinical Infectious Diseases* 54 (5): S385–90.

Opelt, K., C. Berg, G. Berg. 2007. "The Bryophyte Genus Sphagnum Is a Reservoir for Powerful and Extraordinary Antagonists and Potentially Facultative Human Pathogens." *FEMS Microbiology Ecology* 6 (11): 38–53.

Oschner, F. 1975. "*Neckera crispa* Hedw., an Pfahlbaufundstellen in der Schweiz." *Phytocoenologia* (Band 2 Heft) 1–2: 9–12.

Otoguro, K., A. Ishiyama, M. Iwatsuki, M. Namatame et al. 2012. "In Vitro Antitrypanosomal Activity of Bis(bibenzyls) and Bibenzyls from Liverworts Against *Trypanosoma brucei*." *Journal of Natural Medicine* 66 (2): 377–82.

Oyesiku, O. O., and O. J. Caleb. 2015. "Antimicrobial Activity of Three Mosses, *Calymperes erosum* Müll. Hal., *Racopilum africanum* Mitt., *Cyclodictyon* Mitt. from Southwest Nigeria." *IOSR Journal of Pharmacy and Biological Sciences* 10 (2): 1–5.

Özdemir, T., O. Ücüncü, T. B. Cansu, N. Kahriman et al. 2010. "Volatile Constituents in Mosses (*Brachythecium albicans* (Hedw.) Schimp., *Bryum pallescens* Schleich, ex Schwagr and *Syntrichia intermedia* Brid.) Grown in Turkey." *Asian Journal of Chemistry* 22 (9): 7285–90.

Özdemir, T., N. Yayli, T. B. Cansu, C. Volga et al. 2009. "Essential Oils in Mosses (*Brachythecium salebrosum*, *Eurhynchium pulchellum* and *Plagiomnium undulatum*) Grown in Turkey." *Asian Journal of Chemistry* 21 (7): 5505–9.

Özerkan, D., A. Erol, E. M. Altuner, K. Canli et al. 2022. "Some Bryophytes Trigger Cytotoxicity of Stem Cell-like Population in 5-Fluorouracil Resistant Colon Cancer Cells." *Nutrition and Cancer* 74 (3): 1012–22.

Oztopcu-Vatan, P., F. Savaroglu, C. Filik-Iscen, S. Kabadere et al. 2011. "Antibacterial and Antiproliferative Activities of *Homalothecium sericeum* (Hedw.) Schimp. Extracts." *Fresenius Environmental Bulletin* 20 (2a): 461.

Painter, T. J. 2003. "Concerning the Wound-Healing Properties of *Sphagnum holocellulose*: The Maillard Rection in Pharmacology." *Journal of Ethnopharmacology* 88: 145–48.

Pandit, S., S. Biswas, U. Jana, R. K. De, et al. 2016. "Clinical Evaluation of Purified Shilajit on Testosterone Levels in Healthy Volunteers." *Andrologia* 48 (5): 570–75.

Pannequin, A, E. Laurini, L. Giordano, A. Muselli et al. 2020. "Caution: Chemical Instability of Natural Biomolecules During Routine Analysis." *Molecules* 25 (14): 3292.

Pannequin, A., J. Quentin-Leclercq, J. Costa, A. Tintaru et al. 2023. "First Phytochemical Profiling and In-Vitro Antiprotozoal Activity of Essential Oil and Extract of *Plagiochila porelloides*." *Molecules* 28 (2): 616.

Panossian, A., E. Gabrielian, C. Schwartner, H. Wagner. 1996. "Marchantin B from the Liverwort *Marchantia polymorpha* Selectively Inhibits the Biosynthesis of 5-Lipoxygenase Products and the Release of Arachidonic Acid in Ca^{+2} Ionophore A 23187 Stimulated Human Granulocytes." *Phytomedicine* 2 (4): 309–11.

Pant, G., and S. D. Tewari. 1989. "Various Human Uses of Bryophytes in the Kumaun Region of Northwest Himalaya." *Bryologist* 9: 120–22.

Park, C., N. Y. Jeong, G. Y. Kim, M. H. Han et al. 2014. "Momilactone B Induces Apoptosis and G1 Arrest of the Cell Cycle in Human Monocytic Leukemia U937 Cells Through Downregulation of pRB Phosphorylation and Induction of the Cyclin-Dependent Kinase Inhibitor p21Waf1/Cip1." *Oncology Reports* 31 (4): 1653–60.

Park, J. Y., H. J. Lee, E. T. Han, J. H. Han Park et al. 2023. "Caffeic Acid Methyl Ester Inhibits Mast Cell Activation Through the Suppression of MAPKs and NF-kB Signaling in RBL-2H3 Cells." *Heliyon* 9 (6): e16529.

Park, S. Y., H. H. Oh, Y. L. Park, H. M. Yu et al. 2017. "Malformin A1 Treatment Alters Invasive and Oncogenic Phenotypes of Human Colorectal Cancer Cells Through Stimulation of the p38 Signaling Pathway." *International Journal of Oncology* 51 (3): 959–66.

Pates, A. L., and G. C. Madsen. 1955. "Occurrence of Antimicrobial Substances in Chlorophyllose Plants Growing in Florida. II." *International Journal of Plant Sciences* 116 (3): 250–61.

Patil, N. S., and J. P. Jadhav. 2015. "Significance of *Penicillium ochrochloron* Chitinase as a Biocontrol Agent Against Pest *Helicoverpa armigera*." *Chemosphere* 128: 231–35.

Paul, C., W. A. Kónig, H. Muhle. 2001. "Pacifigorgianes and Tamariscene as Constituents of *Frullania tamarisci* and *Valeriana officinalis*." *Phytochemistry* 57 (2): 307–13.

Pavletic, Z., and B. Stilinovic. 1963. "Untersuchungen über die antibiotische Wirking von Mooseextrakten auf einige Bacterien." *Acta Botanica Croatica* 22: 133–39.

Pejin, B., A. Bianco, S. Newmaster, M. Sabovlijevic et al. 2012. "Fatty Acids of *Rhodobryum ontariense* (Bryaceae)." *Natural Product Research* 26 (8): 696–702.

Pejin, B., and J. Bogdanovic-Pristov. 2012. "ABTS Cation Scavenging Activity and Total Phenolic Content on Three Moss Species." *Hemijska Industrija* 66 (5): 723–26.

Pejin, B., J. Bogdanovic-Pristov, I. Pejin, M. Sabovljevic. 2013. "Potential Antioxidant Activity of the Moss *Bryum moravicum*." *Natural Products Research* 27 (10): 900–902.

Pejin, B., C. Iodice, G. Tommonaro, M. Sabovlijevic et al. 2012. "Sugar Composition of the Moss *Rhodobryum ontariense* (Kindb.) Kindb." *Natural Product Research* 26 (3): 209–15.

Pejin, B, Y. Kien-Thai, B. Stanimirovic, G. Vuckovic et al. 2012. "Heavy Metal Content of a Medicinal Moss for Hypertension." *Natural Product Research* 26 (23): 2239–42.

Pejin, B., L. Vujisic, M. Sabovljevic, V. Tesevic et al. 2011. "Preliminary Data on Essential Oil Composition of the Moss *Rhodobryum ontariense* (Kindb.) Kindb." *Cryptomgamie, Bryologie* 32 (2): 113–17.

Perry, N. B., E. J. Burgess, S. H. Baek, R. T. Weavers. 2001. "The First Atisane Diterpenoids from a Liverwort: Polyls from *Lepidolaena clavigera*." *Organic Letters* 3: 4243–45.

Perry, N. B., E. J. Burgess, S. H. Baek, R. T. Weavers et al. 1999. "11-Oxygenated Cytotoxic 8,9-Secokauranes from a New Zealand Liverwort, *Lepidolaena taylorii*." *Phytochemistry* 50 (3): 423–33.

Perry, N. B., E. J. Burgess, L. M. Foster, P. J. Gerard. 2003. "Insect Antifeedant Sesquiterpene Acetals from the Liverwort *Lepidolaena clavigera*." *Tetrahedron Letters* 44: 1651–53.

Perry, N. B., E. J. Burgess, R. S. Tangney. 1996. "Cytotoxic 8,9-Secokaurane Diterpenes from a New Zealand Liverwort, *Lepidolaena taylorii*." *Tetrahedron Letters* 37 (51): 9387–90.

Perry, N. B., and L. M. Foster. 1995. "Sesquiterpene/Quinol from a New Zealand Liverwort, *Riccardia crassa*." *Journal of Natural Products* 58 (7): 1131–35.

Perry, N. B., L. M Foster, S. D. Lorimer, B. C. H. May et al. 1996. "Isoprenyl Phenyl Ethers from Liverworts of the Genus *Trichocolea*: Cytotoxic Activity, Structural Corrections and Synthesis." *Journal of Natural Products* 59 (8): 729–33.

Petersen, M. 2003. "Cinnamic Acid 4-Hydroxylase from Cell Cultures of the Hornwort *Anthoceros agrestis*." *Planta* 217: 96–101.

Petpiroon, N., N. Bhummaphan, S. Tungsukruthai, T. Pinkhien et al. 2019. "Chrysotobibenzyl Inhibition of Lung Cancer Cell Migration Through Caveolin-1-Dependent Mediation of the Integrin Switch and the Sensitization of Lung Cancer Cells to Cisplatin-Mediated Apoptosis." *Phytomedicine* 58: 152888.

Pfeifer, L., K. K. Mueller, B. Classen. 2022. "The Cell Wall of Hornworts and Liverworts: Innovations in Early Land Plant Evolution?" *Journal of Experimental Botany* 73 (13): 4454–72.

Pingali, U., and C. Nutalapati. 2022. "Shilajit Extract Reduces Oxidative Stress, Inflammation and Bone Loss to Dose-Dependently Preserve Bone Mineral Density in Postmenopausal Women with Osteopenia: A Randomized, Double-Blind, Placebo-Controlled Trial." *Phytomedicine* 105: 154334.

Pinheiro, M., R. Lisboa, R. Brazäo. 1989. "*Contribuicão ao estudo de briófitas como fontes de antibióticos*." *Acta Amazonica* 19: 139–45.

Piotrowska, D., A. Dlugosz, K. Witkiewicz, J. Pajak. 2000. "The Research on Antioxidative Properties of TOŁPA Peat Preparation and Its Fractions." *Acta Poloniae Pharmaceutica* 57: 127–29.

Pokharkar, O., H. Lakshmanan, G. Zyryanov, M. Tsurkan. 2022. "In Silico Evaluation of Antifungal Compounds from Marine Sponges against COVID-19 Associated Mucormycosis." *Marine Drugs* 20 (3): 215.

Popper, Z. A., Ian H. Sadler, and Stephen C. Fry. 2003. "α-d-Glucuronosyl-(1→3)-l-Galactose, an Unusual Disaccharide from Polysaccharides of the Hornwort *Anthoceros caucasicus*." *Phytochemistry* 64 (1): 325–35.

Pornpakakul, S., S. Suwancharoen, A. Petsom et al. 2009. "A New Sesquiterpenoid Metabolite from *Psilocybe samuiensis*." *Journal of Asian Natural Products Research* 11: 12–17.

Pouliot, R., L. Rochefort, M. D. Graf. 2012. "Impacts of Oil Sands Process Water on Fen Plants: Implications for Plant Selection in Required Reclamation Projects." *Environmental Pollution* 167: 132–37.

Prateeksha, G., T. S. Rana, A. K. Ashthana, S. K. Barik et al. 2021. "Screening of Cryptogamic Secondary Metabolites as Putative Inhibitors of SARS-CoV-2 Main Protease and Ribosomal Binding Domain of Spike Glycoprotein by Molecular Docking and Molecular Dynamics Approaches." *Journal of Molecular Structure* 1240: 130506.

Preziuso, F., V. A. Taddeo, S. Genovese, F. Epifano et al. 2018. "Phytochemistry of the Genus *Trichocolea*." *Natural Product Communications* 13 (9): 1205–7.

Provenzano, F., J. L. Sánchez, E. Rao, R. Santonocito et al. 2019. "Water Extract of *Cryphaea heteromalla* (Hedw.) D. Mohr Bryophyte as a Natural Powerful Source of Biologically Active Compounds." *International Journal of Molecular Sciences* 20 (22): 5560.

Przybylska-Balcerek, A., T. Szablewski, L. Szwajkowska-Michalek, D. Swierk et al. 2021. "*Sambucus nigra* Extracts-Natural Antioxidants and Antimicrobial Compounds." *Molecules* 26 (10): 2910.

Purkon, D. B., M. I. Iwo, A. A. Soemardji, S. F. Rahmawati et al. 2021. "Immunostimulant Activity *of Marchantia paleacea* Bertol. Herb Liverwort Ethanol Extract in *BALB*/c Mice." *Indonesian Journal of Pharmacy* 32 (4): 464–73.

Qiao, Y., H. B. Zheng, L. Li, J.Z. Zhang et al. 2018. "Terpenoids with Vasorelaxant Effects from the Chinese Liverwort *Scapania carinthiaca*." *Bioorganic and Medicinal Chemistry* 26 (14): 4320–28.

Qiao, Y. N., X. Y. Jin, J. C. Zhou, J. Z. Zhang et al. 2020. "Terpenoids from the Liverwort *Plagiochila fruticosa* and Their Antivirulence Activity Against *Candida albicans*." *Journal of Natural Products* 83 (6): 1766–77.

Qiao, Y. N., Y. Sun, T. Shen, J. Z. Zhang et al. 2019. "Diterpenoids from the Chinese *Frullania hamatiloba* and Their Nrf2 Inducing Activities." *Phytochemistry* 158: 77–85.

Qiu, Y., X. J. Xue, G. Liu, M. M Shen et al. 2021. "Perillaldehyde Improves Cognitive Function In Vivo and In Vitro by Inhibiting Neuronal Damage via Blocking TRPM2/NMDAR Pathway." *Chinese Medicine* 16 (1): 136.

Qu, J., C. Xie, H. Guo, W. Yu et al. 2007. "Antifungal Dibenzofuran Bis(Bibenzyl)s from the Liverwort *Astrella angusta*." *Phytochemistry* 68: 1767–74.

Qu, J. B., R. L. Zhu, Y. L. Zhang, H. F. Guo et al. 2008. "Ent-kaurane Diterpenoids from the Liverwort *Jungermannia atrobrunnea*." *Journal of Natural Products* 71 (8): 1418–22.

Quan, N. V., T. D. Xuan, H. D. Tran, A. Ahmad et al. 2019. "Contribution of Momilactones A and B to Diabetes Inhibitory Potential of Rice Bran: Evidence from In Vitro Assays." *Saudi Pharmaceutical Journal* 27 (5): 643–49.

Quang, D. N., and Y. Asakawa. 2010. "Chemical Constituents of the Vietnamese Liverwort *Porella densifolia*." *Fitoterapia* 81 (6): 659–61.

Radulovic, N. S., S. I. Filipovic, M. S. Nesic, N. M. Stojanovic et al. 2020. "Immunomodulatory Constituents of *Conocephalum conicum* (Snake Liverwort) and the Relationship of Isolepidozenes to Germacranes and Humulanes." *Journal of Natural Products* 83 (12): 3554–63.

Radwan, S. S. 1991. "Sources of C_{20}- Polyunsaturated Fatty Acids for Biotechnological Use." *Applied Microbiology and Biotechnology* 35: 421–30.

Ramírez, M., N. Kamiya, S. Popich, Y. Asakawa et al. 2010. "Insecticidal Constituents from the Argentine Liverwort *Plagiochila bursata*." *Chemistry and Biodiversity* 7 (7): 1855–61.

Ramírez, M., N. Kamiya, S. Popich, Y. Asakawa et al. 2017. "Constituents of the Argentine Liverwort *Plagiochila diversifolia* and Their Insecticidal Activities." *Chemistry and Biodiversity* 14 (12).

Reis, M. H., D. Antunes, L. H. Santos, A. C. Guimarães et al. 2020. "Sharing Binding Mode of Perrottetinene and Tetrahydrocannabinol Diastereomers Inside the CB1 Receptor May Incentivize Novel Medicinal Drug Design: Findings from an In Silico Assay." *ACS Chemical Neuroscience* 11 (24): 4289–300.

Remesh, M., and C. N. Manju. 2009. "Ethnobryological Notes from Western Ghats, India." *Bryologist* 112: 532–37.

Rempt, M., and G. Pohnert. 2010. "Novel Acetylenic Oxylipins from the Moss *Dicranum scoparium* with Antifeeding Activity Against Herbivorous Slugs." *Angewardte Chemic International Edition* (English) 49 (28): 4755–58.

Renner, M. A. M. 2021. "The Typification of Australasian *Plagiochila* Species (Plagiochilaceae: Jungermanniidae): A Review with Recommendations." *New Zealand Journal of Botany* 59: 323–75.

Renu, G., V. V. Divya Rani, S. V. Nair, K. R. V. Subramanian et al. 2012. "Development of Cerium Oxide Nanoparticles and Its Cytotoxicity in Prostate Cancer Cells." *Advanced Science Letters* 6: 17–25.

Rezende-Moraes, E., R. de Cassia Pereira dos Santos, T. G. Miranda, R. J. M. Alves et al. 2023. "Volatile Chemical Constituents of Two Species of Bryophytes (Bryophyta) Occurring in the Brazilian Amazon." *Research Square.*

Rodrigo, G., G. R. Almanza, Y. J. Cheng, J. N. Peng et al. 2010. "Antiproliferative Effects of Curcuphenol, a Sesquiterpene Phenol." *Fitoterapia* 81 (7): 762–66.

Rodrigues, C. K., E. L. Junior, E. M. Ethur, T. Scheibel et al. 2020. "Evaluation of the Antimicrobial Activity of Ethanol Extracts from *Orthostichella rigida* (Mull. Hal.) B.H. Allen & Magill (Bryophyta) on Pathogenic Microorganisms." *Journal of Medicinal Plants Research* 14 (3): 98–104.

Rodriguez-Rodriguez, J. C, I. J. P. Samudio-Echeverry, L. G. Sequeda-Castaneda. 2012. "Evaluation of the Antibacterial Activity of Four Ethanolic Extracts of Bryophytes and Ten Fruit Juices of Commercial Interest in Columbia against Four Pathogenic Bacteria." *Acta Horticulturae* 964: 251–58.

Rogers, R. 2016. *Mushroom Essences: Vibrational Healing from the Kingdom Fungi.*" Berkeley, CA: North Atlantic Books.

Rogers, R. 2017. *Herbal Allies: My Journey with Plant Medicine.* Berkeley, CA: North Atlantic Books.

Rogers, R. 2025. *Medicinal Lichens: Indigenous Knowledge and Modern Pharmacology.* Rochester, VT: Healing Arts Press.

Rol, C. K., T. Y. Joon, C. M. Yoke, T. J. Shun et al. 2022. "Preliminary Assessment of *Polytrichum commune* Extract as an Antimicrobial Soap Ingredient." *Journal of Experimental Biology and Agricultural Sciences.* 10 (4): 894–901.

Rosales, J. 2020. "Volatile Metabolites in Liverworts of Ecuador." *Metabolites* 10 (3): 92.

Roscetto, E., M. Masi, M. Esposito, R. di Lecce et al. 2020. "AntiBiofilm Activity of the Fungal Phytotoxin Sphaeropsidin A Against Clinical Isolates of Antibiotic-Resistant Bacteria." *Toxins* (Basel) 12 (7): 444.

Ruiz-Molina, N., I. Ortega-Bedoya, M. Arias-Zabala. 2019. "Protonema Suspension Cultures of *Polytrichum juniperinum* as a Potential Production Platform for Bioactive Compounds." *Journal of Herbs, Spices & Medicinal Plants* 25 (2): 114–27.

Russel, M. 2010. "Antibiotic Activity of Extracts from Some Bryophytes in South Western British Columbia." *Medical Student Journal of Australia* 2 (1): 9–14.

Russo, A., V. Cardile, A. C. E. Graziano, R. Avola et al. 2019. "Antigrowth Activity and Induction of Apoptosis in Human Melanoma Cells by *Drymis winteri* Forst Extract and Its Active Components." *Chemico-Biological Interactions* 305: 79–85.

Rycroft, D. S. and W. J. Cole 2001. "Hydroquinone Derivatives and Monoterpenoids from the Neotropical Liverwort *Plagiochila rutilans*." *Phytochemistry* 57 (3): 479–88.

Saad, S. B., M. A. Ibrahim, I. D. Jatau, M. N. Shuaibu. 2019. "Trypanostatic Activity of Geranylacetone: Mitigation of *Trypanosoma congolense*-Associated Pathological Perturbations and Insight into the Mechanism of Anaemia Amelioration Using In Vitro and In Silico Models." *Experimental Parasitology* 201: 49–56.

Sabharwal, H., G. Shukla, K. K. Kondepudi et al. 2023. "Phytochemical Analysis and *in Vitro* Assessment of Extracts of *Rhodobryum roseum* for Antioxidant, Antibacterial and Anti-Inflammatory Activities." *Journal of Herbs, Spices & Medicinal Plants* 29 (4): 419–37.

Sabovljevic, A., M. Sokovic, J. Glamoclija, A. Ciric et al. 2011. "Bio-activities of Extracts from Some Axenically Farmed and Naturally Grown Bryophytes." *Journal of Medicinal Plants Research* 5: 565–71.

Sabovljevic, A., M. Sokovic, M. Sabovlijevic, D. Grubisic. 2006. "Antimicrobial Activity of *Bryum argenteum*." *Fitoterapia* 77 (2): 144–45.

Sakai, K., T. Ichikawa, K. Yamada, M. Yamashita et al. 1988. "Antitumor Principles in Mosses: The First Isolation and Identification of Maytansinoids, Including a Novel 15-Methoxyansamitocin P-3." *Journal of Natural Products* 51 (5): 845–50.

Sakurai, K., K. Tomiyama, Y. Kawakami, N. Ochiai et al. 2016. "Volatile Components Emitted from the Liverwort *Marchantia paleacea* subsp. *diptera*." *Natural Product Communications* 11 (2): 263–64.

Sakurai, K., K. Tomiyama, Y. Kawakami, Y. Yaguchi et al. 2018. "Characteristic Scent from the Tahitian Liverwort, *Cyathodium foetidissimum*." *Journal of Oleo Science* 67 (10): 1265–69.

Sakurai, K., K. Tomiyama, Y. Yaguchi, Y. Asakawa. 2020. "Characteristic Odor of Japanese Liverwort (*Leptolejeunea elliptica*)." *Journal of Oleo Science* 68 (7): 767–70.

Salehi, M., H. Piri, A. Farasat, B. Pakbin et al. 2022. "Activation of Apoptosis and G0/G1 Cell Cycle Arrest Along with Inhibition of Melanogenesis by Humic Acid and Fulvic Acid: *BAX/BCL-2* and *Tyr* Genes Expression and Evaluation of Nanomechanical Properties in A375 Human Melanoma Cell Line." *Iranian Journal of Basic Medical Sciences* 25 (4): 489–96.

Samir, N., D. Özerkan, F. Danisman-Kalindemirtas, I.A. Kariper et al. 2023. "Synthesis and Anticancerogenic Effect of New Generation Ruthenium-Based Nanoparticle from *Homalothecium sericeum* with Eco-Friendly Method." *Journal of Pharmaceutical Innovation*. 18: 756–67.

Sandu, M., H. M. Irfan, S. A. Shah, M. Ahmed et al. 2022. "Friedelin Attenuates Neuronal Dysfunction and Memory Impairment by Inhibition of the Activated JNK/NF-kB Signalling Pathway in Scopolamine-Induced Mice Model of Neurodegeneration." *Molecules* 27 (24): 4513.

Sangeetha, D. 2019. "Phytochemicals and Antimicrobial Activity of Bryophytes." *International Journal of Life Sciences* 7 (1): 115–19.

Sansores-Peraza, P., M. Rosado-Vallado, W. Brito-Loeza, G. J. Mena-Rejón et al. 2000. "Cassine, an Antimicrobial Alkaloid from *Senna racemose*." *Fitoterapia* 71 (6): 690–92.

Saritas, Y., M. M. Sonwa, H. Iznaguen, W. A. König et al. 2001. "Volatile Constituents in Mosses (Musci)." *Phytochemistry* 57 (3): 443–57.

Sauerwein, M., and H. Becker. 1990. "Growth, Terpenoid Production and Antibacterial Activity of an In Vitro Culture of the Liverwort *Fossombronia pusilla*." *Planta Medica* 56 (4): 364–67.

Savaroglu, F., S. Ilhan, C. Filik-Iscen. 2011. "An Evaluation of the Antimicrobial Activity of Some Turkish Mosses." *Journal of Medicinal Plants Research* 5 (14): 3286–92.

Savaroglu, F., C. Iscen, F. P. Oztopeu-Vaton, S. Kadabree et al. 2011. "Determination of the Antimicrobial and Antiproliferative Activity of the Aquatic Moss *Fontanilis antipyretica* Hedw." *Turkish Journal of Botany* 35: 361–69.

Sawant U. J., B. A. Karadge. 2010. "Antimicrobial Activity of Some Bryophytes (Liverworts and a Hornwort) from Kolhapur District." *Pharmacognosy Journal* 2: 25–28.

Saxena, D. K., and Harinder. 2004. "Uses of Bryophytes." *Resonance* 9 (6): 55–65.

Saxena, K., and U. Yadav. 2018. "In Vitro Assessment of Antimicrobial Activity of Aqueous and Alcoholic Extracts of Moss *Atrichum undulatum* (Hedw.) P. Beauv." *Physiology and Molecular Biology of Plants* 24 (6): 1203–8.

Scher, J. C., J. B. Speakman, J. Zapp, H. Becker. 2004. "Bioactivity Guided Isolation of Antifungal Compounds from the Liverwort *Bazzania trilobata* (L.) S.F. Gray." *Phytochemistry* 65 (18): 2583–88.

Scher, J. M., E. J. Burgess, S. D. Lorimer, N. B. Perry. 2002. "A Cytotoxic Sesquiterpene and Unprecedented Sesquiterpene-Bibisbenzyl Compounds from the Liverwort *Schistochila glaucescens*." *Tetrahedron* 59: 7875–82.

Scher, J. M., A. Schinkovitz, J. Zapp, Y. Wang et al. 2010. "Structure and Anti-TB Activity of Trachylobanes from the Liverwort *Jungermannia exsertifolia* ssp. *cordifolia*." *Journal of Natural Products* 73 (4): 656–63.

Scher, J. M., J. Zapp, H. Becker. 2003. "Lignan Derivatives from the Liverwort *Bazzania trilobata*." *Phytochemistry* 62 (5): 769–77.

Scher, J. M., J. Zapp, A. Schmidt, H. Becker 2003. "Bazzanins L-R, Chlorinated Macrocyclic Bisbibenzyls from the Liverwort *Lepidozia incurvata*." *Phytochemistry* 64 (3): 791–96.

Schofield, W. B. 2001. *Introduction to Bryology*. Caldwell, NJ: Blackburn Press.

Scholten, J. 2018. *Fairylike Mosses*. Utrecht, Netherlands: Stichting Alonnissos Pub.

Schwartner, C., C. Michel, K. Stettmaier, H. Wagner et al. 1996. "Marchantins and related Polyphenols from Liverwort: Physico-Chemical Studies of Their Radical-Scavenging Properties." *Free Radical Biology and Medicine* 20 (2): 237–44.

Schwenckfeld, C. von, 1600. *Stirpium et Fossilium Silesiae Catalogus in quo practer etymon, Natales, tempus, natura et vires cum variis Expermentis assignatur*. Leipzig, Germany: Impensis Davidis Alberti.

Science Daily. 2010. "Brain Structure Corresponds to Personality." July 23.

Sevim, E., Y. Bas, G. Celik, M. Pinarbas et al. 2017. "Antibacterial Activity of Bryophyte Species Against Paenibacillus Larvae Isolates." *Turkish Journal of Veterinary and Animal Sciences* 41 (4): 521–31.

Shaaban, R., M. S. Elnaggar, N. Khalil, A. N. B. Singab. 2023. "A Comprehensive Review on the Medicinally Valuable Endosymbiotic Fungi *Penicillium chrysogenum*." *Archives in Microbiology* 205 (6): 240.

Shadid, K. A., A. K. Shakya, R. R. Naik, T. S. Al-Qaisi et al. 2023. "Exploring the Chemical Constituents, Antioxidant, Xanthine Oxidase and COX Inhibitory Activity of *Commiphora gileadensis* Commonly Grown Wild in Saudi Arabia." *Molecules* 28 (5): 2321.

Shafreen, R. M. B., S. Seema, S. A. Lakshmi, A. Srivathsan et al. 2022. "In Vitro and In Vivo Antibiofilm Potential of Eicosane Against *Candida albicans*." *Applied Biochemistry and Biotechnology* 194 (10): 4800–4816.

Sharma, C., A. Sharma, M. Katoch. 2013. "Comparative Evaluation of Antimicrobial Activity of Methanolic Extract and Phenolic Compounds of a Liverwort, *Reboulia hemispherica*." *Archives in Bryology* 193: 1–6.

Sharma, A., S. Slathia, D. Gupta, N. Handa. 2014. "Antifungal and Antioxidant Profile of Ethnomedicinally Important Liverworts (*Pellia endivaefolia* and *Plagiochasma appendiculatum*) Used by Indigenous Tribes of District Reasi: North West Himalayas." *Proceedings of the National Academy of Sciences. India-Section B: Biological Sciences* 85: 571–79.

Sharma, R., S. Singh, A. Alam. 2022. "Pharmacological, Cytotoxic, Immunostimulant, and Auto-Immune Activity of Thalloid Liverworts: An Overview." *Critical Reviews in Immunology* 42 (5): 9–19.

Sheikh-Zeinoddin, M., T. M. Perehinic, S. E. Hill, and C. E. Rees. 2000. "Maillard Reaction Causes Suppression of Virulence Gene Expression in *Listeria* Monocytogenes." *International Journal of Food Microbiology* 61 (1): 41–9.

Shen, Y. C., Y. B. Cheng, Y. C. Lin, J. H. Guh et al. 2004. "New Prostanoids with Cytotoxic Activity from Taiwanese Octocoral *Clavularia viridis*." *Journal of Natural Products* 67 (4): 542–46.

Shi, B., S. X. Liu, A. Huang, M. Y. Zhou et al. 2021. "Revealing the Mechanism of Friedelin in the Treatment of Ulcerative Colitis Based on Network Pharmacology and Experimental Verification." *Evidence Based Complementary and Alternative Medicine* 2021: 4451779.

Shi, Y. Q., Y. X. Liao, X. J. Qu, et al. 2008. "Marchantin C, a Macrocyclic Bisbibenzyl, Induces Apoptosis of Human Glioma A172 Cells." *Cancer Letters* 262: 173–82.

Shi, Y. Q., X. J. Qu, Y. X. Laio et al. 2008. "Reversal Effect of a Macrocyclic Bisbibenzyl Plagiochin E on Multi-Drug Resistance in Adriamycin-Resistant K562/A02 Cells." *European Journal of Pharmacology* 584: 66–71.

Shi, Y. Q., C. Zhu, H. Yuan, B. Li et al. 2009. "Marchantin C, a Novel Microtubule Inhibitor from Liverwort with Anti-Tumor Activity Both in Vivo and in Vitro." *Cancer Letters* 276: 160–70.

Shin, K. O, K. S. Choi, Y. H. Kim. 2016. "In Vitro Antioxidative Activity of Moss Extract, and Effect of Moss on Serum Lipid Level of Mice Fed with High-Fat Diet." *Tropical Journal of Pharmaceutical Research* 15 (6): 1215–24.

Shirsat, R. P. 2008. "Ethnomedicinal Uses of Some Common Bryophytes and Pteridophytes Used by Tribals of Melghat Region (Ms)." *Indian Ethnobotanical Leaflet* 1: 92.

Shivom, S., R. Kajals, K. D. Raj. 2020. "Impact of Aqueous and Organic Extracts of *Rhodobryum roseum* on Inhibition of Fungal and Bacterial Growth." *Environment Conservation Journal* 21 (1–2): 151–61.

Shu, Y. F., H. C. Wei, C. L. Wu. 1994. "Sesquiterpenoids from Liverworts *Lepidozia vitrea* and *L. fauriana*." *Phytochemistry* 37: 773–76.

Simsek, O., K. Canli, A. Benek, D. Turu et al. 2023. "Biochemical, Antioxidant Properties and Antimicrobial Activity of Epiphytic Leafy Liverwort *Frullania dilatata* (L.) Dumort." *Plants* (Basel) 12 (9): 1877.

Simsek, O., K. Canli, G. Gürsu. 2006. "Karasal Yasamin Baslangicunda Briyofitler." *Anatolian Bryology* 1 (2): 70–74.

Sim-Sim, M., M. Abreu, C. Garcia, C. Sergio et al. 2017. "Essential Oil Composition of Two *Shagnum* Species Grown in Portugal and Their in Vitro Culture Establishment." *Natural Product Communications* 12 (8): 1307–10.

Singh, A. P., A. Asthana, V. Nath. 2000. "Medicinal Importance of Bryophytes—a Review" [in Hindi]. *Bharteey Vaigyanik evam Audyogik Anusandhan Patrika* 8 (2): 55–61.

Singh, M., R. Govindarajan, V. Nath, A. K. S. Rawat et al. 2006. "Antimicrobial, Wound Healing and Antioxidant Activity of *Plagiochasma appendiculatum* Lehm. et Lind." *Journal of Ethnopharmacology* 107 (1): 67–72.

Singh, M., A. K. S. Rawat, R. Govindarajan. 2007. "Antimicrobial Activity of Some Indian Mosses." *Fitoterapia* 78 (2): 156–58.

Singh, M., S. Singh, V. Nath, V. Sahu et al. 2011. "Antibacterial Activity of Some Bryophytes Used Traditionally for the Treatment of Burn Infections." *Pharmaceutical Biology* 49 (5): 526–30.

Singh, M., R. Govindarajan, V. Nath, A.K.S. Rawat et. al. 2006. "Antimicrobial, Wound Healing and Antioxidant Activity of *Plagiochasma appendiculatum* Lehm. et Lind." *Journal of Ethnopharmacology* 107 (1): 67–72.

Singh, V., A. Alam, A. Sharma. 2016. "Evaluation of Phytochemicals, Antioxidant and Antibacterial Activity of *Hyophila involuta* (Hook.) Jaeg. and *Entodon plicatus* C. Muell. (Bryophyta) from Rajasthan, India." *International Journal of Scientific Research in Knowledge* 4 (3): 56–63.

Siregar, E. S., N. Pasaribu, M. Z. Sofyan. 2021. "Antioxidant Activity of Liverworts *Marchantia paleacea* Bertol. from North Sumatra Indonesia." In *IOP Conference Series: Earth and Environmental Science*, vol. 713. Bristol, UK: IOP Publishing.

Sivasankari, S., and T. Vinotha. 2014. "In Vitro Degradation of Plastics (Plastic Cup) Using *Micrococcus luteus* and *Masoniella* Sp." *Scholars Academic Journal of Biosciences* 2 (2): 85–89.

Smith, H. H. 1932. "Ethnobotany of the Ojibwe Indians." *Bulletin of the Public Museum Milwaukee* 4 (3): 327–525.

Smolinska-Kondla, D., M. Zych, P. Ramos, S. Waclawek et al. 2022. "Antioxidant Potential of Various Extracts from 5 Common European Mosses and Its Correlation with Phenolic Compounds." *Herba Polonica* 68 (2): 54–68.

Söderström, L., A. Hagborg, M. von Konrat, S. Bartholomew-Began et al. 2016. "World Checklist of Hornworts and Liverworts." *PhytoKeys* 59: 1–828.

Song, J. H., T. J. Humphrey, A. Zhang, J. K. Czerwein et al. 2021. "A Rare *Streptomyces griseus* Infection of the Sacroiliac Joint: A Case Report." *Cureus* 13 (12): e20078.

Song, M. H., J. W. Lee, M. S. Kim, J. K. Yoon et al. 2012. "A Flucytosine-Responsive Mbp1/Swi4-Like Protein, Mbs1 Plays Pleiotropic Roles in Antifungal Drug Resistance, Stress Response and Virulence of *Cryptococcus neoformans*." *Eukaryotic Cell* 11 (1): 53–67.

Speicher, A, J. Holz, A. Hoffmann. 2011. "Syntheses of Marchantins C, O, and P as Promising Highly Bioactive Compounds." *Natural Product Communications* 6 (3): 393–402.

Spjut, R. W., J. M. Cassady, T. McCloud, M. Suffness et al. 1988. "Variation in Cytotoxicity and Antitumor Activity among Samples of the Moss *Claopodium crispifolium* (Thuidiaceae)." *Economic Botany* 42 (1): 62–72.

Spjut, R. W., M. Suffness, G. M. Cragg, D. H. Norris. 1986. "Mosses, Liverworts and Hornworts Screened for Antitumor Agents." *Economic Botany* 40(3): 310–38.

Spörle, J., H. Becker, N. S. Allen, M. P. Gupta. 1991. "Spiroterpenoids from *Plagiochila moritziana*." *Phytochemistry* 30: 3043–47.

Spörle, J., H. Becker, M. P. Gupta, M. Veith et al. 1989. "Novel C-35 Terpenoids from the Panamanian Liverwort *Plagiochila moritziana*." *Tetrahedron* 45 (16): 5003–14.

Stebel, A., H. D. Smolarz, M. Jankowska-Blaszczuk, M. Trylowski et al. 2016. "Seasonal Variation in Antioxidant Activity of Selected Mosses from Poland." *Fragmenta Naturae* 49: 65–73.

Stelmasiewicz, M., L. Swiatek, S. Gibbons, A. Ludwiczuk. 2023. "Bioactive Compounds Produced by Endophytic Microorganisms Associated with Bryophytes—The "Bryendophytes." *Molecules* 28 (7): 3246.

Stelmasiewicz, M., L. Swiatek, A. Ludwiczuk. 2021. "Phytochemical Profile and Anticancer Potential of Endophytic Microorganisms from Liverwort Species, *Marchantia polymorpha* L." *Molecules* 27 (1): 153.

Stelmasiewicz, M., L. Swiatek, A. Ludwiczuk. 2023. "Chemical and Biological Studies of Endophytes Isolated from *Marchantia polymorpha*." *Molecules* 28 (5): 2202.

Stivers, N. S., A. Islam, E. M. Reyes-Reyes et al. 2018. "Plagiochilin A Inhibits Cytokinetic Abscission and Induces Cell Death." *Molecules* 23 (6): 1418.

Sturtevant, W. 1954. *The Mikasuki Seminole: Medical Beliefs and Practices*. Ph.D. diss., Yale University.

Subhisha, S., A. Subranomiam. 2007. "Promising Antifungal Activities of *Hyophila involuta*, a Moss." *Biomedicine* 27: 117–22.

Subin, K., P. A. Jose, B. Tom, B. Nair et al. 2021. "GC-MS Analysis of a Fragrant Epipyllous Liverwort *Leptolejeunea balansae* from Western Ghats, India." *Research Journal of Pharmacognosy and Phytochemistry* 13 (3).

Sugawa, S. 1960. "Nutritive Values of Mosses as a Food for Domestic Animals and Fowls." *Hikobia* 2: 119–24.

Suhail, M. 2010. "Na^+, K^+-ATPase: Ubiquitous Multifunctional Transmembrane Protein and Its Relevance to Various Pathophysiological Conditions." *Journal of Clinical Medicine Research* 2 (1): 1–17.

Suire, C., G. Bourgeois, T. Koponen. 2000. "Some Chemical Constituents of Thirteen Mosses from the Traditional Mniaceae Family." *Journal of the Hattori Botanical Laboratory* 89: 233–46.

Sun, B., J. Liu, Y. Gao, H. Zheng et al. 2017. "Design, Synthesis and Biological Evaluation of Nitrogen-Containing Macrocyclic Bisbibenzyl Derivatives as Potent Anticancer Agents by Targeting the Lysosome." *European Journal of Medicinal Chemistry* 136: 603–18.

Sun, C., Y. Zhang, X. Xue, Y. Cheng et al. 2011. "Inhibition of Angiogenesis Involves in Anticancer Activity of Riccardin D, a Macrocyclic Bisbibenzyl, in Human Lung Carcinoma." *European Journal of Pharmacology* 667: 136–43.

Sun, Y., Y. Qiao, Y. Liu, J. C. Zhou et al. 2021. "Ent-Kaurane Diterpenoids Induce Apoptosis and Ferroptosis Through Targeting Redox Resetting to Overcome Cisplatin Resistance." *Redox Biology* 43: 101977.

Surendran, S., F. Qassadi, G. Surendran, D. Lilley et al. 2021. "Myrcene—What Are the Potential Health Benefits of This Flavouring and Aroma Agent?" *Frontiers in Nutrition* 8: 699666.

Suwanborirux, K., C. J. Chang, R. W. Spjut, J. M. Cassady. 1990. "Ansamitocin P-3, a Maytansinoid, from *Claopodium crispifolium* and *Anomodon attenuatus* or Associated Actinomycetes." *Experientia* 46 (1): 117–20.

Suzuki, I., M. Kondoh, M. Harada, N. Koizumi et al. 2004. "An Ent-Kaurene Diterpene Enhances Apoptosis Induced by Tumor Necrosis Factor in Human Leukemia Cells." *Planta Medica* 70: 723–27.

Suzuki, T., N. Tamehiro, Y. Sato, T. Kobayashi et al. 2008. "The Novel Compounds that Activate Farnesoid X Receptor: the Diversity of Their Effects on Gene Expression." *Journal of Pharmacological Sciences* 107: 285–94.

Sweeney, J. D., P. J. Silk, J. M. Gutowski, J. P. Wu et al. 2010. "Effect of Chirality, Release Rate, and Host Volatiles on Response of *Tetropium fuscum* (F.), *Tetropium cinnamopterum* Kirby, and *Tetropium castaneum* (L.) to the Aggregation Pheromone, Fuscumol." *Journal of Chemical Ecology* 36 (12): 1309–21.

Tachibana, S., and B. J. Meeuse. 1960. "Isolation of Trans-Aconitic Acid from the Moss *Mnium affine*." *Science* 132 (3440): 1671.

Tag, H., A. K. Das, H. Loyi. 2007. "Anti-Inflammatory Plants Used by the Khamti Tribe of Lohit District in Eastern Arunachal Pradesh India." *Natural Product Radiance* 6 (4): 334–40.

Taira, Z., M. Takei, K. Endo, T. Hashimoto et al. 1994. "Marchantin A Trimethyl Ether: Its Molecular Structure and Tubocurarine-Like Skeletal Muscle Relaxation Activity." *Chemical and Pharmaceutical Bulletin* 42 (1): 52–56.

Takeda, R., and K. Katoh. 1981. "Growth and Sesquiterpenoid Production by *Calypogeia granulata* I Cells in Suspension Culture." *Planta* 151 (6): 525–30.

Takei, M., A. Umeyama, S. Arihara. 2006. "T-cadinol and Calamenene Induce Dendritic Cells from Human Monocytes and Drive Th1 Polarization." *European Journal of Pharmacology* 537 (1–3): 190–99.

Tamehiro, N., Y. Sato, T. Hashimoto, Y. Asakawa et al. 2005. "Riccardin C: A Natural Product That Functions as a Liver XR (LXR)*a* Agonist and LXRß Antagonist." *FEBS Letters* 579: 5299–304.

Tan, C. Y., M. Inagaki, H. B. Chai, M. K. Lambrechts et al. 2017. "Phytochemical and Cytotoxic Investigations of Pinguisanoids from Liverwort *Porella cordaeana*." *Phytochemistry Letters* 19: 77–82.

Tazaki, H., T. Hayashida, M. Ito., S. Minoshima et al. 1999. "Erimopyrone, a Lignan Derivative from the Liverwort *Moerckia erimona*." *Bioscience Biotechnology and Biochemistry* 63 (7): 1238–41.

Tazaki, H., M. Ito, M. Miyoshi, J. Kawabata et al. 2002. "Subulatin, an Antioxidic Caffeic Acid Derivative Isolated from the In Vitro Cultured Liverworts, *Jungermannia subulata*, *Lophocolea heterophylla*, and *Scapania parvitexta*." *Bioscience Biotechnology and Biochemistry* 66 (2): 255–61.

Tedela, P. O., A. O. Adebiyl, A. Aremu, O. M. David. 2014. "In Vitro Antibacterial Activity of Two Mosses: *Calymperes erosum* C. Mull and *Bryum coronatum* Schwaegr from South-Western Nigeria." *Journal of Biology and Life Science* 5 (2): 77.

Téllez-Rocha, N., B. Moncada, L. M. Pombo-Ospina, O. E. Rodríguez-Aguirre. 2021. "Antioxidant Activity of the Mosses *Breutilia subdisticha, Leptodontium viticulosoides* and *Pylaisia falcata*." *Ciencia en Desarrollo* 12 (2): 1–20.

Teodoro, A. L. S., M. H. S. Ramada, M. L. B. Paciencia, S. Dohms et al. 2024. "Antarctic Bryophyte *Sanionia uncinate* (Hedw.) Loeske, Amblystegiaceae, Antimicrobial, Antioxidant, Cytotoxic, and Acetylcholinesterase Activities." *Anais da Academia Brasileira de Ciencias* 96 (suppl 2): e20240678.

Tesso, H., W. A. König, Y. Asakawa. 2005. "Composition of the Essential Oil of the Liverwort *Radula perrottetii* of Japanese Origin." *Phytochemistry* 66 (8): 941–49.

Thadhani, V. M., and V. Karunaratne. 2017. "Potential of Lichen Compounds as Antidiabetic Agents with Antioxidative Properties: A Review." *Oxidative Medicine and Cellular Longevity* 2017: 2079697.

The, S. N., A. L. Tuan, T. D. T. Thu, L .N. Dinh et al. 2021. "Essential Oils of *Uvaria boniana*—Chemical Composition, in Vitro Bioactivity, Docking and in Silico ADMET Profiling of Selective Major Compounds." *Zeitschrift für Naturforschung C Journal of Bioscience* 77 (5–6): 207–18.

Thieret, J. W. 1956. "Bryophytes as Economic Plants." *Economic Botany* 10: 75–91.

Tian, X. L., R. Wang, T. X. Gu, F. Y. Ma et al. 2022. "Costunolide Is a Dual Inhibitor of MEK1 and AKT1/2 That Overcomes Osimertinib Resistance in Lung Cancer." *Molecular Cancer* 21 (1): 193.

Tintelnot, J., Y. Xu, T. R. Lesker, M. Schönlein et al. 2023. "Microbiota-Derived 3-IAA Influences Chemotherapy Efficacy in Pancreatic Cancer." *Nature* 615 (7950): 168–74.

Tochio, T., Y. Kadota, T. Tanaka, Y. Koga. 2018. "1-Kestose, the Smallest Fructo-oligosaccharide Component, Which Efficiently Stimulates *Faecalibacterium prausnitzii* as Well as Bifidobacteria in Humans." *Foods* 7 (9): 140.

Tominaga, K., A. Tsuchlya, O. Nakano, Y. Kuroki et al. 2021. "Increase in Muscle Mass Associated with the Prebiotic Effects of 1-kestose in Super-Elderly Patients with Sarcopenia." *Bioscience of Microbiota Food and Health* 40 (3): 150–55.

Tori, M., M. Aoki, Y. Asakawa. 1994. "Chenopodene, Marchantin P, and Riccardin G from the Liverwort *Marchantia chenopoda*." *Phytochemistry* 36 (1): 73–76.

Tosun, A., E. K. Akkol, I. Suntar, H. O. Kiremit et al. 2013. "Phytochemical Investigations and Bioactivity Evaluation of Liverworts as a Function of Anti-Inflammatory and Antinociceptive Properties in Animal Models." *Pharmaceutical Biology* 51 (8): 1008–13.

Tosun, G., B. Yayh, T. Özdemir, N. Batan et al. 2015. "Volatiles and Antimicrobial Activity of the Essential Oils of the Mosses *Pseudoscleropodium purum, Eurhynchium striatum,* and *Eurhynchium angustirete* Grown in Turkey." *Records of Natural Products* 9 (2): 237–42.

Toyota, M, F. Nagashima, Y. Asakawa. 1988. "Labdane type diterpenoids from the liverwort *Frullania hamachiloba*." *Phytochemistry* 27 (6): 1789–93.

Toyota, M. 2000. "Phytochemical Study of Liverworts *Conocephalum conicum* and *Chiloscyphus polyanthos*." *Yakugaku Zasshi* 120 (12): 1359–72.

Toyota, M., Y. Asakawa, J. P. Frahm. 1990. "Ent-sesquiterpenoids and Cyclic Bis(bibenzyls) from the German Liverwort *Marchantia polymorpha*." *Phytochemistry* 29: 1577–84.

Toyota, M., and Y. Asakawa. 1993. "Diterpenoid Constituents of the Liverwort *Nardia subclavata*." *Phytochemistry* 34 (3): 751–53.

Toyota, M., R. Ikeda, H. Kenmoku, Y. Asakawa. 2013. "Activity-Guided Isolation of Cytotoxic Bis-benzyl Constituents from *Dumortiera hirsuta*." *Journal of Oleo Science* 62 (2): 105–8.

Toyota, M, I. Omatsu, J. Braggins, Y. Asakawa. 2009. "Pungent Aromatic Compound from New Zealand liverwort *Hymenophyton flabellatum*." *Chemical and Pharmaceutical Bulletin* 57 (9): 1015–18.

Toyota, M., H. Koyama, Y. Asakawa. 1997. "Volatile components of the liverworts *Archilejeunea olivacea, Cheilolejeunea imbricata* and *Leptolejeunea elliptica*." *Phytochemistry* 44 (7): 1261–64.

Toyota, M., I. Omatsu, J. Braggins, Y. Asakawa. 2004. "New Humulane-Type Sesquiterpenes from the Liverworts *Tylimanthus tenellus* and *Marchantia emarginata* subsp. *tosana*." *Chemical and Pharmaceutical Bulletin* 52 (4): 481–84.

Toyota, M., T. Shimamura, H. Ishii, M. Renner et al. 2002. "New Bibenzyl Cannabinoid from the New Zealand Liverwort *Radula marginata*." *Chemistry and Pharmaceutical Bulletin* 50 (10): 1390–92.

Toyota, M., K. Tanimura, Y. Asakawa. 1998. "Cytotoxic 2,3-Secoaromadendrane-Type Sesquiterpenoids from the Liverwort *Plagiochila ovalifolia*." *Planta Medica* 64 (5): 462–64.

Trennheuser, F., G. Burkhard, H. Becker. 1994. "Anthocerodiazonin an Alkaloid from *Anthoceros agrestis*." *Phytochemistry* 37 (3): 899–03.

Trevisan, V. 1874. *Rendiconti. Reale istituto lombardo di scienze e lettere.* Volume 7. Milano, Italy: Tipografia di Giuseppe Bernardoni.

Tripathi, J., S. Gupta, S. Gautam. 2023. "Alpha-Cadinol as a Potential ACE-Inhibitory Volatile Compound Identified from *Phaseolus vulgaris* L. Through In Vitro and In Silico Analysis." *Journal of Biomolecular Structure and Dynamics* 41 (9): 3847–61.

Trofimova, E. S., M. V. Zykova, E. Y. Sherstoboev, M. G. Danilets et al. 2020. "Effects of Humic Acids, Isolated from High-Moor Pine-Peat Moss-Cotton Grass Peat on the Production of Cytokines by Mouse and Human Immunocompetent Cells and on Humoral Immune Response." *Bulletin of Experimental Biology and Medicine* 168 (5): 651–53.

Trofimova, E. S., M. V. Zykova, E. Y. Sherstoboev, M. G. Danilets et al. 2022. "Influence of Humic Acids Isolated from Raised Bog Sphagnum Peat on Development of Th1/Th2 Immune Response." *Bulletin of Experimental Biology and Medicine* 174 (2): 236–40.

Trybus, W., T. Król, E. Trybus, A. Stachurska. 2021. "Physcion Induces Potential Anticancer Effects in Cervical Cancer Cells." *Cells* 10 (8): 2029.

Turmel, M., A. Bélanger, C. Otis, C. Lemieux. 2020. "Complete Mitogenomes of the Chlorophycean Green Algae *Bulbochaete rectangularis* var. *biloensis* (Oedogoniales) and *Stigeoclonium helveticum* (Chaetophorales) Provide Insight into the Sequence of Events That Led to the Acquisition of a Reduced-Derived Pattern of Evolution in the Chlamydomonadales and Sphaeropleales." *Mitochondrial DNA* Part B 5 (1): 611–13.

Turner, N. J. 1973. "The Ethnobotany of the Bella Coola Indians of British Columbia." *Economic Botany* 25 (1): 63–104.

Turner, N. J., B. S. Efrat. 1982. *Ethnobotany of the Hesquiat Indians of Vancouver Island.* Cultural Recovery Paper, vol 2. Hesquiat Cultural Committee. Victoria, Canada: British Columbia Provincial Museum.

Turner, N. J., and R. J. Hebda. 2012. *Saanich Ethnobotany.* Victoria, Canada: Royal BC Museum Publishing.

Turner, N. J., J. Thomas, B. F. Carlson, R. T. Ogilvie. 1983. *Ethnobotany of the Nitinaht Indians of Vancouver Island.* Victoria, Canada: British Columbia Provincial Museum.

Turner, N. J., L. C. Thompson, M. T. Thompson, A. Z. York. 1990. *Thompson Ethnobotany. Knowledge and Usage of Plants by the Thompson Indians of British Columbia.* Memoir no. 3. Victoria Canada: Royal British Columbia Museum.

Tyagi, A. K., D. Bukvicki, D. Gottardi, M. Veljic et al. 2013. "Antimicrobial Potential and Chemical Characterization of Serbian Liverwort (*Porella arboris-vitae*): SEM and TEM Observations." *Evidence Based Complementary and Alternative Medicine* 2013: 382927.

Tzeng, C. Y., W. S. Lee, K. F. Liu, H. K. Tsou et al. 2022. "Allantoin Ameliorates Amyloid ß-Peptide-Induced Memory Impairment by Regulating the PI3K/Akt/GSK-3ß Signaling Pathway in Rats." *Biomedicine and Pharmacotherapy* 153: 113389.

Ücüncü, O., T. B. Cansu, T. Ozdemir, S. A. Karaoglu et al. 2010. "Chemical Composition and Antimicrobial Activity of the Essential Oils of Mosses (*Tortula muralis* Hedw., *Homalothecium lutescens* (Hedw.) H. Rob., *Hypnum cupressiforme* Hedw., and *Pohlia nutans* (Hedw.) Lindb.) from Turkey." *Turkish Journal of Chemistry* 34: 825–34.

Ul Haq, I., M. Imran, M. Nadeem, T. Tufail et al. 2021. "Piperine: A Review of Its Biological Effects." *Phytotherapy Research* 35 (2): 680–700.

University of Exeter. 2018. "Peatlands Will Store More Carbon as Planet Warms." News Archive Exeter (website), September 10.

Valarezo, E., V. Vidal, J. Calva, S.P. Jaramillo et al. 2018. "Essential Oil Constituents of Mosses Species from Ecuador." *Journal of Essential Oil Bearing Plants* 21 (1): 189–97.

Valarezo, E., O. Tandazo, K. Galán, J. Rosales et al. 2020. "Volatile Metabolites in Liverworts of Ecuador." *Metabolites* 10 (3): 92.

Valcic, S., J. Zapp, H. Becker. 1997. "Plagiochilines and Other Sesquiterpenoids from Plagiochila (Hepaticae)." *Phytochemistry* 44: 89–99.

Valeeva, L. R., A. L. Dague, M. H. Hall, A. E. Tikhonova et al. 2022. "Antimicrobial Activities of Secondary Metabolites from Model Mosses." *Antibiotics* (Basel) 11 (8): 1004.

van Klink, J. W., J. Zapp, H. Becker. 2002. "Pinguisane-Type Sesquiterpenes from the South American Liverwort *Porella recurva* (Taylor) Kuhnemann." *Zeitschrift für Naturforschung C Journal of Biosciences* 57 (5–6): 413–17.

Varley, S. J., and S. E. Barnett. 1987. "Sphagnum Moss and Wound Healing." *Clinical Rehabilitation* 1 (2).

Vashistha, H., R. C. Dubey, N. Pandey. 2007. "Antimicrobial Activity of Three Bryophytes Against Human Pathogens." In *Current Trends in Bryology*, edited by V. Nath and A. K. Asthana. Dehra Dun, India: Bishen Singh Mahendra Pal Singh.

Veljic, M., A. Ciric, M. Sokovic, P. Janackovic et al. 2010. "Antibacterial and Antifungal Activity of the Liverwort (*Ptilidium pulcherrimum*) Methanol Extract." *Archives of Biological Sciences* 62: 381–85.

Veljic, M., A. Duric, M. Sokovic, A. Ciric et al. 2009. "Antimicrobial Activity of Methanol Extracts of *Fontinalis antipyretica, Hypnum cupressiforme,* and *Ctenidium molluscum.*" *Archives of Biological Sciences* 61: 225–29.

Venkatesan, R., M. A. Hussein, L. Moses, J. S. Liu et al. 2022. "Polygodial, a Sesquiterpene Dialdehyde, Activates Apoptotic Signaling in Castration-Resistant Prostate Cancer Cell Lines by Inducing Oxidative Stress." *Cancers* (Basel) 14 (21): 5260.

Verlag, N. 2021. *Mosses and Ferns: Spectrum of Homeopathy*. Germany: Homeopathic Book Company.

Verma, V. K., K. B. Kumar, K. Sagar, S. Majumdar et al. 2021. "Amelioration of Immune and Digestive System Through Weed Supplemented Feed Against *Aeromonas hydrophila* in *Clarias gariepinus*." *Fish and Shellfish Immunology* 115: 124–33.

Vermeulen, F. and L. Johnston. 2011. *Plants: Homeopathic and Medicinal Uses from a Botanical Family Perspective, Volume 3*. Glasgow, Scotland: Saltire Books Limited.

Vicherová, E., R. Glinwood, T. Hájek, P. Šmilauer et al. 2020. "Bryophytes Can Recognize Their Neighbours Through Volatile Organic Compounds." *Scientific Reports* 10 (1): 7405.

Vidal, C. A., E. O. Sousa, F. F. G. Rodrigues, A. R. Campos et al. 2012. "Phytochemical Screening and Synergistic Interactions between Aminoglycosides, Selected Antibiotics and Extracts from the Bryophyte *Octoblepharum albidum* Hedw (Calymperaceae)." *Archives of Biological Sciences* 64: 465–70.

Vogelsang, K., B. Schneider, M. Petersen. 2006. "Production of Rosmarinic Acid and a New Rosmarinic Acid 3'-O-beta-D-glucoside in Suspension Cultures of the Hornwort *Anthoceros agrestis* Paton." *Planta* 223 (2): 369–73.

Vollár, M., A. Gyovai, P. Szücs, I. Zupkó et al. 2018. "Antiproliferative and Antimicrobial Activities of Selected Bryophytes." *Molecules* 23 (7): 1520.

von Marilaun, A. K. 1863. "*Das pflanenleben der Donauländer.*" 9th edition, 2019.

von Reuss, S. H., and W. A König. 2004. "Corsifurans A-C, 2-Arylbenzofurans of Presumed Stilbenoid Origin from *Corsinia coriandrina* (Hepaticae)." *Phytochemistry* 65 (23): 3113–18.

von Reuss, S. H., C. L. Wu, H. Muhle, W. A. König. 2004. "Sesquiterpene Constituents from the Essential Oils of the Liverworts *Mylia taylorii* and *Mylia nuda.*" *Phytochemistry* 65 (15): 2277–91.

Vroom, R. J. E., R. J. M. Temmink, G. van Dijk, H. Joosten et al. 2020. "Nutrient Dynamics of Sphagnum Farming on Rewetted Bog Grassland in NW Germany." *Science of the Total Environment* 726: 138470.

Wada, K., and K. Munakata. 1971. "Insect Feeding Inhibitors in Plants." *Agricultural and Biological Chemistry* 35 (1): 115–18.

Wagner, C., J. de Gezelle, S. Komarnytsky. 2020. "Celtic Provenance in Traditional Herbal Medicine of Medieval Wales and Classical Antiquity." *Frontiers in Pharmacology* 11: 105.

Wakeford, T. 2001. *Liasons of Life: From Hornworts to Hippos, How the Unassuming Microbe Has Driven Evolution.* New York: John Wiley & Sons.

Wandry, F., B. Henes, F. Zulli, R. Reski. 2018. "Biotechnologically Produced Moss Active Improves Skin Resilence." *SOFW Journal* vol. 144: 34–37.

Wang, B., P. Liu, Y. M. Shen, C. Dai. 2005. "Studies on the Chemical Constituents from Herb of *Rhodobryum roseum.*" *Zhongguo Zhong Yao Za Zhi* 30 (12): 895–97.

Wang, D., R. L. Zhu, L. Qu. 2006. "Antibacterial Activity in Extracts of *Cylindrocolea recurvifolia* (Cephaloziellaceae, Marchantiophyta) and *Pleurozia subinflata* (Pleuroziaceae, Marchantiophyta)." *Cryptogamie Bryologie* 27: 343–48.

Wang, K. Q., Y. Y. Chen, S. Gao, M. Wang et al. 2021. "Norlichexanthone Purified from Plant Endophyte Prevents Postmenopausal Osteoporosis by Targeting ER Alpha to Inhibit RANKL Signaling." *Acta Pharmaceutica Sinica* B 11 (2): 442–55.

Wang, L. N., J. Z. Zhang, X. Li, X. N. Wang, et al. 2012. "Pallambins A and B, Unprecendented Hexacyclic 19-nor-secolabdane Diterpenoids from the Chinese Liverwort *Pallavicinia ambigua.*" *Organic Letters* 14 (4): 1102–5.

Wang, S., R. J. Li, R. X. Zhu, X. Y. Hu et al. 2014. "Notolutesins A-J, Dolabrane-Type Diterpenoids from the Chinese Liverwort *Notoscyphus lutescens.*" *Journal of Natural Products* 77: 2081–87.

Wang, S., S. S. Liu, Z. M. Lin, R. J. Li et al. 2013. "Terpenoids from the Chinese Liverwort *Plagiochila pulcherrima* and Their Cytotoxic Effects." *Journal of Asian Natural Products Research* 15 (5): 473–81.

Wang, X., J. G. Cao, X. L. Dai, J. B. Xiao et al. 2017. "Total Flavonoid Concentrations of Bryophytes from Tianmu Mountain, Zhejiang Province (China): Phylogeny and Ecological Factors." *PLoS One* 12 (3): e0173003.

Wang, X., J. G. Cao, Y. H. Wu, Q. X. Wang et al. 2016. "Flavonoids, Antioxidant Potential, and Acetylcholinesterase Inhibition Activity of the Extracts from the Gametophyte and Archegoniophore of *Marchantia polymorpha* L." *Molecules* 21 (3): 360.

Wang, X., X. Y. Jin, J. C. Zhou, R. X. Zhu et al. 2020. "Terpenoids from the Chinese Liverwort *Heteroscyphus coalitus* and Their Anti-Virulence Activity Against *Candida albicans*." *Phytochemistry* 174: 112324.

Wang, X., L. Li, R. X. Zhu, J. Z. Zhang et al. 2017. "Bibenzyl-Based Meroterpenoid Enantiomers from the Chinese Liverwort *Radula sumatrana*." *Journal of Natural Products* 80 (12): 3143–50.

Wang, X., L. L. Qian, Y. Qiao, X. Y. Jin et al. 2022. "Cembrane-Type Diterpenoids from the Chinese Liverwort *Chandonanthus birmensis*." *Phytochemistry* 203: 113376.

Wang, X., J. Z. Zhang, J. C. Zhou, T. Shen et al. 2016. "Terpenoids from *Diplophyllum taxifolium* with Quinone Reductase-Inducing Activity." *Fitoterapia* 109: 1–7.

Wang, X. J., Z. Yang, Y. Liu, X. H. Wang et al. 2022. "Structural Characteristic of Polysaccharide Isolated from *Nostoc commune*, and Their Potential as Radical Scavenging and Antidiabetic Activities." *Scientific Reports* 12 (1): 22155.

Wang, X. N., B. P. Bashyal, E. M. K. Wijeratne, J. M. U'Ren et al. 2011. "Smardaesidins A-G, Isopimarane and 20-nor-isopimarane Diterpenoids from Smardaea sp., a Fungal Endophyte of the Moss *Ceratodon purpureus*." *Journal of Natural Products* 74 (10): 2052–61.

Wang, X. N., W. T. Yu, H. X. Lou. 2005. "Antifungal Constituents from the Chinese Moss *Homalia trichomanoides*." *Chemistry & Biodiversity* 2 (1): 139–45.

Wang, Y. Y., Y. Ji, Z. Y. Hu, H. M. Jiang et al. 2013. "Riccardin D Induces Cell Death by Activation of Apoptosis and Autophagy in Osteosarcoma Cells." *Toxicology In Vitro* 27 (6): 1928–36.

Wang, Y., X. B. Nie, S. J. Liu, W. H. Bian. 2022. "Curcumol Attenuates Endometriosis by Inhibiting the JAK2/STAT3 Signaling Pathway." *Medical Science Monitor* 28:e934914.

Wang, Z., F. Liu, J. J. Yu, J. Z. Jin. 2018. "ß-Bouronene Attenuates Proliferation and Induces Apoptosis of Prostate Cancer Cells." *Oncology Letters* 16 (4): 4519–25.

Warmers, U., K. Wihstutz, M. Bülow, C. Fricke et al. 1998. "Sesquiterpene Constituents of the Liverwort *Calypogeia muelleriana*." *Phytochemistry* 49 (6): 1723–31.

Watanabe, A., T. Tochio, Y. Kadota, M. Takahashi et al. 2021. "Supplementation of 1-Kestose Modulates the Gut Microbiota Composition to Ameliorate Glucose Metabolism in Obesity-Prone Hosts." *Nutrients* 13 (9): 2983.

Waterman, M. J., A. S. Nugraha, R. Hendra, G. E. Ball et al. 2017. "Antarctic Moss Bioflavonoids Show High Antioxidant and Ultraviolet-Screening Activity." *Journal of Natural Products* 80 (8): 2224–31.

Wawrzyniak, R., W. Wasiak, B. Jasiewicz, A. Ludwiczuk et al. 2018. "High Correlation of Chemical Composition with Genotype in Cryptic Species of the Liverwort *Aneura pinguis*." *Phytochemistry* 152: 134–47.

Wei, H., Y. M. Xu, P. Espinosa-Artiles, M. P. X. Liu et al. 2015. "Sesquiterpenes and Other Constituents of *Xylaria* sp. NC1214, a Fungal Endophyte of the Moss *Hypnum* sp." *Phytochemistry* 118: 102–8.

Wei, M. Y., J. J. Li, J. H. Qiu, Y. Y. Yan et al. 2020. "Costunolide Induces Apoptosis and Inhibits Migration and Invasion in H1299 Lung Cancer Cells." *Oncology Reports* 43 (6): 1986–94.

Wei, W., A. Rasul, A. Sadiqa, I. Sarfraz et al. 2019. "Curcumol: From Plant Roots to Cancer Roots." *International Journal of Biological Sciences* 15 (8): 1600–1609.

Weinberger, P., and R. Greenhaigh. 1985. "The Sorptive Capacity of an Aquatic Macrophyte for the Pesticide Aminocarb." *Journal of Environment Science and Health B.* 20 (2): 263–73.

Wellman, C. H., P. L. Osterloff, U. Mohiuddin. 2003. "Fragments of the Earliest Land Plants." *Nature* 425: 282–85.

White, G. 1837. *The Natural History And Antiquities of Selborne*. London: Chiswick Press.

Whiteman, N. 2023. *Most Delicious Poison*. New York: Little, Brown Spark.

Wilson, R. M., A. M. Hopple, M. M. Tfaily, S. D. Sebestyen et al. 2016. "Stability of Peatland Carbon to Rising Temperatures." *Nature Communications* 7: 13723.

Witthauer, J., R. Klöcking, B. Helbig, P. Drabke. 1976. "Chemical and Physicochemical Characterization of Antivirally Active Humic Acids." In *Proceedings of the 5th International Peat Congress*. Vol. 1, *Peat and Peatlands in the Natural Environment Protection*, 456–66. Poznabn, Poland.

Wohl, J., and M. Petersen. 2020. "Functional Expression and Characterization of Cinnamic Acid 4-hydroxylase from the Hornwort *Anthoceros agrestis* in *Physcomitrella patens*." *Plant Cell Reports* 39 (5): 597–607.

Wolski, G. J., P. Nowicka-Krawczyk, and W. R. Buck. 2022. "*Plagiothecium talbotii*, a New Species from the Aleutian Islands (Alaska, U.S.A.)." *PhytoKeys* 194: 63–73.

Wolski, G. J., B. Sadowska, M. Fol, A. Podsedek et al. 2021. "Cytotoxicity, Antimicrobial and Antioxidant Activities of Mosses Obtained from Open Habitats." *PLoS One* 16 (9): e0257479.

Wolters, B. 1966. "*Zur wirkung von antimycotica auf das wachstum des luftmycels bei einigen pilzen*." *Archiv für Mikrobiologie* 53: 389–95; *Planta Medica* 14 (4): 392–401.

Wu, C., A. A. L. Gunatilaka, F. L. McCabe, R. K. Johnson et al. 1997. "Bioactive and Other Sesquiterpenes from *Chiloscyphus rivularis*." *Journal of Natural Products* 60: 1281–86.

Wu, C. L., and Y. Asakawa. 1987. "The Chemical Constituents of the Liverwort *Mylia Nuda*." *Journal of the Chinese Chemical Society* 34 (3): 219–23.

Wu, C. L., and C. L. Chen. 1992. "Oxygenated Sesquiterpenes from the Liverwort *Bazzania tridens*." *Phytochemistry* 31 (2): 4213–17.

Wu, C. L., and J. R. Jong. 2001. "A Cyclic Peroxide of Clerodenoic Acid from the Taiwanese Liverwort *Schistochila acuminata*." *Journal of Asian Natural Products Research* 3 (3): 241–46.

Wu, C. X., A. Q. Lyu, S. J. Shan. 2023. "Fulvic Acid Attenuates Atopic Dermatitis by Downregulating CCL17/22." *Molecules* 28 (8): 3507.

Wu, X. Z., A. X. Cheng, L. M. Sun, H. X. Lou. 2008. "Effect of Plagiochin E, an Antifungal Macrocyclic Bis(Bibenzyl), on Cell Wall Chitin Synthesis in *Candida albicans*." *Acta Pharmacologica Sinica* 29 (12): 1478–85.

Wu, J. G., W. Peng, P. Y. Zeng, Y. B. Wu et al. 2013. "Antimicrobial Activity and Cytotoxicity of Endophytes from *Scapania verrucosa* Heeg." *Genetics and Molecular Research* 12 (2): 916–24.

Wu, J. Y., X. Wang, J. Z. Zhang, J. C. Zhou et al. 2016. "Notolutesin K-P, Dolabrane-Type Diterpenoids from the Chinese Liverwort *Notoscyphus collenchymatosus*." *Phytochemistry Letters* 17: 226–31.

Wu, P. C. 1977. "*Rhodobryum giaganteum* (Schwaegr.) Par Can be Used for Curing Cardiovascular Disease." *Acta Phytotaxonomica Sinica* 15: 93.

Wu, P. C., 1982. "Some Uses of Mosses in China." *Bryology Times* 13: 5.

Wu, P. C., and Y. Jia. 2003. "The Medicinal Uses of Bryophytes." *Acta Botanica Yunnanica* Suppl. 14: 51–55.

Wu, X. Z., W. Q. Chang, A. X. Cheng, L. M. Sun et al. 2010. "Plagiochin E, an Antifungal Active Macrocylic Bis(bibenzyl), Induced Apoptosis in *Candida albicans* Through a Metacapase-Dependent Apoptotic Pathway." *Biochimica et Biophysica Acta* 1800 (4): 439–47.

Xavier, J. K., N. S. F. Alves, W. N. Setzer, J. K. R da Silva. 2020. "Chemical Diversity and Biological Activities of Essential Oils from *Licaria, Nectrandra* and *Ocotea* Species (Lauraceae) with Occurrence in Brazilian Biomes." *Biomolecules* 10 (6): 869.

Xi, G., B. Sun, H. Jiang, F. Kong et al. 2010. "Bisbibenzyl Derivatives Sensitize Vincristine-Resistant KB/VCR Cells to Chemotherapeutic Agents by Retarding P-Gp Activity." *Bioorganic and Medicinal Chemistry* 18: 6725–33.

Xiao, J. B., X. Q. Chen, Y. W. Zhang, X. Y. Jiang et al. 2006. "Cytotoxicity of *Marchantia convoluta* Leaf Extracts to Human Liver and Lung Cancer Cells." *Brazilian Journal of Medical and Biological Research* 39 (6): 731–38.

Xie, C. F., J. B. Qu, X. Z. Wu, N. Liu et al. 2010. "Antifungal Macrocyclic Bis(bibenzyls) from the Chinese Liverwort *Plagiochasm intermedium* L." *Natural Product Research* 24 (6): 515–20.

Xie, F., X. B. Li, J. C. Zhou, Q. Q. Xu et al. 2015. "Secondary Metabolites from *Aspergillus fumigatus*, an Endophytic Fungus from the Liverwort *Heteroscyphus tener* (Steph.) Schiffn." *Chemistry and Biodiversity* 12 (9): 1313–21.

Xiu, Z. R., Y. L. Zhu, J. C. Han, Y. R. Li et al. 2022. "Caryophyllene Oxide Induces Ferritinophagy by Regulating the NCOA4/FTH1/LC3 Pathway in Hepatocellular Carcinoma." *Frontiers in Pharmacology* 13: 930958.

Xu, A. H., Z. M. Hu, J. B. Qu, S. M. Liu et al. 2010. "Cyclic Bisbibenzyls Induce Growth Arrest and Apoptosis of Human Prostate Cancer PC3 Cells." *Acta Pharmacologica Sinica* 31: 609–15.

Xu, C. L., J. X. Wang, H. L. Li. 2016. "Two New Cyclic Bisbibenzyl Derivatives from *Herbertus dicranus*." *Chinese Journal of Natural Medicine* 14 (6): 457–61.

Xu, H. H., L. Yang, M. X. Tang, A. P. Ye et al. 2022. "From Cis-Lobeline to Trans-Lobeline: Study on the Pharmacodynamics and Isomerization Factors." *Molecules* 27 (19): 6253.

Xu, T., L. H. Huang, Z. Q. Liu, D. W. Ma et al. 2019. "Totarol, a Natural Diterpenoid, Induces Selective Antitumor Activity in SGC-7901 Human Gastric Carcinoma Cells by Triggering Apoptosis, Cell Cycle Disruption and Suppression of Cancer Cell Migration." *Journal of the Balkan University of Oncology* 24 (2): 686–92.

Xu, Z. Q., S. Krajewski, T. Weindl, R. Loeffler et al. 2020. "Application of Totarol as Natural Antibacterial Coating on Dental Implants for Prevention of Peri-Implantitis." *Materials Science and Engineering C: Materials for Biological Applications* 110: 110701.

Xue, X., X. J. Qu, Z. H. Gao, C. C. Sun et al. 2012. "Riccardin D, a Novel Macrocyclic Bisbibenzyl, Induces Apoptosis of Human Leukemia Cells by Targeting DNA Topoisomerase II." *Investigational New Drugs* 30: 212–22.

Xue, X., D. F. Sun, C. C. Sun, H. P. Liu et al. 2012. "Inhibitory Effect of Riccardin D on Growth of Human Non-Small Cell Lung Cancer: In Vitro and In Vivo studies." *Lung Cancer* 76 (3): 300–308.

Yaglioglu, M. S., G. Abay, I. Demirtas, A. S. Yaglioglu. 2017. "Phytochemical Screening, Antiproliferative and Cytotoxic Activities of the Mosses *Rhytidiadelphus triquetrus* (Hedw.) Warnst. and *Tortella tortuosa* (Hedw.) Limpr." *Anatolian Bryology* 3 (1): 31–42.

Yakir, M., and P. Theriault. 2020. "Crescent Cup Liverwort" in *Mosses and Ferns: Spectrum of Homeopathy* by N. Verlag.

Yamada, P., H. Isoda, J. K. Han, T. P. Talorate et al. 2007. "Inhibitory Effect of Fulvic Acid Extracted from Canadian Sphagnum Peat on Chemical Mediator Release by RBL-2H3 and KU812 Cells." *Bioscience Biotechnology and Biochemistry* 71: 1294–305.

Yan, X. G, W. G. Li, D. M. Liang, O. Caiyin et al. 2021. "*De nova* Assembly of the *Mylia taylorii* Transcriptome and Identification of Sesquiterpene Synthases." *Archives of Biochemistry and Biophysics* 698: 108742.

Yang, H., E. M. Jung, C. Ahn, G. S. Lee et al. 2015. "Elemol from *Chamaecyparis obtusa* Ameliorates 2,4-Dinitrochlorobenzene-Induced Atopic Dermatitis." *International Journal of Molecular Medicine* 36 (2): 463–72.

Yang, H., X. Y. Liu, P. L. Zhang, H. M. Gao et al. 2020. "New Terpenoids and Triketides from Culture of the Fungus *Botrysphaeria laricina*." *Fitoterapia* 147: 104758.

Yang, X., S. H. M. Lim, J. C. Lin, J. Wu et al. 2022. "Oxygen Mediated Oxidative Couplings of Flavones in Alkaline Water." *Nature Communications* 13: 6424.

Yang, Y. Y., S. Y. Hong, J. Z. Xu, C. Li et al. 2022. "*Enterobacter cloacae*: A Villain in CaOx Stone Disease?" *Urolithasis* 50 (2): 177–88.

Yayintas, O. T., D. Alpasian, Y. K. Yuceer, S. Yilmaz et al. 2017. "Chemical Composition, Antimicrobial, Antioxidant and Anthocyanin Activities of Mosses (*Cinclidotus fontinaloides* (Hedw.) P. Beauv. and *Palustriella communtata* (Hedw.) Ochyra) Gathered from Turkey." *Natural Product Research* 31 (18): 2169–73.

Yayintas, O. T., B. M. Yapici. 2009. "In Vitro Antimicrobial Activity of *Brachythecium campestre* and *Eurhynchium pulchellum* Extracts." *Asian Journal of Chemistry* 21: 2193–97.

Yayintas, O. T., S. Yilmaz, M. Sokmen. 2019. "Determination of Antioxidant, Antimicrobial and Antitumor Activity from Mount Ida, Canakkale, Turkey." *Indian Journal of Traditional Knowledge* 18 (2): 395–401.

Yen, P. L., S. S. Cheng, C. C. Wei, H. Y. Lina et al. 2016. "Antioxidant Activities and Reduced Amyloid-ß Toxicity of 7-Hydroxycalamenene Isolated from the Essential Oil of *Zelkova serrata* Heartwood." *Natural Product Communications* 11 (9): 1357–62.

Yong, L. K., S. Tsuboyama, R. Kitamura, T. Kurokura et al. 2021. "Chloroplast Relocation Movement in the Liverwort *Apopellia endiviifolia*." *Physiologia Plantarum* 173 (3): 775–87.

Yongabi, K. A., M. Novakovic, D. Bukvicki, Y. Asakawa. 2016. "Bis-bibenzyls from the Cameroon Liverwort *Marchantia debilis*." *Natural Product Communications* 11 (9): 1317–18.

Yongabi, K. A., M. Novakovie, D. Bukvicki, C. Reeb et al. 2016. "Management of Diabetic Bacterial Foot Infections with Organic Extracts of Liverwort *Marchantia debilis* from Cameroon." *Natural Products Communications* 11 (9): 1333–36.

Yoshida, T., T. Hashimoto, S. Takaoka, Y. Kan et al. 1996. "Phenolic Constituents of the Liverwort: For Novel Bisbenzyl Dimers from *Blasia pusila*." *Tetrahedron* 52: 14487–500.

Yoyota, M., H. Koyama, Y. Asakawa. 1997. "Sesquiterpenoids from the Three Japanese Liverworts *Lejeunea aquatica, L. flava* and *L. japonica*." *Phytochemistry* 46 (1): 145–50.

Yuan, W. J., X. X. Cheng, P. Wang, Y. Jia et al. 2015. "*Polytrichum commune* L. ex Hedw Ethyl Acetate Extract-Triggered Perturbations in Intracellular Ca2+ Homeostasis Regulates Mitochondrial-Dependent Apoptosis." *Journal of Ethnopharmacology* 172: 410–20.

Yuan, Y. H., M. Y. Gao. 2015. "Genomic Analysis of a Ginger Pathogen *Bacillus pumilis* Providing the Understanding to the Pathogenesis and the Novel Control Strategy." *Scientific Reports* 5: 10259.

Yuan, Z. H., H. Wang, Z. Y. Hu, Y. Q. Huang et al. 2015. "Quercitin Inhibits Proliferation and Drug Resistance in KB/VCR Oral Cancer Cells and Enhances Its Sensitivity to Vincristine." *Nutrition and Cancer* 67 (1): 126–36.

Yücel, T. B. 2021. "Chemical Composition and Antimicrobial and Antioxidant Activities of Essential Oils of *Polytrichum commune* (Hedw.) and *Antitrichia curtipendula* (Hedw.) Brid. Grown in Turkey." *International Journal of Secondary Metabolites* 8 (3): 272–83.

Yücel, T. B., and H. Erata. 2021. "Antimicrobial and Antioxidant Activities and Volatile Constituents of *Eurhynchium angustirete* (Broth.) T. J. Kop. and *Isothecium alopecuroides* (Lam. ex Dubois) Isov. from Turkey." *Natural Volatiles and Essential Oils* 8 (3): 64–74.

Yue, B., Y. S. Zhang, H. M. Xu, C. R. Zhao et al. 2013. "Riccardin D-26, a Synthesized Macrocyclic Bisbibenzyl Compound, Inhibits Human Hepatocellular Carcinoma Growth Through Induction of Apoptosis in p53-Dependent Way." *Cancer Letters* 328 (1): 104–13.

Yue, B., C. R. Zhao, H. M. Xu, Y. Y. Li et al. 2013. "Riccardin D-26, a Synthesized Macrocyclic Bisbibenzyl Compound, Inhibits Human Oral Squamous Carcinoma Cells KB and KB/VCR: In Vitro and in Vivo studies." *Biochimica et Biophysica Acta* 1830 (1): 2194–203.

Yue, X. F., J. X. Han, Z. M. Shen, W. Y. Yang et al. 1992. "Cytotoxic Activity of Trewiasine in 4 Human Cancer Cell Lines and 5 Murine Tumors." *Acta Pharmacologica Sinica* 13: 252–55.

Yue, Z. W., X. H. Xiao, J. B. Wu et al. 2018. "Ent-Jungermannenone C Triggers Reactive Oxygen Species-Dependent Cell Differentiation in Leukemia Cells." *Journal of Natural Products* 81 (2): 298–306.

Yusup, S., S. Sundberg, M. K. J. Ooi, M. M. Zhang et al. 2023. "Smoke Promotes Germination of Peatland Bryophyte Spores." *Journal of Experimental Botany* 74 (1): 251–54.

Zaitseva, N., 2009. "A Polysaccharide Extracted from Sphagnum Moss as Antifungal Agent in Archeological Conservation." Thesis for Master of Art Conservation, Queen's University, Kingston, Ontario.

Zakirova, E. Y., I. B. Chastukhina, L. R. Valeeva, V. V. Vorobev et al. 2019. "Stable Co-Cultivation of the Moss *Physcomitrella patens* with Human Cells in Vitro as a New Approach to Support Metabolism of Diseased Alzheimer Cells." *Journal of Alzheimer's Disease* 70 (1): 75–89.

Zandi, M., F. Hosseini, A. H. Adli, S. Salmanzadeh et al. 2022. "State-of-the-Art Cerium Nanoparticles as Promising Agents Against Human Viral Infections." *Biomedicine and Pharmacotherapy* 156: 113868.

Zeng, P. Y., J. G. Wu, L. M. Liao, T. Q. Chen et al. 2011. "In Vitro Antioxidant Activities of Endophytic Fungi Isolated from the Liverwort *Scapania verrucosa*." *Genetics and Molecular Research* 10 (4): 3169–79.

Zhan, X., Y. H. Zhang, D. F. Chen, H. T. Simonsen. 2014. "Metabolic Engineering of the Moss *Physomitrella patens* to Produce the Sesquiterpenoids Patchoulol and *a*/ß-Santalene." *Frontiers in Plant Science* 5: 536.

Zhang, C. Y., Z. J. Chu, J. C. Zhou, S. G. Liu et al. 2021. "Cytotoxic Activities of 9,10-Seco-Cycloartane-Type Triterpenoids from the Chinese Liverwort *Lepidozia reptans*." *Journal of Natural Products* 84: 3020–28.

Zhang, C. Y., Y. Gao, J. C. Zhou, Z. J. Xu et al. 2021. "Diverse Prenylated Bibenzyl Enantiomers from the Chinese Liverwort *Radula apiculata* and Their Cytotoxic Activities." *Journal of Natural Products* 84: 1459–68.

Zhang, C. Y., Y. Gao, R. X. Zhu, Y. N. Qiao et al. 2019. "Prenylated Bibenzyls from the Chinese Liverwort *Radula constricta* and Their Mitochondria-Derived Paraptotic Cytotoxic Activities." *Journal of Natural Products* 82 (7): 1741–51.

Zhang, C. Y. J. C. Zhou, H. X. Lou. 2022. "Prenylated Bibenzyls from the Chinese Liverwort *Radula apiculata*." *Journal of Asian Natural Products Research* 24 (9): 803–9.

Zhang, J., P. Fan, R. Zhu, R. Li et al. 2014. "Marsupellins A-F, Ent-longipinane-Type Sesquiterpenoids from the Chinese Liverwort *Marsupella alpina* with Acetylcholinesterase Inhibitory Activity." *Journal of Natural Products* 77 (4): 1031–36.

Zhang, J., Y. Li, R. Zhu, Y. Wang et al. 2015. "Scapairrins A-Q Labdane-Type Diterpenoids from the Chinese Liverwort *Scapania irrigua* and Their Cytotoxic Activity." *Journal of Natural Products* 78: 2087–94.

Zhang, J. Z., Y. N. Qiao, L. Li, Y. J. Wang et al. 2016. "Ent-Eudesmane-Type Sesquiterpenoid from the Chinese Liverwort *Chiloscyphus polyanthos* var. *rivularis*." *Planta Medica* 82 (11–12): 1128–33.

Zhang, J. Z., Y. J. Wang, R. X. Zhu, Y. Li et al. 2018. "Cyperane and Eudesmane-Type Sesquiterpenoids from Chinese Liverwort and Their Anti-Diabetic Nephropathy Potential." *Royal Society of Chemistry Advances* 8 (68): 39091–97.

Zhang, K. F., H. K. Cao, Y. Gao, M. L. Zhong et al. 2022. "*Marchantia polymorpha* L. Flavonoids Protect Liver from CCl_4-Induced Injury by Antioxidant and Gene-Regulatory Effects." *Alternative Therapies in Health and Medicine* 28 (3): 34–41.

Zhang, P., X. He, Y. H. Ma, K. Lu et al. 2012. "Distribution and Bioavailability of Ceria Nanoparticles in an Aquatic Ecosystem Model." *Chemosphere* 89: 530–35.

Zhang, R. L., Y. Han, L. T. Zhang, X. L. Wang et al. 2017. "Botrysphones A-C and Botrysphins A-F, Triketides and Diterpenoids from the Fungus *Botrysphaeria laricina*." *Journal of Natural Products* 80 (6): 1791–97.

Zhang, T. W., L. Xing, J. L. Tang et al. 2015. "Marchantin M Induces Apoptosis of Prostate Cancer Cells Through the Endoplasmic Reticulum Stress." *Medical Science Monitor* 21: 3570–76.

Zhang, W., H. X. Lou, G. Y. Li, H. M. Wu. 2003. "A New Triterpenoid from *Entodon okamurae* Broth." *Journal of Asian Natural Products Research* 5 (3): 189–95.

Zhao, M., J. J. Cheng, B. Guo, J. Duan et al. 2018. "Momilactone and Related Diterpenoids as Potential Agricultural Chemicals." *Journal of Agricultural and Food Chemistry* 66 (30): 7859–72.

Zhao, M. M., W. L. Yang, F. Y. Yang, L. Zhang et al. 2021. "Cathepsin L Plays a Key Role in SARS-CoV-2 Infection in Humans and Humanized Mice and Is a Promising Target for New Drug Development." *Signal Transduction and Targeted Therapy* 6 (1): 134.

Zhao, Y., X. S Wen, R. Ni, A. Cheng et al. 2022. "Tissue Culture of *Plagiochasma appendiculatum* and the Effect of Callus Differentiation on Types and Content of Bisbibenzyls." *Natural Product Communications* 17 (9): 1–8.

Zhao, Z. J., Y. L. Sun, X. F. Ruan. 2023. "Bornyl Acetate: A Promising Agent in Phytomedicine for Inflammation and Immune Modulation." *Phytomedicine* 114: 154781.

Zheng, G. Q., C. J. Chang, T. J. Stout, J. Clardy et al. 1993. "Ohioensins: Novel Benzonaphthoxanthenones from *Polytrichum ohioense*." *Journal of Organic Chemistry* 58 (2): 366–72.

Zheng, G. Q., D. K. Ho, P. J. Elder et al. 1994. "Ohioensins and Pallidesetins: Novel Cytotoxic Agents from the Moss *Polytrichum pallidisetum*." *Journal of Natural Products* 57: 32–41.

Zheng, S., W. Q. Chang, M. Zhang, H. Z. Shi et al. 2018. "Chiloscyphenol A Derived from Chinese Liverworts Exerts Fungicidal Action by Eliciting Both Mitochondrial Dysfunction and Plasma Membrane Destruction." *Scientific Reports* 8 (1): 326.

Zhernov, Y. V., A. I. Konstantinov, A. Zherebker, E. Nikolaev et al. 2021. "Antiviral Activity of Natural Human Substances and Shilajit Materials Against HIV-1: Relation to Structure." *Environmental Research* 193: 110312.

Zhong Hua Ben Cao. 1999. *Chinese Materia Medica*, edited by Federal Department of Medicine. Vol. 2. Shanghai: Shanghai Science and Technology Press.

Zhou, F. F., A. Aipire, L. J. Xia, X. R. G. Halike et al. 2021. "*Marchantia polymorpha* L. Ethanol Extract Induces Apoptosis in Hepatocellular Carcinoma Cells via Intrinsic- and Endoplasmic Reticulum Stress-Associated Pathways." *Chinese Medicine* 16 (1): 94.

Zhou, H. B., L. Y. Li, W. Wang, Q. Che et al. 2015. "Chrodrimanins I and J from the Antarctic Moss-Derived Fungus *Penicillium funiculosum* GWT2-24." *Journal of Natural Products* 78 (6): 1442–45.

Zhou, H. B, L. Y Li, C. M. Wu, T. Kurtán et al. 2016. "Penipyridones A-F, Pyridone Alkaloids from *Penicillium funiculosum*." *Journal of Natural Products* 79 (7): 1783–90.

Zhu, M. Z., C. He, J. C. Zhou, Y. Li et al. 2023. "Liverwort-Derived Metabolites Retard Endophyte Growth and Inspire Antifungal Application." *Journal of Agricultural and Food Chemistry* 71 (12): 4863–75.

Zhu, M. Z., Y. Li, J. C. Zhou, T. Wang, X.B. Li et al. 2022. "Pinguisane Sesquiterpenoids from the Chinese Liverwort *Trocholejeunea sandvicensis* and Their Anti-Inflammatory Activity." *Journal of Natural Products* 85 (1): 205–14.

Zhu, M. Z., Y. Li, J. C. Zhou, T. Wang, L. L. Qian et al. 2022. "Unprecedented 4,9-Seco-Oplopanane and Seven Drimane Sesquiterpenoids from the Chinese Liverwort *Lejeunea flava* (Sw.) Nees." *Chemistry and Biodiversity* 19 (9): e202200559.

Zhu, R. L., D. Wang, L. Xu, R. P. Shi et al. 2006. "Antibacterial Activity in Some Bryophytes from China and Mongolia." *Journal of the Hattori Botanical Laboratory* 100: 603–13.

Zykova, M. V., K. S. Brazovski, K. A. Bratishko, E. E. Buyko et al. 2022. "Quantitative Structure-Activity Relationship, Ontology-Based Model of the Antioxidant and Cell Protective Activity of Peat Humic Acids." *Polymers* (Basel) 14 (16): 3293.

Index of Bryophytes and Medicinal Applications

Bryophytes listed under medical conditions represent the most relevant genus entries for that condition. Other passing references to these conditions can be found in the text.